Cardiovascular Emergencies

Editors

SEMHAR Z. TEWELDE
JOSHUA C. REYNOLDS

EMERGENCY MEDICINE CLINICS OF NORTH AMERICA

www.emed.theclinics.com

Consulting Editor
AMAL MATTU

August 2015 • Volume 33 • Number 3

ELSEVIER

1600 John F. Kennedy Boulevard • Suite 1800 • Philadelphia, Pennsylvania, 19103-2899

http://www.theclinics.com

EMERGENCY MEDICINE CLINICS OF NORTH AMERICA Volume 33, Number 3
August 2015 ISSN 0733-8627, ISBN-13: 978-0-323-39330-0

Editor: Patrick Manley
Developmental Editor: Casey Jackson

Emergency Medicine Clinics of North America (ISSN 0733-8627) is published quarterly by Elsevier Inc., 360 Park Avenue South, New York, NY, 10010-1710. Months of issue are February, May, August, and November. Business and Editorial Offices: 1600 John F. Kennedy Boulevard, Suite 1800, Philadelphia, PA 19103-2899. Customer Service Office: 6277 Sea Harbor Drive, Orlando, FL 32887-4800. Periodicals postage paid at New York, NY, and additional mailing offices. Subscription prices are $155.00 per year (US students), $315.00 per year (US individuals), $523.00 per year (US institutions), $220.00 per year (international students), $450.00 per year (international individuals), $642.00 per year (international institutions), $220.00 per year (Canadian students), $385.00 per year (Canadian individuals), and $642.00 per year (Canadian institutions). International air speed delivery is included in all *Clinics'* subscription prices. All prices are subject to change without notice. **POSTMASTER:** Send address changes to *Emergency Medicine Clinics of North America*, Elsevier Periodicals Customer Service, 11830 Westline Industrial Drive, St. Louis, MO 63146. Customer Service (orders, claims, online, change of address): Elsevier Periodicals **Customer Service, 11830 Westline Industrial Drive, St. Louis, MO 63146. Tel: 1-800-654-2452 (U.S. and Canada); 314-453-7041 (outside U.S. and Canada). Fax: 314-453-5170. E-mail: journalscustomerservice-usa@elsevier.com (for print support); journalsonlinesupport-usa@elsevier.com (for online support).**

Reprints. For copies of 100 or more of articles in this publication, please contact the Commercial Reprints Department, Elsevier Inc., 360 Park Avenue South, New York, NY 10010-1710. Tel.: 212-633-3874; Fax: 212-633-3820; E-mail: reprints@elsevier.com.

Emergency Medicine Clinics of North America is covered in *MEDLINE/PubMed (Index Medicus)*, *Current Contents/Clinical Medicine*, *EMBASE/Excerpta Medica*, *BIOSIS*, *SciSearch*, *CINAHL*, *ISI/BIOMED*, and *Research Alert*.

Contributors

CONSULTING EDITOR

AMAL MATTU, MD
Professor and Vice Chair, Department of Emergency Medicine, University of Maryland School of Medicine, Baltimore, Maryland

EDITORS

SEMHAR Z. TEWELDE, MD
Assistant Professor, Department of Emergency Medicine, University of Maryland School of Medicine, Baltimore, Maryland

JOSHUA C. REYNOLDS, MD, MS
Assistant Professor, Department of Emergency Medicine, Michigan State University College of Human Medicine, Grand Rapids, Michigan

AUTHORS

OMOYEMI ADEBAYO, MD
Chief Resident, Clinical Instructor, Administrative and Teaching Fellow, Department of Emergency Medicine, University of Maryland School of Medicine, Baltimore, Maryland

MICHAEL G. ALLISON, MD
Division of Pulmonary and Critical Care Medicine, Department of Medicine; Department of Emergency Medicine, University of Maryland School of Medicine, Baltimore, Maryland

LAURA J. BONTEMPO, MD, MEd
Assistant Professor, Department of Emergency Medicine, University of Maryland, Maryland

ANKUR A. DOSHI, MD
Assistant Professor, Department of Emergency Medicine, University of Pittsburgh, Pittsburgh, Pennsylvania

SARAH B. DUBBS, MD
Assistant Professor, Department of Emergency Medicine, University of Maryland School of Medicine, Baltimore, Maryland

ADAM FRISCH, MD, MS
Assistant Professor, Department of Emergency Medicine, Albany Medical Center, Albany, New York

ERIC GORALNICK, MD, MS
Assistant Professor; Instructor, Department of Emergency Medicine, Brigham and Women's Hospital, Harvard Medical School, Boston, Massachusetts

JOHN C. GREENWOOD, MD
Assistant Professor, Department of Emergency Medicine; Department of Anesthesiology and Critical Care, Perelman School of Medicine at the University of Pennsylvania, Philadelphia, Pennsylvania

FRANCIS X. GUYETTE, MD, MPH
Associate Professor, Department of Emergency Medicine, University of Pittsburgh, Pittsburgh, Pennsylvania

JOSHUA KEEGAN, MD
Resident Physician, Department of Emergency Medicine, Yale University School of Medicine, New Haven, Connecticut

ANDREW M. KING, MD
Assistant Professor, Department of Emergency Medicine, Detroit Medical Center, Children's Hospital of Michigan Regional Poison Control Center, Detroit Receiving Hospital, Wayne State University School of Medicine, Detroit, Michigan

BENJAMIN J. LAWNER, DO, EMT-P
Assistant Professor, Department of Emergency Medicine, University of Maryland School of Medicine, Baltimore, Maryland

ZACHARY D. LEVY, MD
Assistant Professor of Emergency Medicine, Department of Emergency Medicine, Hofstra North Shore-LIJ School of Medicine, Hempstead, New York

LE N. LU, MD
Department of Emergency Medicine, University of Maryland School of Medicine, Baltimore, Maryland

HANEY A. MALLEMAT, MD
Department of Emergency Medicine, University of Maryland School of Medicine, Baltimore, Maryland

EVIE G. MARCOLINI, MD, FACEP, FAAEM
Assistant Professor, Division of Surgical Critical Care, Department of Emergency Medicine; Division of Neurocritical Care and Emergency Neurology, Assistant Professor, Department of Neurology, Yale University School of Medicine, New Haven, Connecticut

NATHAN B. MENKE, MD, PhD
Division of Medical Toxicology, Department of Emergency Medicine, University of Pittsburgh Medical Center, Pittsburgh, Pennsylvania

JOSHUA B. MOSKOVITZ, MD, MPH, MBA
Assistant Professor of Emergency Medicine, Department of Emergency Medicine, Hofstra North Shore-LIJ School of Medicine; Adjunct Assistant Professor of Public Health, Hofstra School of Health Sciences and Human Services, Hempstead, New York

JOSE V. NABLE, MD, NRP
Attending Physician, Department of Emergency Medicine, MedStar Georgetown University Hospital, Georgetown University School of Medicine, Washington, DC

THUY VAN PHAM, MD
Clinical Instructor, Chief Resident, Department of Emergency Medicine, University of Maryland School of Medicine, Baltimore, Maryland

JOSHUA C. REYNOLDS, MD, MS
Assistant Professor, Department of Emergency Medicine, Michigan State University College of Human Medicine, Grand Rapids, Michigan

JON C. RITTENBERGER, MD, MS
Associate Professor, Department of Emergency Medicine, University of Pittsburgh, Pittsburgh, Pennsylvania

ROBERT L. ROGERS, MD
Department of Emergency Medicine, University of Maryland School of Medicine, Baltimore, Maryland

MICHAEL C. SCOTT, MD
Fellow, Emergency Medicine/Internal Medicine/Critical Care Program, Departments of Emergency Medicine and Medicine, University of Maryland Medical Center, Baltimore, Maryland

TODD L. SLESINGER, MD
Associate Professor of Emergency Medicine and Surgery, Department of Emergency Medicine, Hofstra North Shore-LIJ School of Medicine, Hempstead, New York

RYAN M. SPANGLER, MD
Clinical Instructor, Department of Emergency Medicine, University of Maryland School of Medicine, Baltimore, Maryland

ASHLEY M. STROBEL, MD
Departments of Emergency Medicine and Pediatrics, University of Maryland Medical Center, Baltimore, Maryland

SEMHAR Z. TEWELDE, MD
Assistant Professor, Department of Emergency Medicine, University of Maryland School of Medicine, Baltimore, Maryland

MERCEDES TORRES, MD
Clinical Assistant Professor, Department of Emergency Medicine, University of Maryland School of Medicine, Baltimore, Maryland

STEVEN J. WALSH, MD, FAAEM
Division of Medical Toxicology, Department of Emergency Medicine, Einstein Medical Center, Philadelphia, Pennsylvania

MICHAEL E. WINTERS, MD, FACEP, FAAEM
Associate Professor of Emergency Medicine and Medicine, Departments of Emergency Medicine and Medicine, University of Maryland School of Medicine, Baltimore, Maryland

Contents

Pregnancy is a complex and dynamic physiologic state, in which the needs of the mother and fetus must achieve a fine balance with one another. Some of the most dreaded and deadly complications that can arise during this period affect the cardiovascular system are hypertensive emergencies (including preeclampsia and eclampsia), acute coronary syndrome, peripartum cardiomyopathy, dysrhythmias, dissection, thromboembolism, and cardiac arrest. This review provides emergency physicians, obstetricians, intensivists, and other health care providers with the most recent information on the diagnosis and management of these deadly cardiovascular complications of pregnancy.

This article presents an approach for identification of infants with congenital heart disorders. These disorders are difficult to diagnose because of the complexity and variety of cardiac malformations; additionally presentation can be complicated by age-dependent physiology. By compiling data from the history and the physical examination, the emergency physician can identify lesion category and initiate stabilization procedures. Critical congenital cardiac lesions can be classified as left-sided obstructive ductal dependent, right-sided obstructive ductal dependent, and shunting or mixing. The simplified approach categorizes infants with these lesions respectively as "pink," "blue," or "gray." The emergency provider can provide life-saving stabilization until specialized care can be obtained.

Blunt cardiac injury encompasses multiple different injuries, including contusion, chamber rupture, and acute valvular disorders. Blunt cardiac injury is common and may cause significant morbidity and mortality; a high index of suspicion is needed for accurate diagnosis. Diagnostic work-up should always include electrocardiogram and cardiac enzymes, and may include echocardiography if specific disorders (ie, tamponade or valvular disorders) are suspected. Patients with myocardial contusion

The imperative for timely reperfusion therapy for patients presenting with ST-segment elevation myocardial infarction (STEMI) underscores the need for clinicians to have an understanding of how to distinguish patterns of STEMI from its imitators. These imitating diagnoses may confound an evaluation, potentially delaying necessary therapy. Although numerous diagnoses may mimic STEMI, several morphologic clues may allow the physician to determine if the pattern is concerning for either STEMI or a mimicking diagnosis. Furthermore, obtaining a satisfactory history, comparing previous electrocardiograms, and assessing serial tests may provide valuable clues.

Hypertension affects approximately one-third of Americans. An additional 30% are unaware that they harbor the disease. Significantly increased blood pressure constitutes a hypertensive emergency that could lead to end-organ damage. When organs such as the brain, heart, or kidney are affected, an intervention that will lower the blood pressure in several hours is indicated. Several pharmacologic options are available for treatment, with intravenous antihypertensive therapy being the cornerstone, but there is no standard of care. Careful consideration of each patient's specific complaint, history, and physical examination guides the emergency physician through the treatment algorithm.

Patients with acute decompensated heart failure are usually critically ill and require immediate treatment. However, most are not volume overloaded. Emergency department (ED) management is based on rapid initiation of noninvasive positive-pressure ventilation and aggressive titration of nitrates. Afterload reduction with an angiotensin-converting enzyme inhibitor can be considered. A diuretic should not be administered before optimal preload and afterload reduction has been achieved. Short-term inotropic therapy can be considered in select patients with cardiogenic shock and acute decompensated heart failure (ADHF) who fail to respond to standard therapy.

Maintaining adequate tissue perfusion depends on a variety of factors, all of which can be influenced by xenobiotics (substances foreign to the body, including pharmaceuticals, chemicals, and natural compounds). Volume status, systemic vascular resistance, myocardial contractility, and cardiac rhythm all play a significant role in ensuring hemodynamic stability and proper cardiovascular function. Direct effects on the nervous system, the vasculature, or the heart itself as well as indirect metabolic effects may play a significant role in the development of cardiotoxicity. This article is dedicated to discussion of the disruption of cardiovascular physiology by xenobiotics.

Atrial fibrillation (AF) is a supraventricular tachyarrhythmia that results from the chaotic depolarization of atrial tissue. AF is the most common sustained cardiac dysrhythmia and the most common dysrhythmia diagnosed in US emergency departments. All patients with AF must have their cardioembolic risk assessed, even if sinus rhythm is restored. Novel oral anticoagulants may be considered instead of vitamin K antagonists for anticoagulation in patients with nonvalvular AF.

Human immunodeficiency virus (HIV) infection and antiretroviral medications are independent risk factors for cardiovascular disease. In the pre–antiretroviral therapy (ART) era, HIV-infected patients had increased morbidity and mortality from opportunistic infections. In the post-ART era, these patients are at increased risk of chronic diseases such as acute coronary syndrome, coronary artery disease, cardiac arrhythmias, and cardiomyopathy. They may present with vague symptoms such as weakness, dyspnea, or fatigue as the initial presentation of their cardiovascular disease. An overview of the clinical presentation, workup, management, and treatment of different cardiovascular disease is provided in this article.

Critically ill patients with pulmonary hypertension (PH) often seem well, but they can decompensate dramatically in a short time. PH has several causes, classes, and complications, but the natural progression eventually leads to right ventricular failure, which can be extraordinarily difficult to manage. The purpose of this review is to discuss the causes, signs, and symptoms of PH as well as its management strategies and emergent complications. Treatment options are often limited, so it is imperative that the emergency department physician can recognize and manage these patients in a timely fashion.

Cardiogenic shock is the leading cause of morbidity and mortality in patients presenting with acute coronary syndrome. Although early reperfusion strategies are essential to the management of these critically ill patients, additional treatment plans are often needed to stabilize and treat the patient before reperfusion may be possible. This article discusses pharmacologic and surgical interventions, their indications and contraindications, management strategies, and treatment algorithms.

Devices such as pacemakers and implantable cardioverter-defibrillators (ICDs) are commonly inserted to treat unstable cardiac rhythm disturbances. Despite the benefits of these devices on mortality and morbidity rates, patients often present to the emergency department with complaints related to device insertion or malfunction. Emergency physicians must be able to rapidly identify potential life threats caused by pacemaker malfunction, ICD firing, and complications associated with implantation of the devices.

Cardiac arrest is a dynamic disease that tests the multitasking and leadership abilities of emergency physicians. Providers must simultaneously manage the logistics of resuscitation while searching for the cause of cardiac arrest. The astute clinician will also realize that he or she is orchestrating only one portion of a larger series of events, each of which directly affects patient outcomes. Resuscitation science is rapidly evolving, and emergency providers must be familiar with the latest evidence and controversies surrounding resuscitative techniques. This article reviews evidence, discusses controversies, and offers strategies to provide quality cardiac arrest resuscitation.

Cardiac arrest afflicts more than 300,000 persons annually in North America alone. Advances in systematic, regimented postresuscitation care have lowered mortality and improved neurologic outcomes in select cohorts of patients over the last decade. Postcardiac arrest care now comprises its own link in the chain of survival. For most patients, high-quality postcardiac arrest care begins in the Emergency Department. This article reviews the evidence and offers treatment strategies for the key components of postcardiac arrest care.

EMERGENCY MEDICINE
CLINICS OF NORTH AMERICA

RELATED INTEREST

Cardiology Clinics, February 2015 (Vol. 33, No. 1)
Vascular Disease
Leonardo C. Clavijo, *Editor*

THE CLINICS ARE NOW AVAILABLE ONLINE!
Access your subscription at:
www.theclinics.com

PROGRAM OBJECTIVE

The goal of *Emergency Medicine Clinics of North America* is to keep practicing emergency medicine physicians and emergency medicine residents up to date with current clinical practice in emergency medicine by providing timely articles reviewing the state of the art in patient care.

LEARNING OBJECTIVES

Upon completion of this activity, participants will be able to:

1. Review unique methods of treatment for cardiovascular emergency in specific populations, such as obstetric and infant populations.
2. Recognize patient management techniques during resuscitation and post-cardiac arrest.
3. Discuss treatment plans for patients with varying sources of cardiac distress, such as blunt trauma, atrial fibrillation, HIV, cardiogenic shock, and pulmonary hypertension.

ACCREDITATION

The Elsevier Office of Continuing Medical Education (EOCME) is accredited by the Accreditation Council for Continuing Medical Education (ACCME) to provide continuing medical education for physicians.

The EOCME designates this enduring material for a maximum of 15 *AMA PRA Category 1 Credit*(s)™. Physicians should claim only the credit commensurate with the extent of their participation in the activity.

All other health care professionals requesting continuing education credit for this enduring material will be issued a certificate of participation.

DISCLOSURE OF CONFLICTS OF INTEREST

The EOCME assesses conflict of interest with its instructors, faculty, planners, and other individuals who are in a position to control the content of CME activities. All relevant conflicts of interest that are identified are thoroughly vetted by EOCME for fair balance, scientific objectivity, and patient care recommendations. EOCME is committed to providing its learners with CME activities that promote improvements or quality in healthcare and not a specific proprietary business or a commercial interest.

The planning committee, staff, authors and editors listed below have identified no financial relationships or relationships to products or devices they or their spouse/life partner have with commercial interest related to the content of this CME activity:

Omoyemi Adebayo, MD; Michael G. Allison, MD; Laura J. Bontempo, MD, MEd; Ankur A. Doshi, MD; Sarah B. Dubbs, MD; Anjali Fortna; Adam Frisch, MD, MS; Eric Goralnick, MD, MS; John C. Greenwood, MD; Francis X. Guyette, MD, MPH; Kristen Helm; Joshua Keegan, MD; Andrew M. King, MD; Indu Kumari; Benjamin J. Lawner, DO, EMT-P; Zachary D. Levy, MD; Le N. Lu, MD; Haney A. Mallemat, MD; Patrick Manley; Evie G. Marcolini, MD, FACEP, FAAEM; Amal Mattu, MD; Nathan B. Menke, MD, PhD; Joshua B. Moskovitz, MD, MPH, MBA; Jose V. Nable, MD, NRP; Thuy Van Pham, MD; Joshua C. Reynolds, MD, MS; Robert L. Rogers, MD; Michael C. Scott, MD; Todd L. Slesinger, MD; Ryan M. Spangler, MD; Ashley M. Strobel, MD; Semhar Z. Tewelde, MD; Mercedes Torres, MD; Steven J. Walsh, MD, FAAEM; Michael E. Winters, MD, FACEP, FAAEM.

The planning committee, staff, authors and editors listed below have identified financial relationships or relationships to products or devices they or their spouse/life partner have with commercial interest related to the content of this CME activity:

Jon C. Rittenberger, **MD, MS** receives research support from the National Institute of Neurological Disorders and Stroke, a part of the National Institutes of Health; Laerdal Medical; and the DSF Charitable Foundation, and has an employment affiliation with UPMC, affiliated with University of Pittsburgh Schools of the Health Sciences.

UNAPPROVED/OFF-LABEL USE DISCLOSURE

The EOCME requires CME faculty to disclose to the participants:

1. When products or procedures being discussed are off-label, unlabelled, experimental, and/or investigational (not US Food and Drug Administration [FDA] approved); and
2. Any limitations on the information presented, such as data that are preliminary or that represent ongoing research, interim analyses, and/or unsupported opinions. Faculty may discuss information about pharmaceutical agents that is outside of FDA-approved labelling. This information is intended solely for CME and is not intended to promote off-label use of these medications. If you have any questions, contact the medical affairs department of the manufacturer for the most recent prescribing information.

TO ENROLL

To enroll in the *Emergency Medicine Clinics* Continuing Medical Education program, call customer service at 1-800-654-2452 or sign up online at http://www.theclinics.com/home/cme. The CME program is available to subscribers for an additional annual fee of $235 USD.

METHOD OF PARTICIPATION

In order to claim credit, participants must complete the following:

1. Complete enrolment as indicated above.
2. Read the activity.
3. Complete the CME Test and Evaluation. Participants must achieve a score of 70% on the test. All CME Tests and Evaluations must be completed online.

CME INQUIRIES/SPECIAL NEEDS

For all CME inquiries or special needs, please contact elsevierCME@elsevier.com.

Foreword

Matters of the Heart

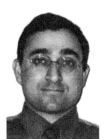

Amal Mattu, MD
Consulting Editor

Cardiac conditions constitute the greatest cause of death in first-world countries. Such "matters of the heart" are also a great source of confusion, controversy, and stress to emergency care providers. Delays in or missed diagnoses of cardiac conditions account for a significant percentage of lawsuits against emergency physicians in the United States. As a result, emergency care providers have a keen interest in learning more about the diagnosis and management of cardiac emergencies.

In this issue of *Emergency Medicine Clinics of North America*, guest editors Drs Joshua Reynolds and Semhar Tewelde have assembled an outstanding group of authors to address many of the high-risk cardiac conditions that we face in the specialty of emergency medicine. Though it may come as a surprise to some readers that there are no articles on low-risk chest pain or acute coronary syndrome, these topics are already discussed ad nauseum at virtually every emergency medicine conference in the world. Instead, the writing group has focused their efforts on addressing other common topics, such as congestive heart failure, atrial fibrillation, and cardiac arrest, all of which have been changing recently in terms of management because of new literature. They also focus on deadly conditions, such as cardiogenic shock, hypertensive emergencies, and blunt cardiac injury. They have emphasized cardiac emergencies in an assortment of special populations, such as pregnant patients, infants, patients with HIV, patients with pulmonary hypertension, and patients with implanted devices. An additional article focuses on the increasingly common, though poorly recognized, condition of cardiotoxicities.

Although this issue of *Emergency Medicine Clinics of North America* may not be a comprehensive treatise on emergency cardiology, it does serve as a fantastic complement to the many other books and to conferences that focus on more common and mundane issues pertaining to the heart. This text is an invaluable addition to the library of emergency physicians and other health care providers that diagnose and manage patients in acute care settings. This issue is must-reading for all of our own residents and faculty. Knowledge and practice of the concepts that are discussed in the

Emerg Med Clin N Am 33 (2015) xv–xvi
http://dx.doi.org/10.1016/j.emc.2015.06.002
0733-8627/15/$ – see front matter © 2015 Published by Elsevier Inc.

following pages are certain to save lives. The guest editors and authors are to be commended for providing this outstanding resource for our specialty.

Amal Mattu, MD
Department of Emergency Medicine
University of Maryland School of Medicine
Baltimore, MD 21201, USA

E-mail addresses:
amattu@smail.umaryland.edu; amalmattu@comcast.net

Preface
Matters of the Heart

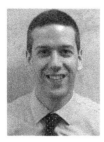
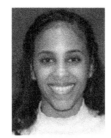

Joshua C. Reynolds, MD, MS   Semhar Z. Tewelde, MD
Editors

Recognizing and treating cardiovascular emergencies are cornerstones of Emergency Medicine, and many defining capabilities of our specialty implicate the cardiovascular system. The circulatory system interfaces with every other organ system in the body, and there is a myriad of pathology to consider.

In light of this, it was particularly challenging to narrow down the list of proposed topics to the final table of contents in this issue of *Emergency Medicine Clinics of North America*. Readers will notice that there are no articles on chest pain, myocardial infarction, or acute coronary syndrome in this particular issue on cardiovascular emergencies. Though these specific topics remain a core component in the practice of Emergency Medicine, it is too often tempting for our clinical focus to stray or devolve into these areas while failing to consider other cardiovascular conditions. Our intentional omission of these topics serves as a bulwark for the reader against this cognitive error and further underscores the diverse content featured in this issue. The material is loosely organized in a chronologic fashion from birth to death, and we feature articles on pregnancy, pediatrics, accumulated injuries and comorbidities of adulthood, and cardiac arrest.

We cannot extend enough appreciation to the nearly 30 individual authors that collaborated on this issue of *Emergency Medicine Clinics of North America*. Likewise, we acknowledge the ceaseless efforts of the editorial staff of *Emergency Medicine Clinics of North America* to assemble and collate individual submissions into a cohesive issue.

We hope you find useful information in this issue that enhances your clinical practice. Thanks for reading!

Joshua C. Reynolds, MD, MS
Department of Emergency Medicine
Michigan State University College of Human Medicine
15 Michigan Street Northeast, Suite 420
Grand Rapids, MI 49503, USA

Emerg Med Clin N Am 33 (2015) xvii–xviii
http://dx.doi.org/10.1016/j.emc.2015.06.001
0733-8627/15/$ – see front matter © 2015 Published by Elsevier Inc.

emed.theclinics.com

Semhar Z. Tewelde, MD
Department of Emergency Medicine
University of Maryland School of Medicine
110 South Paca Street
6th Floor, Suite 200
Baltimore, MD 21201, USA

E-mail addresses:
reyno406@msu.edu (J.C. Reynolds)
stewe001@umaryland.edu (S.Z. Tewelde)

Cardiovascular Catastrophes in the Obstetric Population

Sarah B. Dubbs, MD*, Semhar Z. Tewelde, MD

KEYWORDS

- Pregnancy • Emergency • Cardiovascular • Eclampsia • Cardiomyopathy
- Dissection • Pulmonary embolism • Cardiac arrest

KEY POINTS

- The absence of proteinuria does not exclude the diagnosis of preeclampsia/eclampsia.
- Severely hypertensive pregnant patients might be paradoxically volume depleted; aggressive pressure control without volume resuscitation can lead to profound hypotension and shock.
- The incidence of pregnancy-related myocardial infarction is accelerating; physicians must be vigilant in screening pregnant patients for this condition.
- Left ventricular (LV) thrombus occurs in up to 30% of patients with peripartum cardiomyopathy (PPCM); it should be sought aggressively and treated if found because the effects of embolization are often devastating.
- In maternal cardiac arrest, the tenets of resuscitation remain the same as for the nonpregnant population, with a few modifications: uterine displacement for aortocaval decompression, compressions higher on the sternum, venous access above the diaphragm, and consideration of perimortem cesarean delivery.

INTRODUCTION

Pregnancy induces immense and profound changes in a woman's body, causing her to undergo many anatomic and physiologic changes in order to accommodate the physical and metabolic demands of carrying, delivering, and nurturing another (or more than one other) human being. These changes affect every system of the body, especially the cardiovascular system; they allow the body to balance the needs of both the fetus and the mother; however, these changes come with a price. These

The authors have nothing to disclose.
Department of Emergency Medicine, University of Maryland School of Medicine, 110 South Paca Street, 6th Floor Suite 200, Baltimore, MD 21201, USA
* Corresponding author.
E-mail address: sdubbs@umem.org

Emerg Med Clin N Am 33 (2015) 483–500
http://dx.doi.org/10.1016/j.emc.2015.04.001
0733-8627/15/$ – see front matter © 2015 Elsevier Inc. All rights reserved.

emed.theclinics.com

changes put both the mother and the fetus at risk for complications—some are less severe than others, some are life altering, and some are life threatening. This article discusses some infrequently seen, but life-threatening cardiovascular complications of the obstetric population that every emergency physician must know.

HYPERTENSIVE EMERGENCIES

Hypertension is one of the most common complications of pregnancy, affecting 10% of all pregnant women.[1] The number of pregnant patients with preexisting hypertension has been growing, and so has the number of pregnant patients (with or without preexisting hypertension) who experience hypertensive emergencies.[2] As a consequence, maternal morbidity and mortality rates related to hypertensive emergencies are also trending upward.[3]

The 4 major hypertensive categories related to pregnancy (**Table 1**), as defined by the American College of Obstetricians and Gynecologists (ACOG) Task Force on Hypertension in Pregnancy,[4] are listed below:

- Preeclampsia-eclampsia
- Chronic hypertension
- Chronic hypertension with superimposed preeclampsia
- Gestational hypertension

Table 1
Classification of hypertensive disorders of pregnancy

Category	Definition
Preeclampsia-eclampsia	• New-onset hypertension (SBP $\geq$140 mm Hg or DBP $\geq$90 mm Hg) accompanied by proteinuria, usually occurring after 20 wk of gestation *or* • New-onset hypertension without proteinuria, but associated with thrombocytopenia, impaired liver function, renal insufficiency, pulmonary edema, cerebral disturbances, or visual disturbances • Eclampsia is defined by the onset of tonic-clonic seizures
Chronic hypertension	• Hypertension (SBP $\geq$140 mm Hg or DBP $\geq$90 mm Hg) that is present and observable before pregnancy or that is diagnosed before the 20th week of gestation *or* • Hypertension that is diagnosed for the first time during pregnancy and does not resolve postpartum
Chronic hypertension with superimposed preeclampsia	Chronic hypertension *and* any of the following: • Sudden worsening of blood pressure elevation • New-onset proteinuria • Thrombocytopenia (platelet <100,000 cells/mm³) • Increase in alanine aminotransferase or aspartate aminotransferase • Renal insufficiency • Pulmonary edema • Right upper quadrant pain, severe headaches
Gestational hypertension	• Hypertension detected for the first time after midpregnancy • No proteinuria or other clinical features of preeclampsia • If blood pressure normalizes by week 12 postpartum, a more specific diagnosis of transient hypertension of pregnancy is made

Abbreviations: DBP, diastolic blood pressure; SBP, systolic blood pressure.
Data from American College of Obstetrics and Gynecologists, Task Force on Hypertension in Pregnancy. Report of the American College of Obstetricians and Gynecologists' Task Force on Hypertension in Pregnancy. Obstet Gynecol 2013;122(5):1122–31.

These categories constitute a continuum of hypertensive disease that can affect pregnant patients, putting them at risk for serious complications (summarized in **Table 2**). Health care providers should note that proteinuria is no longer required to make the diagnosis of preeclampsia. The 2013 ACOG Task Force publication provides a new definition of preeclampsia: new-onset hypertension without proteinuria, but associated with thrombocytopenia, impaired liver function, renal insufficiency, pulmonary edema, cerebral disturbances, or visual disturbances.[4]

From a cardiovascular standpoint, during pregnancy, afterload is increased because of increased systemic vascular resistance (SVR), preload is decreased because of diminished volume expansion, and intravascular fluid shifts into third spaces (especially the lungs) because of endothelial injury related to hypertension.[5] Prolonged, uncontrolled hypertension puts the patient at increased risk of aortic or coronary artery dissection[6,7] and PPCM[8] (both are discussed later in this article). Blunted volume expansion,[9] in addition to renal artery vasospasm,[10] significantly decreases renal flow and glomerular filtration rate, causing impressive oliguria. Furthermore, subendothelial deposits of proteins and fibrins in the glomeruli lead to the protein leakage recognized as a sign of preeclampsia.[11,12] The most infamous neurologic complication of obstetric hypertensive emergencies is eclampsia, characterized by tonic-clonic seizure, which can lead to coma and death if not treated effectively. Less-common complications include intracranial hemorrhage, infarction, and posterior reversible encephalopathy syndrome (PRES). Finally, hypertension in pregnancy can compromise uterine and placental blood flow by limiting spiral artery remodeling.[13] The compromised blood flow can lead to fetal growth retardation, oligohydramnios, placental abruption, and fetal death.

Pharmacologic treatment of hypertension in pregnancy depends on the category of disease. The pharmacologic choices for patients with chronic hypertension or gestational hypertension include methyldopa, labetalol, hydrochlorothiazide, nifedipine, and hydralazine.[14] The antihypertensives that are contraindicated during pregnancy include angiotensin-converting enzyme (ACE) inhibitors, angiotensin receptor

Table 2	
Complications of hypertension in pregnancy	
System	**Effect**
Cardiovascular/Pulmonary	• Increased systemic vascular resistance ->decreased afterload • Decreased preload • Interstitial edema • Pulmonary edema • Increased risk of aortic or coronary artery dissection • Peripartum cardiomyopathy
Renal	• Decreased renal flow and GFR • Oliguria • Proteinuria
Neurologic	• Eclampsia • Intracranial hemorrhage • Ischemic stroke • PRES
Obstetric	• Fetal growth retardation • Oligohydramnios • Increased risk of placental abruption and fetal death

Abbreviations: GFR, glomerular filtration rate; PRES, posterior reversible encephalopathy syndrome.

blockers, and direct renin inhibitors.[14] Emergency physicians should be cognizant of these contraindications when treating pregnant patients with chronic hypertension or diagnosing new pregnancy in hypertensive patients.

Several options are available for the parenteral treatment of uncontrolled hypertension during pregnancy. For preeclampsia-eclampsia, magnesium sulfate remains the drug of choice, followed by the ultimate cure of delivery. When blood pressure is refractory to magnesium sulfate, additional antihypertensive agents are required. Hypertensive emergencies that do not meet the definition of preeclampsia-eclampsia (eg, aortic dissection, PRES, or acute pulmonary edema) must be treated with parenteral medications. These medications include intravenous hydralazine, labetalol, nicardipine, and sodium nitroprusside.[14–18] Dosing recommendations, indications, and adverse effects are listed in **Table 3**.

It is extremely important to remember that, because of the unique physiology of the pregnant state (increased SVR and afterload as well as decreased preload), hypertensive patients might actually be volume depleted. Aggressive blood pressure control without volume resuscitation can lead to profound hypotension and shock. At the same time, fluid resuscitation must be managed carefully, because the pregnant state predisposes patients to pulmonary edema.[19]

ACUTE CORONARY SYNDROME

Pregnancy-related deaths are not common, but, when they do occur, cardiovascular disease (CVD) is the leading culprit.[20] In the United States, CVD accounts for roughly 15% of maternal deaths, followed by cardiomyopathy (12%), hypertensive emergencies (10%), and thromboembolic diseases (10%).[21–23] The prevalence of CVD is being amplified by the exponential growth in the number of people with diabetes, hypertension, hyperlipidemia, obesity, and metabolic syndrome, compounded by the trend for women to delay pregnancy until later in their reproductive years. These conditions and circumstances, coupled with the inherent physiologic stress of pregnancy, are contributing to increased morbidity and mortality rates during pregnancy. At present, the United States has a higher maternal death rate than 50 other countries.[24,25]

The incidence of acute coronary syndrome (ACS) and pregnancy-related myocardial infarction is accelerating. ACS occurs most frequently during the third trimester and within the 6-week period after delivery.[26] Risk factors include older maternal age (>35 years), oral contraceptive use, preeclampsia, infection, diabetes, hypertension, hyperlipidemia, smoking, and thrombocytosis. Atherosclerosis accounts for fewer than half of the cases of ACS among pregnant women (different from the general population with ACS). Most cases during pregnancy are related to causes other than atherosclerosis: coronary artery dissection, thromboembolism without atherosclerosis, and vasospasm.[27,28] The presentation of ACS in women, especially during pregnancy, can include gastrointestinal complaints and nonspecific symptoms such as fatigue and dizziness. One study from the United Kingdom found that among pregnant women who presented with symptoms of ACS, some were never assessed with an electrocardiogram (ECG) or cardiac biomarkers.[29] Almost half the women in this study who died of ACS were thought to have received substandard care.[29]

The diagnosis and management of ACS during pregnancy is essentially unchanged from standard protocol, with a few exceptions. ECGs obtained during pregnancy frequently show axis deviation, nonspecific T-wave inversions, and an increased R/S ratio in leads V_1 and V_2, making the diagnosis of ischemia challenging.[30] If ECG and cardiac biomarkers are nondiagnostic, provocative testing should be pursued with an exercise stress test or echocardiogram.[31] Myocardial perfusion imaging

Table 3
Preferred medications for hypertensive emergency in pregnancy

Drug	Route	Starting Dose	Titration	Maximum Dose	Mode	Onset	Duration of Action	Comorbid Indications	Adverse Effects
Hydralazine	IV (intermittent)	5 mg IV push or IM	5–10 mg IV every 20–40 min	30 mg	Direct smooth muscle relaxation	10 min	12 h	Preeclampsia/eclampsia—(first line)	Headaches, aggravation of angina, tachycardia, nausea, flushing, hypotension, lupuslike syndrome
Labetalol	IV (intermittent)	10–20 mg IV (over 2 min)	20–80 mg IV, every 20–30 min	300 mg	α_1 and nonselective β-blockade	5–10 min	2–6 h	Preeclampsia/eclampsia—(first line) acute pulmonary edema—diastolic dysfunction Acute myocardial infarction Hypertensive encephalopathy	Fetal/maternal bradycardia, heart block, postural hypotension, cold extremities, sleep disturbances, rebound hypertension, bronchospasm, and masking of hypoglycemia
	IV (infusion)	1–2 mg/min	Increase 1 mg/min every 10 min	300 mg	—	—	—	Aortic dissection Hypertensive encephalopathy Ischemic or hemorrhagic stroke	—

(continued on next page)

anc 488

Table 3 *(continued)*

Drug	Route	Starting Dose	Titration	Maximum Dose	Mode	Onset	Duration of Action	Comorbid Indications	Adverse Effects
Esmolol	IV (infusion)	Bolus: 500 μg/kg Maintenance: 50 μg/kg/min	Increase by 50 μg/kg/min every 4 min	300 μg/kg/min	β-blockade	<1 min	15–30 min	Acute myocardial infarction Aortic dissection	First-degree heart block, maternal bradycardia, congestive heart failure, and bronchospasm Crosses the placenta; may cause fetal bradycardia, persistent fetal β-blockade
Nifedipine	Oral	10–20 mg	Repeat in 30 min if needed	30 mg	Calcium channel blocker	5–10 min	2–4 h	—	Uncontrolled hypotension, stroke, myocardial infarction, flushing, headache, and reflex tachycardia

Nicardipine	IV (infusion)	5 mg/h	Increase by 2.5 mg/h every 5–15 min	15 mg/h	Calcium channel blocker	1–5 min	4–6 h	Preeclampsia/eclampsia (second line) acute pulmonary edema—systolic dysfunction Hypertensive encephalopathy Acute renal failure Ischemic or hemorrhagic stroke	Tachycardia, flushing, and headache
Sodium nitroprusside	IV (infusion)	0.25 μg/kg/min	Increase by 0.25–0.5 μg/kg/min every 2–3 min	5 μg/kg/min	Nonselective direct NO inhibitor	<1 min	2–3 min	Aortic dissection Acute pulmonary edema	Nausea, vomiting Potential risk for maternal and fetal cyanide and thiocyanate toxicity if use >4 h LV dysfunction

Abbreviations: IM, intramuscular; IV, intravenous.
From Too GT, Hill JB. Hypertensive crisis during pregnancy and postpartum period. Semin Perinatol 2013;37(4):284–5; with permission.

should not be used because of its inherent radiation and the concomitant risk of teratogenicity.[31] Percutaneous coronary intervention (PCI) is the first-line therapy for ST-elevation myocardial infarction.[31] If PCI is unavailable, transfer of the patient to a facility with the appropriate clinical capabilities should be considered, particularly in the antepartum period. Thrombolytics are relatively contraindicated in pregnancy, because they potentiate bleeding and can lead to miscarriage, abruption, and placenta previa.[31] Heparin is a less-potent agent that does not cross the placenta; it should be considered in pregnant patients with ACS but must be used with caution given its potential to induce hemorrhage.[32] Aspirin, β-blockers, and nitrates are all safe, unlike the other commonly used cardiovascular agents such as ACE inhibitors, angiotensin II receptor blockers, and statins.[32] Ultimately, early consultation and aggressive management by both cardiology and obstetrics is paramount in the care of the mother and the infant.

CARDIOMYOPATHY

PPCM is a life-threatening idiopathic form of heart failure that begins during the last month of pregnancy or within 5 months after delivery. PPCM affects approximately 1 in 3000 pregnancies in the United States,[33] but its incidence seems to be much higher in developing nations such as South Africa (1 in 1000) and Haiti (1 in 300).[33–35] The clinical course of PPCM is highly unpredictable. Some patients progress rapidly to end-stage heart failure over days, and others experience a short course with full recovery within weeks. Risk factors for the development of PPCM include ethnicity (highest incidence in certain African ethnic groups[36]), advanced maternal age, chronic hypertension, gestational hypertension, pre-eclampsia, multiparity, history of multiple gestations, obesity, and prolonged use of tocolytics.[8,33,37]

Patients might present with complaints that are common in pregnancy, such as shortness of breath, dyspnea on exertion, fatigue, and lower extremity edema. Symptoms that should induce greater concern are palpitations, dizziness, and chest pain.[38] At the time of initial presentation, most patients have New York Heart Association class III or IV symptoms.[38] When the disease is complicated by LV thrombus, patients can present with embolic events such as cerebral or coronary infarcts.[39–41]

In addition to a basic laboratory evaluation searching for anemia, electrolyte disturbances, and liver, renal, and thyroid dysfunction, the initial workup for PPCM should include measurement of levels of serum B-type natriuretic peptide (BNP) or its N-terminal fragment (NT-proBNP), an ECG, a chest radiograph, and an echocardiogram. As with other forms of cardiomyopathy, the BNP or NT-proBNP levels are commonly elevated.[42] However, BNP or NT-proBNP levels can also be elevated in preeclampsia,[43] so they cannot be relied upon as specific markers of cardiomyopathy. ECG findings in PPCM tend to be even more nonspecific, showing sinus tachycardia and nonspecific ST-segment and T-wave changes. Sometimes, patients have conduction delays or ECG evidence of LV hypertrophy.[44] Chest radiographs can demonstrate cardiomegaly, pulmonary venous congestion, pulmonary edema, and pulmonary effusion.[44] The echocardiogram serves as the most essential diagnostic tool to evaluate anatomy, systolic function, diastolic function, and valvular function and to rule out LV thrombus. PPCM is echocardiographically indistinguishable from other forms of dilated cardiomyopathy, its main features being global cardiac dilation, reduced LV ejection fraction, a restrictive pattern of LV diastolic function, and severe mitral and tricuspid regurgitation.[45,46] The incidence of LV thrombus has been reported as 10% to 30%.[41,47–49] Because of the devastating effects of embolization, it is critical to diagnose and treat LV thrombus as early as possible. **Table 4** summarizes all of these diagnostic findings.

The management of PPCM should involve a highly coordinated, multidisciplinary team effort among the emergency physicians who initiate treatment and the cardiologists, obstetricians, intensivists, and neonatologists who will care for the patient and child in the hospital and after their eventual discharge. The current method of treatment is similar to that of other forms of nonischemic cardiomyopathy—oxygen supplementation, fluid restriction, diuretics, and antihypertensives. Of course, each pharmacologic agent must be chosen carefully to limit harm to the fetus. Anticoagulation of patients with PPCM with a known thrombus should be achieved with heparin or low-molecular-weight heparin, because warfarin is contraindicated in pregnancy. Prophylactic anticoagulation is recommended for cases complicated by atrial fibrillation and for patients without an identified thrombus but a depressed LV ejection fraction of less than 35%.[8,38,50,51] Patients with hemodynamically unstable, low cardiac output might require inotropes such as dobutamine or milrinone, and those with significant pulmonary edema might require noninvasive positive pressure ventilation or intubation and mechanical ventilation. More recently, severely ill patients with PPCM have benefited from interventions such as intra-aortic balloon pumps, extracorporeal membrane oxygenation, LV assist devices, and heart transplant.[52–56] Several experimental treatment strategies are currently undergoing research and validation, including immunosuppressive agents, intravenous immunoglobulin, bromocriptine, and pentoxifylline.[51] These agents are not currently recommended but could play a role in PPCM treatment in the future.

DYSRHYTHMIAS

Of all the aforementioned cardiac conditions, dysrhythmias are quite common during pregnancy. Symptomatic supraventricular tachycardia (SVT) is present in up to 40% of patients.[57] Palpitations are a common complaint during pregnancy and often not associated with true dysthymias.[57] Even in patients with true dysrhythmias, the majority are benign, but they do provoke anxiety. Identifying structural heart disease is paramount when assessing a pregnant woman; for women with known structural heart

Table 4	
Characteristic findings in peripartum cardiomyopathy	
Modality	**Findings**
BNP or NT proBNP	• Elevated BNP or NT proBNP levels
ECG	• Sinus tachycardia • Nonspecific ST-segment or T-wave changes • Conduction delays • Voltage criteria for LV hypertrophy
Chest radiograph	• Cardiomegaly • Pulmonary vascular congestion • Pulmonary edema • Pulmonary effusion
Echocardiogram	• Global cardiac dilation • Decreased LV ejection fraction • LV diastolic dysfunction in a restrictive pattern • Mitral regurgitation • Tricuspid regurgitation • LV thrombus

disease, an arrhythmia is 1 of 5 independent predictors of having a cardiac event during the pregnancy and should therefore be treated seriously.[58] Most critical for the identification of an arrhythmia in pregnancy, just as with any other patient population, are an ECG, a thorough history, and a physical examination. A thorough family history that concentrates on sudden premature or unexplained deaths might indicate a genetic propensity for life-threatening dysrhythmias. Diagnoses to consider in addition to structural heart disease are electrolyte imbalances, thyroid derangements, pulmonary embolism (PE), infection, and hemorrhage.

Treatment of sustained dysrhythmias in pregnancy is similar to that in the nonpregnant population. The choice depends on the frequency, duration, and tolerability of the arrhythmia, specifically its symptoms or hemodynamic compromise. During pregnancy, the clinician must balance the benefit of arrhythmia termination with the side effects of any drug treatment on the mother and the fetus. Sinus tachycardia is common in pregnancy and often nonspecific; however, identifying a culprit (eg, pain, fever, anxiety) and providing symptomatic treatment are key to management. SVT should be approached with nonpharmacologic therapy (ie, vagal maneuvers) before initiation of adenosine.[59] If adenosine is used, as with any other medication, the smallest recommended dose should be administered initially while the cardiac function of the mother and fetus is monitored continuously. Atrial fibrillation and flutter are uncommon in pregnancy. These dysthymias are most commonly associated with congenital or valvular heart disease as well as metabolic disturbances.[59] Treatment of any hemodynamic instability, just as with ventricular arrhythmias, is electrical cardioversion. For patients who are hemodynamically stable, the preferred agents are β-blockers (sotalol, atenolol), procainamide, and flecainide.[59] If rate control is required rather than restoration of sinus rhythm, β-blockers, verapamil, and digoxin are the preferred drugs along with adequate anticoagulation.[59]

Bradycardia occurs less frequently compared with tachycardia during pregnancy. Often, it is encountered in patients with congenital heart disease.[60] Symptomatic treatment in the pregnant patient does not deviate from the standard Advanced Cardiac Life Support (ACLS) protocol. Both transcutaneous and transvenous pacemakers are safe and recommended when appropriate.[60]

Coronary Artery and Aortic Dissection

The obstetric population is at risk for dissection of the coronary arteries or aorta. Arterial dissection during pregnancy is thought to occur through several mechanisms. Progesterone causes structural changes in the vascular walls of the intima and media.[61] The hemodynamic stress of pregnancy increases both the blood volume and cardiac output, causing sheer stress on the vasculature.[62] Undiagnosed connective tissue or vasculitic disorders such as Ehlers-Danlos syndrome and Takayasu arteritis also contribute to risk in this population.[28]

Coronary artery dissection, although rare, is one of the primary causes of ACS during pregnancy; this poses a diagnostic dilemma, given the recommendation of PCI for treatment of the other causes of ACS (atherosclerosis and thromboembolism). In patients who are at low risk and hemodynamically stable, noninvasive risk stratification with echocardiography should be considered before PCI to preclude worsening dissection.[31] Myocardial infarction often involves the anterior wall because the most common artery affected is the left anterior descending artery, followed by the right coronary artery, the left circumflex artery, and the left mainartery.[63–65]

The diagnosis and treatment of coronary dissection are difficult. Based on case reports and an increasing number of publications on this topic, coronary angiography and intravascular ultrasonography are the safest recommended diagnostic modalities.[65] Management remains controversial and can range from conservative medical management to coronary artery bypass; the optimal therapy is yet to be determined.[65] The prognosis is quite poor but has improved over recent years with early identification and aggressive management.

Dissections are not limited to the coronary vasculature; they also occur in the aorta but are less common and often secondary to accelerated aortic dilation.[30] In contrast to coronary artery dissection, the guidelines for management of aortic dissection are well defined, with a better prognosis for affected patients. For hemodynamically stable pregnant patients, MRI is preferred over computed tomography, which is associated with ionizing radiations (which is the first-line imaging modality for the nonpregnant patient).[66] In the unstable patient, an alternative modality, if available, is transesophageal echocardiography.[66] Management does not differ in the pregnant versus nonpregnant patient: in both groups, it consists of controlling both the blood pressure and sheer stressors with β-blockers and vasodilators.[66] For type A dissections, just as with the nonpregnant patient, surgical repair is the treatment of choice; however, because cardiac surgery is associated with fetal loss, cesarean section with concomitant thoracic surgery is recommended if fetal maturation can be confirmed.[67]

THROMBOEMBOLISM

The physiologic changes in pregnancy increase the risk of thromboembolism; therefore, deep vein thrombosis (DVT) and PE occur more frequently in pregnant and postpartum women than in nonpregnant women. Pregnant or recently pregnant women carry 4 to 5 times the risk of thromboembolism compared with their nonpregnant counterparts.[68,69] Furthermore, a Centers for Disease Control and Prevention analysis of maternal deaths occurring in the United States between 2006 and 2009 revealed that 9.4% were caused by pulmonary thromboembolism.[21]

When lower extremity DVT is suspected, the initial diagnostic test should be compression ultrasonography of the proximal veins. If the ultrasonography yields negative result, but iliac vein thrombosis is suspected, the ACOG recommends proceeding to MRI[70] (non–gadolinium-enhanced magnetic resonance venography[71]).

Clinical prediction rules for PE have been developed and extensively studied in the general population, but they have not been validated in the pregnant population. Until a prediction model is created and validated specifically for pregnant women, clinicians must rely more heavily on testing modalities to diagnose PE. D-dimer levels carry a high negative predictive value in nonpregnant patients with low to moderate pretest probability[72,73]; however, evidence to support the routine use of D-dimers to rule out PE in pregnancy has not yet reached a critical mass. Chest radiographs impart minimal radiation to the patient. It is rare that they show signs that suggest PE, but they can reveal an alternative diagnosis. Fetal radiation exposure from a ventilation/perfusion (V/Q) scan is higher than that from multidetector CT pulmonary angiogram, and the radiation doses for both are much less than ACOG's acceptable limit of 5 rad.[74] V/Q scans also have the advantage of exposing the maternal breast tissue to less ionizing radiation[75]; however, clinicians must also consider that the nondiagnostic V/Q scan rate in pregnancy is between 7% and 21%.[76,77] These patients need additional testing and therefore probably will have more radiation exposure. MRI, as a diagnostic modality for PE, is limited in pregnancy because of the need for gadolinium enhancement. Gadolinium is known to cross the placenta,[78] and its effects and safety profile in pregnancy are not well understood.

Once DVT or PE is diagnosed, or if it is highly suspected and imaging is equivocal or not available, anticoagulation therapy should be initiated promptly. Heparins (unfractionated and low-molecular-weight heparin) are the primary pharmacologic agents used for this condition. Heparins do not cross the placenta, so patients can be assured that there is no direct risk to the fetus. Treatment should be initiated at the standard nonpregnant doses but must be monitored closely, because the pharmacokinetics of heparin are different in pregnant patients. Warfarin is contraindicated in pregnancy but may be used in lactating mothers because concentrations are negligible in breast milk.[79] The more recently developed oral anticoagulants, which include dabigatran, rivaroxaban, and apixaban, are currently not recommended for pregnant or lactating women.[80–82]

CARDIAC ARREST

Few cases are more medically, ethically, and emotionally challenging than a pregnant woman in cardiac arrest. The emergency physician is faced with 2 patients: the mother and the fetus. The physiology of the mother and the fetus is intertwined, with fetal survival highly depending on maternal survival. The altered physiologic state of pregnancy makes the resuscitation of these patients seem like an extremely complex and challenging task; however, use of the following few key principles affords these patients the best chance of survival and quality of life.

The steadfast tenets of resuscitation in cardiac arrest remain the same: continuous, effective chest compressions with minimization of interruptions and early defibrillation of shockable rhythms. As detailed in the following paragraphs, patient positioning and the location of chest compressions must be adjusted for gravid patients. Defibrillation, however, needs no adjustments and should be performed at the recommended ACLS doses.[83,84]

After approximately 20 weeks of gestation (or as early as 12–14 weeks[85]), the uterus begins to displace and compress intra-abdominal and intrathoracic organs and structures, causing hemodynamic changes. Two of the critical structures affected by the gravid uterus are the aorta and inferior vena cava. Compression of the vena cava impedes venous return, which then decreases stroke volume and cardiac output (whether native or produced by chest compressions). Several techniques have been described to relieve the aortocaval compression and subsequently improve maternal hemodynamics and fetal parameters. The 2010 American Heart Association Guidelines for Cardiopulmonary Resuscitation and Emergency Cardiovascular Care recommend manual left uterine displacement in the supine position first. This technique can be accomplished by using 2 hands to pull the gravid abdomen upward and to the patient's left if standing on the left side (2-handed technique) or using 1 hand to push the abdomen upward and to the patient's left if standing on the right side (1-handed technique). It is important to ensure that the person performing the maneuver does not inadvertently push the uterus down and make the compression worse. If this technique is not successful, the patient should be placed in a left lateral tilt of 27° to 30° using a firm wedge,[83] although it should be noted that chest compressions in this position are less effective than when the patient is supine.[86] When aortocaval decompression and resuscitation efforts do not achieve return of spontaneous circulation (ROSC) within 4 minutes after arrest, a perimortem cesarean section should be considered if the gestational age is greater than 20 weeks.[83] Delivery of the fetus will fully relieve the aortocaval compression and can be life saving for both the mother and the fetus.

Other adjustments necessitated by the mass effect of the gravid abdomen are that chest compressions should be performed slightly higher on the sternum and intravenous access should be obtained above the diaphragm.[83]

Proper management of airway and breathing during the resuscitation of a pregnant patient also demands that the provider be familiar with the anatomic and physiologic changes of pregnancy. These changes result in more rapid desaturation, higher rates of aspiration, and increased risk of failed intubation.[87,88] Hormonal changes during pregnancy lead to edema, increased secretions, and friability in the upper airway. This combination reduces visibility and increases the risk of bleeding during airway manipulation.[89] These changes also contribute to a decrease in airway diameter[90]; thus, the provider must be prepared with a range of smaller endotracheal tubes. Furthermore, decreased lung volumes and increased oxygen consumption lead to a depressed pulmonary reserve and quick desaturation in pregnant patients. The functional residual capacity decreases by 20% during pregnancy, with an additional 25% decrease when changing from the sitting to supine position.[89] During rapid sequence intubation, an approach similar to handling a morbidly obese patient should be used. Preoxygenation and apneic oxygenation should be maximized, and the patient should be positioned in a semirecumbent position if possible (maintaining alignment of the ear with the sternal notch). Finally, these patients are at higher risk for aspiration because of lower esophageal sphincter tone as a physiologic consequence of pregnancy.

In the 2010 American Heart Association Guidelines for Cardiopulmonary Resuscitation and Emergency Cardiovascular Care,[83,91] and in Part 12, Cardiac Arrest in Special Situations,[83] an algorithm for maternal cardiac arrest is mentioned (See figure 1 from *Ref.* 83). The latter document also presents a mnemonic for possible contributing factors in maternal cardiac arrest: BEAU-CHOPS (bleeding/disseminated intravascular coagulation, embolism, anesthetic complications, uterine atony, cardiac disease, hypertension/preeclampsia-eclampsia, other, placenta abruption/previa, and sepsis).

If ROSC is achieved, the patient should be placed in the left lateral decubitus position so that aortocaval compression can continue to be minimized, preventing a decline in hemodynamics.

Postcardiac arrest hypothermia for maternal cardiac arrest without delivery of the fetus is considered safe and effective, with favorable maternal and fetal outcomes.[92,93] The decision to initiate hypothermia should be based on the current recommendations for the nonpregnant patient, and the fetus should be monitored continuously for potential complications such as bradycardia.[83]

SUMMARY

The cardiovascular complications of pregnancy can be catastrophic, but when they are suspected and diagnosed early, aggressive management and a multidisciplinary effort by emergency physicians, obstetricians, cardiologists, intensivists, and neonatologists can improve outcomes for both the mother and the child.

REFERENCES

1. Wagner SJ, Barac S, Garovic VD. Hypertensive pregnancy disorders: current concepts. J Clin Hypertens (Greenwich) 2007;9(7):560–6.
2. Kuklina EV, Ayala C, Callaghan WM. Hypertensive disorders and severe obstetric morbidity in the United States. Obstet Gynecol 2009;113(6):1299–306.
3. Hutcheon JA, Lisononkova S, Joseph KS. Epidemiology of pre-eclampsia and the other hypertensive disorders of pregnancy. Best Pract Res Clin Obstet Gynaecol 2011;25(4):391–403.
4. American College of Obstetricians and Gynecologists, Task Force on Hypertension in Pregnancy. Hypertension in pregnancy. Report of the American College of

Obstetricians and Gynecologists' Task Force on Hypertension in Pregnancy. Obstet Gynecol 2013;122(5):1122–31.

5. Alexander JM, Wilson KL. Hypertensive emergencies of pregnancy. Obstet Gynecol Clin North Am 2013;40(1):89–101.

6. Buppajarntham S, Junpaparp P, Shah M, et al. Spontaneous coronary artery dissection following a preeclampsia pregnancy. Int J Cardiol 2014;173(2):e3–4.

7. Thalmann M, Sodeck GH, Domanovits H, et al. Acute type A aortic dissection and pregnancy: a population-based study. Eur J Cardiothorac Surg 2011;39(6):e159–63.

8. Shah T, Ather S, Bavishi C, et al. Peripartum cardiomyopathy: a contemporary review. Methodist Debakey Cardiovasc J 2013;9(1):38–43.

9. Zeeman GG, Cunningham FG, Pritcahrd JA. The magnitude of hemoconcentration with eclampsia. Hypertens Pregnancy 2009;28(2):127–37.

10. Lindheimer MD, Conrad KP, Karumanchi SA. Renal physiology and disease in pregnancy. In: Alpern RJ, Hebert SC, editors. Seldin and Giebisch's the kidney; physiology and pathophysiology. 4th edition. San Diego (CA): Academic Press, Elsevier; 2008. p. 2339–98.

11. Karumanchi SA, Maynaard SE, Stillman IE, et al. Preeclampsia: a renal perspective. Kidney Int 2005;67(6):2101–13.

12. Spargo B, McCartney CP, Winemiller R. Glomerular capillary endotheliosis in toxemia of pregnancy. Arch Pathol 1959;68:593–9.

13. Stevens DU, Al-Nasiry S, Bulten J, et al. Decidual vasculopathy and adverse perinatal outcome in preeclamptic pregnancy. Placenta 2012;33(8):630–3.

14. Jim B, Sharma S, Kebede T, et al. Hypertension in pregnancy: a comprehensive update. Cardiol Rev 2010;18(4):178–89.

15. Duley L, Meher S, Jones L. Drugs for treatment of very high blood pressure during pregnancy. Cochrane Database Syst Rev 2013;(7):CD001449.

16. Elatrous S, Nouira S, Ouanes Besbes L, et al. Short-term treatment of severe hypertension of pregnancy: prospective comparison of nicardipine and labetalol. Intensive Care Med 2002;28(9):1281–6.

17. ACOG Committee on Practice Bulletins–Obstetrics. ACOG practice bulletin #33: diagnosis and management of preeclampsia and eclampsia. Obstet Gynecol 2002;99(1):159–67.

18. Too GT, Hill JB. Hypertensive crisis during pregnancy and postpartum period. Semin Perinatol 2013;37(4):280–7.

19. Thornton CE, von Dadelszen P, Makris A, et al. Acute pulmonary oedema as a complication of hypertension during pregnancy. Hypertens Pregnancy 2011;30(2):169–79.

20. Hogan MC, Foreman KJ, Naghavi M, et al. Maternal mortality for 181 countries, 1980–2008: a systematic analysis of progress towards Millennium Development Goal 5. Lancet 2010;375(9726):1609–23.

21. Pregnancy Mortality Surveillance System. Trends in pregnancy-related deaths. Available at: www.cdc.gov/reproductivehealth/maternalinfanthealth/pmss.html. Accessed June 30, 2014.

22. Marelli AJ, Mackie AS, Ionescu-Ittu R, et al. Congenital heart disease in the general population: changing prevalence and age distribution. Circulation 2007;115(2):163–72.

23. Drenthen W, Boersma E, Balci A, et al. Predictors of pregnancy complications in women with congenital heart disease. Eur Heart J 2010;31(17):2124–32.

24. Hill K, Thomas K, AbouZahr C, et al. Estimates of maternal mortality worldwide between 1990 and 2005: an assessment of available data. Lancet 2007;370(9595):1311–9.

25. Gaskin IM. Maternal death in the United States: a problem solved or a problem ignored? J Perinat Educ 2008;17(2):9–13.
26. Ladner HE, Danielsen B, Gilbert WM. Acute myocardial infarction in pregnancy and the puerperium: a population-based study. Obstet Gynecol 2005;105(3): 480–4.
27. Roth A, Elkayam U. Acute myocardial infarction associated with pregnancy. J Am Coll Cardiol 2008;52(3):171–80.
28. James AH, Jamison MG, Biswas MS, et al. Acute myocardial infarction in pregnancy: a United States population-based study. Circulation 2006;113(12): 1564–71.
29. Cantwell R, Clutton-Brock T, Cooper G, et al. Saving Mothers' Lives: reviewing maternal deaths to make motherhood safer: 2006–2008. The Eighth Report of the Confidential Enquiries into Maternal Deaths in the United Kingdom. BJOG 2011;118(suppl 1):1–203.
30. Sahni G. Chest pain syndromes in pregnancy. Cardiol Clin 2012;30(3):343–67.
31. European Society of Gynecology, Association for European Paediatric Cardiology, German Society for Gender Medicine, et al. ESC Guidelines on the management of cardiovascular diseases during pregnancy: the Task Force on the Management of Cardiovascular Diseases during Pregnancy of the European Society of Cardiology (ESC). Eur Heart J 2011;32(24):3147–97.
32. Gibson PS, Powrie R. Anticoagulants and pregnancy: when are they safe? Cleve Clin J Med 2009;76(2):113–27.
33. Mielniczuk LM, Williams K, Davis DR, et al. Frequency of peripartum cardiomyopathy. Am J Cardiol 2006;97(12):1765–8.
34. Pearson GD, Veille JC, Rahimtoola S, et al. Peripartum cardiomyopathy: National Heart, Lung, and Blood Institute and Office of Rare Diseases (National Institutes of Health) workshop recommendations and review. JAMA 2000; 283(9):1183–8.
35. Brar SS, Khan SS, Sandhu GK, et al. Incidence, mortality, and racial differences in peripartum cardiomyopathy. Am J Cardiol 2007;100(2):302–4.
36. Gentry MB, Dias JK, Luis A, et al. African-American women have a higher risk for developing peripartum cardiomyopathy. J Am Coll Cardiol 2010;55(7):654–9.
37. Heider AL, Kuller JA, Strauss RA, et al. Peripartum cardiomyopathy: a review of the literature. Obstet Gynecol Surv 1999;54(8):526–31.
38. Sliwa K, Hilfiker-Kleiner D, Petrie MC, et al. Current state of knowledge on aetiology, diagnosis, management, and therapy of peripartum cardiomyopathy: a position statement from the Heart Failure Association of the European Society of Cardiology Working Group on peripartum cardiomyopathy. Eur J Heart Fail 2010;12(8):767–78.
39. Box LC, Hanak V, Arciniegas JG. Dual coronary emboli in peripartum cardiomyopathy. Tex Heart Inst J 2004;31(4):442–4.
40. Helms AK, Kittner SJ. Pregnancy and stroke. CNS Spectr 2005;10(7):580–7.
41. Napporn AG, Kane A, Damorou JM, et al. Intraventricular thrombosis complicating peri-partum idiopathic myocardiopathy. Ann Cardiol Angeiol (Paris) 2000;49(5):309–14 [in French].
42. Hameed AB, Chan K, Ghamsary M, et al. Longitudinal changes in the B-type natriuretic peptide levels in normal pregnancy and postpartum. Clin Cardiol 2009;32(8):E60–2.
43. Resnik JL, Hong C, Resnik R, et al. Evaluation of B-type natriuretic peptide (BNP) levels in normal and preeclamptic women. Am J Obstet Gynecol 2005;193(2): 450–4.

44. Elkayam U, Jalnapurkar S, Barakat M. Peripartum cardiomyopathy. Cardiol Clin 2012;30(3):435–40.
45. Ain DL, Narula J, Sengupta PP. Cardiovascular imaging and diagnostic procedures in pregnancy. Cardiol Clin 2012;30(3):331–41.
46. Blauwet LA, Cooper LT. Diagnosis and management of peripartum cardiomyopathy. Heart 2011;97(23):1970–81.
47. Sakamoto A. Case report: peripartum cardiomyopathy with biventricular thrombus which led to massive cerebral embolism. J Cardiol Cases 2014;9(2):71–4.
48. Amos AM, Jaber WA, Russell SD. Improved outcomes in peripartum cardiomyopathy with contemporary. Am Heart J 2006;152(3):509–13.
49. Kane A, Mbaye M, Ndiaye MB, et al. Évolution et complications thromboemboliques de la myocardiopathie idiopathique du péripartum au CHU de Dakar: étude prospective à propos de 33 cas. J Gynecol Obstet Biol Reprod (Paris) 2010; 39(6):484–9.
50. Karaye KM, Henein MY. Peripartum cardiomyopathy: a review article. Int J Cardiol 2013;164(1):33–8.
51. Bhattacharyya A, Basra SS, Sen P, et al. Peripartum cardiomyopathy: a review. Tex Heart Inst J 2012;39(1):8–16.
52. Gevaert S, Van Belleghem Y, Bouchez S, et al. Acute and critically ill peripartum cardiomyopathy and 'bridge to' therapeutic options: a single center experience with intra-aortic balloon pump, extra corporeal membrane oxygenation and continuous-flow left ventricular assist devices. Crit Care 2011;15(2):R93.
53. Keogh A, Macdonald P, Spratt P, et al. Outcome in peripartum cardiomyopathy after heart transplantation. J Heart Lung Transplant 1994;13:202–7.
54. Yang HS, Hong YS, Rim SJ, et al. Extracorporeal membrane oxygenation in a patient with peripartum cardiomyopathy. Ann Thorac Surg 2007;84:262–4.
55. Palanzo DA, Baer LD, El-Banayosy A, et al. Successful treatment of peripartum cardiomyopathy with extracorporeal membrane oxygenation. Perfusion 2009; 24:75–9.
56. Smith IJ, Gillham MJ. Fulminant peripartum cardiomyopathy rescue with extracorporeal membranous oxygenation. Int J Obstet Anesth 2009;18:186–8.
57. Silversides CK, Harris L, Haberer K, et al. Recurrence rates of arrhythmias during pregnancy in women with previous tachyarrhythmia and impact on fetal and neonatal outcomes. Am J Cardiol 2006;97(8):1206–12.
58. Siu SC, Sermer M, Harrison DA, et al. Risk and predictors for pregnancy-related complications in women with heart disease. Circulation 1997;96(9):2789–94.
59. Gowda RM, Khan IA, Mehta NJ, et al. Cardiac arrhythmias in pregnancy: clinical and therapeutic considerations. Int J Cardiol 2003;88(2–3):129–33.
60. Hidaka N, Chiba Y, Kurita T, et al. Is intrapartum temporary pacing required for women with complete atrioventricular block? An analysis of seven cases. BJOG 2006;113(5):605–7.
61. Bonnet J, Aumailley M, Thomas D, et al. Spontaneous coronary artery dissection: case report and evidence for a defect in collagen metabolism. Eur Heart J 1986; 7(10):904–9.
62. Elkayam U, Gleicher N. Cardiac problems in pregnancy: diagnosis and management of maternal and fetal disease. 3rd edition. New York: Wiley-Liss; 1998.
63. Maeder M, Ammann P, Drack G, et al. Pregnancy-associated spontaneous coronary artery dissection: impact of medical treatment: case report and systematic review. Z Kardiol 2005;94(12):829–35.

64. Appleby CE, Barolet A, Ing D, et al. Contemporary management of pregnancy-related coronary artery dissection: a single-centre experience and literature review. Exp Clin Cardiol 2009;14(1):e8–16.
65. Sheikh AS, O'Sullivan M. Pregnancy-related spontaneous coronary artery dissection: two case reports and a comprehensive review of literature. Heart Views 2012;13(2):53–65.
66. Hiratzka LF, Bakris GL, Beckman JA, et al. 2010 ACCF/AHA/AATS/ACR/ASA/SCA/SCAI/SIR/STS/SVM guidelines for the diagnosis and management of patients with Thoracic Aortic Disease: a report of the American College of Cardiology Foundation/American Heart Association Task Force on Practice Guidelines, American Association for Thoracic Surgery, American College of Radiology, American Stroke Association, Society of Cardiovascular Anesthesiologists, Society for Cardiovascular Angiography and Interventions, Society of Interventional Radiology, Society of Thoracic Surgeons, and Society for Vascular Medicine. Circulation 2010;121(13):e266–369.
67. Immer FF, Bansi AG, Immer-Bansi AS, et al. Aortic dissection in pregnancy: analysis of risk factors and outcome. Ann Thorac Surg 2003;76(1):309–14.
68. Pomp ER, Lenselink AM, Rosendaal FR, et al. Pregnancy, the postpartum period and prothrombotic defects: risk of venous thrombosis in the MEGA study. J Thromb Haemost 2008;6(4):632–7.
69. Heit JA, Kobbervig CE, James AH, et al. Trends in the incidence of venous thromboembolism during pregnancy or postpartum: a 30-year population-based study. Ann Intern Med 2005;143(10):697–706.
70. James A, Committee on Practice Bulletins—Obstetrics. Practice bulletin no. 123: thromboembolism in pregnancy. Obstet Gynecol 2011;118(3):718–29.
71. Miller MA, Chalhoub M, Bourjeily G. Peripartum pulmonary embolism. Clin Chest Med 2011;32(1):147–64.
72. Kline JA, Runyon MS, Webb WB, et al. Prospective study of the diagnostic accuracy of the simplify D-dimer assay for pulmonary embolism in emergency department patients. Chest 2006;129(6):1417–23.
73. van Belle A, Büller HR, Huisman MV, et al. Effectiveness of managing suspected pulmonary embolism using an algorithm combining clinical probability, D-dimer testing, and computed tomography. JAMA 2006;295(2):172–9.
74. ACOG Committee on Obstetric Practice. ACOG Committee Opinion No. 299, September 2004 (replaces No. 158, September 1995). Guidelines for diagnostic imaging during pregnancy. Obstet Gynecol 2004;104:647–51.
75. Groves AM, Yates SJ, Win T, et al. CT pulmonary angiography versus ventilation-perfusion scintigraphy in pregnancy: implications from a UK survey of doctors' knowledge of radiation exposure. Radiology 2006;240(3):765–70.
76. Chan WS, Ray JG, Murray S, et al. Suspected pulmonary embolism in pregnancy: clinical presentation, results of lung scanning, and subsequent maternal and pediatric outcomes. Arch Intern Med 2002;162(10):1170–5.
77. Scarsbrook AF, Bradley KM, Gleeson FV. Perfusion scintigraphy: diagnostic utility in pregnant women with suspected pulmonary embolic disease. Eur Radiol 2007;17(10):2554–60.
78. Lin SP, Brown JJ. MR contrast agents: physical and pharmacologic basics. J Magn Reson Imaging 2007;25(5):884–99.
79. Yurdakok M. Fetal and neonatal effects of anticoagulants used in pregnancy: a review. Turk J Pediatr 2012;54(3):207–15.

80. Highlights of prescribing information: Eliquis. 2012. Available at: www. accessdata.fda.gov/drugsatfda_docs/label/2012/202155s000lbl.pdf. Accessed June 30, 2014.
81. Highlights of prescribing information: Pradaxa. 2014. Available at: www. accessdata.fda.gov/drugsatfda_docs/label/2013/022512s017lbl.pdf. Accessed June 30, 2014.
82. Highlights of prescribing information: Xarelto. 2011. Available at: www. accessdata.fda.gov/drugsatfda_docs/label/2011/202439s001lbl.pdf. Accessed June 30, 2014.
83. Vanden Hoek TL, Morrison LJ, Shuster M, et al. Part 12: cardiac arrest in special situations: 2010 American Heart Association Guidelines for Cardiopulmonary Resuscitation and Emergency Cardiovascular Care. Circulation 2010;122(18 suppl 3):S829–61.
84. Nanson J, Elcock D, Williams M, et al. Do physiological changes in pregnancy change defibrillation energy requirements? Br J Anaesth 2001;87(2):237–9.
85. McLennan CE. Antecubital and femoral venous pressure in normal and toxemic pregnancy. Am J Obstet Gynecol 1943;45(4):568–91.
86. Rees GA, Willis BA. Resuscitation in late pregnancy. Anaesthesia 1988;43(5): 347–9.
87. Hobbs A, Cockerham R. Obstetric anaesthesia: general anaesthesia for operative obstetrics. Anaesth Intensive Care Med 2013;14:346–9.
88. Quinn AC, Milne D, Columb M, et al. Failed tracheal intubation in obstetric anaesthesia: 2 yr national case–control study in the UK. Br J Anaesth 2013;110(1): 74–80.
89. Vasdev GM, Harrison BA, Keegan MT, et al. Management of the difficult and failed airway in obstetric anesthesia. J Anesth 2008;22(1):38–48.
90. Izci B, Vennelle M, Liston WA, et al. Sleep-disordered breathing and upper airway size in pregnancy and post-partum. Eur Respir J 2006;27(2):321–7.
91. Field JM, Hazinski MF, Sayre MR, et al. Part 1: executive summary: 2010 American Heart Association Guidelines for Cardiopulmonary Resuscitation and Emergency Cardiovascular Care. Circulation 2010;122(18 suppl 3):S640–56.
92. Rittenberger JC, Kelly E, Jang D, et al. Successful outcome utilizing hypothermia after cardiac arrest in pregnancy: a case report. Crit Care Med 2008;36(4): 1354–6.
93. Chauhan A, Musunuru H, Donnino M, et al. The use of therapeutic hypothermia after cardiac arrest in a pregnant patient. Ann Emerg Med 2012;60(6):786–9.

The Critically Ill Infant with Congenital Heart Disease

Ashley M. Strobel, MD[a,b], Le N. Lu, MD[c,*]

KEYWORDS

- Congenital heart disease • Cyanotic cardiac disease • Pediatric cardiology
- Critically ill neonate • Decompensated neonate

KEY POINTS

- Neonates presenting with acute and profound systemic hypoperfusion or cyanosis have a ductal-dependent cardiac lesion until proven otherwise.
- Ductal-dependent lesions typically present within the first 2 weeks of life, whereas shunting lesions with heart failure present within 1 to 6 months of life.
- Prostaglandin E1 is a life-saving medication. Be wary of its adverse effects of apnea and hypotension.
- Essential elements in the evaluation of a critically ill infant with congenital cardiac disease include (1) right upper and lower extremity blood pressure, (2) pulse oximetry, (3) brachial–femoral pulse differential, (4) electrocardiography, (5) chest radiography, (6) brain natri-uretic peptide, and (7) bedside echocardiogram.

INTRODUCTION

Critically ill infants presenting to the emergency department (ED) inherently produce anxiety for emergency physicians (EPs). They often have nonspecific or subtle findings, making timely accurate diagnosis and implementation of life-saving interventions fraught with difficulty. The differential diagnosis for an ill neonate is best remembered by the mnemonic THE MISFITS (**Box 1**).[1] Children with congenital cardiac disease are especially challenging to diagnose and manage because of their complex physiology

Disclosures: The authors have no relevant financial relationships to disclose.
[a] Department of Emergency Medicine, University of Maryland Medical Center, 110 South Paca Street, 6th Floor, Suite 200, Baltimore, MD 21201, USA; [b] Department of Pediatrics, University of Maryland Medical Center, 22 South Greene Street, North Hospital, 5th floor, Baltimore, MD 21201, USA; [c] Department of Emergency Medicine, University of Maryland School of Medicine, 110 South Paca Street, 6th Floor, Suite 200, Baltimore, MD 21201, USA
* Corresponding author.
E-mail address: dr.mimi@gmail.com

Emerg Med Clin N Am 33 (2015) 501–518
http://dx.doi.org/10.1016/j.emc.2015.04.002
0733-8627/15/$ – see front matter © 2015 Elsevier Inc. All rights reserved.

Box 1
THE MISFITS

- *T*rauma (accidental and nonaccidental)
- *H*eart disease and hypovolemia
- *E*ndocrine (congenital adrenal hyperplasia and thyrotoxicosis)
- *M*etabolic (hypocalcemia, hypoglycemia, etc)
- *I*nborn errors of metabolism
- *S*epsis
- *F*ormula dilution
- *I*ntestinal catastrophes (necrotizing enterocolitis, volvulus, intussusception)
- *T*oxins
- *S*eizures

---

and age-dependent variability. This article discusses the tools necessary for the identification and initial ED management of the infant with undifferentiated decompensated congenital heart disease (CHD).

Critical congenital cardiac lesions can be classified into 3 broad categories based on physiology: left-sided obstructive ductal dependent, right-sided obstructive ductal dependent, and shunting or mixing lesions. As with all pediatric cases, physiology is age dependent, so the child's age at presentation is among the most important variables to consider. Infants who present early—in the first month of life—most likely have a ductal-dependent lesion. They might be cyanotic from an obstructive right heart lesion or, more commonly, profoundly hypoperfused from an obstructive left heart lesion. After 1 month of age, infants most likely present in respiratory distress or congestive heart failure caused by a left-to-right shunt.[2] A rapid compilation of data obtained from the history and physical examination, focusing on essential elements (**Box 2**), can provide clues to the presence and physiology of the cardiac lesion. Subsequent interventions, such as use of supplemental oxygen, initiation of prostaglandin E1 (PGE1), or administration of fluid boluses can then be tailored to fit the patient's unique physiology.

Box 2
Toolkit for identification of a congenital cardiac disease

- Hyperoxia test
- Weight gain, murmur, hepatomegaly, brachial–femoral pulse differential
- Right upper and lower extremity blood pressure differential of greater than 10 mm Hg
- Pulse oximetry differential of greater than 3%, or less than 94% in lower extremity, or less than 90% in any extremity
- Electrocardiography (ECG)
- Chest radiography (CXR)
- Brain natriuretic peptide (BNP)
- Bedside limited echocardiography by the emergency physician (BLEEP)

Epidemiology

The true incidence of CHD is difficult to determine because of the variability in its definition. Some studies have broadly included physiologically trivial atrial septal defects (ASDs) and ventricular septal defects (VSDs); others have specifically defined critical CHD (CCHD). A CCHD lesion is defined as one that requires surgical repair or intervention to prevent significant morbidity and mortality within the first year of life. In the United States and the United Kingdom, it is estimated that 6 in 1000 live-born infants have a serious congenital heart defect.[3–6] A more recent review, with clear definition of CCHD, by The Tennessee Task Force on Screening Newborn Infants for Critical Congenital Heart Disease, estimated the incidence of CCHD to be approximately 1.7 in 1000 live births.[7] Among those, nearly 1 infant in 1000 was discharged home from the nursery with a missed critical left heart obstructive lesion.[7]

Screening

Overreliance on the newborn screening examination to rule out CCHD is commonplace. At 1 pediatric cardiology referral center, 8% of all neonates admitted for CHD were diagnosed after discharge from the hospital.[8] The most common lesions presenting after discharge are left obstructive lesions, which include coarctation of the aorta, interruption of the aortic arch, aortic valve stenosis, total anomalous pulmonary venous return (TAPVR), and hypoplastic left heart syndrome (HLHS).[6,8] A study of missed congenital cardiac lesions found that more than one-half of infants with a missed diagnosis of CCHD died at home or in the ED. Their median age at death was 13.5 days, and the most common delayed diagnoses were HLHS and coarctation of the aorta.[9]

The use of fetal echocardiography to detect cardiac lesions in the prenatal period has certainly lowered morbidity and mortality rates, but fetal ultrasonography still has limitations. Chew and colleagues[10] found that CCHD was diagnosed before birth in only about one-fourth of their study population.

Unfortunately, the screening physical examination in the newborn nursery is inadequate to detect many critical congenital heart defects. There are even fewer opportunities to diagnose CCHD in the newborn nursery, because infants are being discharged earlier than in the past. It is estimated that 8% to 44% of infants with CCHD are being discharged undiagnosed.[2,4,5,8,11–14] In the patient series studied by Wren and colleagues,[6] only 50% of infants with CHD had an abnormal nursery examination finding (usually a murmur) and 65% had abnormal findings during the 6-week examination. Left obstructive lesions are even less likely to be detected during the nursery physical examination. Fewer than one-third of 108 neonatal examinations of children with left-obstructive lesions were abnormal over a 4-year period.[5] Undiagnosed children with CCHD frequently present to nontertiary EDs for initial management before transfer for subspecialist care.[15] It is therefore critical for all EPs to be prepared to recognize and manage undiagnosed congenital cardiac lesions in the critically ill infant.

In 2009, the American Heart Association and the American Academy of Pediatrics published a joint statement noting the potential for pulse oximetry to improve clinicians' ability to identify CCHD before discharge from the nursery.[16,17] Since 2011, many states have adopted legislation calling for mandatory pulse oximetry screening of all newborns before discharge. Screening entails obtaining a pulse oximetry measurement (saturation of peripheral oxygen [SpO_2]) from the preductal right upper extremity (RUE) and either postductal lower extremity (LE; **Box 3**). Normal newborns have a median SpO_2 of 98% after 24 hours of life. A positive screen is indicated by

> **Box 3**
> **CCHD screening pulse oximetry**
>
> - SpO_2 of less than 90% RUE or either LE → echocardiography
> - SpO_2 of 94% or less RUE and either LE → echocardiography
> - SpO_2 difference of greater than 3% between RUE and LE → echocardiography
>
> *Abbreviations:* LE, lower extremity; RUE, right upper extremity; SpO_2, saturation of peripheral oxygen.

a RUE or LE SpO_2 of less than 90%, both preductal and postductal SpO_2 of 94% or less, or a difference of greater than 3% between the preductal and postductal SpO_2 (see **Box 3**). Any patient with a positive screen is either referred for echocardiogram before discharge or scheduled for a diagnostic follow-up with the local pediatric cardiology referral center. The ability of this CCHD pulse oximetry screening protocol to lower the false-positive rate was demonstrated by Granelli and colleagues,[18] who documented a rate of 0.17% compared with 1.9% achieved with physical examination alone. The CCHDs targeted in the pulse oximetry screening are HLHS, pulmonary atresia, tetralogy of Fallot, TAPVR, transposition of the great arteries (TGA), tricuspid atresia, and truncus arteriosus. The timing of the screen allows assessment for HLHS, but not for other left-obstructive lesions such as coarctation of the aorta. Interestingly, many patients with false-positive pulse oximetry screens have an urgent disease process, such as persistent pulmonary hypertension.[19]

Cyanosis

Cyanosis becomes apparent when the oxygen saturation drops below 80% or the concentration of deoxygenated hemoglobin is 5 g/dL or greater. Central cyanosis involves the lips, tongue, and mucous membranes, as opposed to acrocyanosis, which affects the hands, feet, and circumoral region. Acrocyanosis is caused typically by cool ambient temperatures, gastroesophageal reflux, sepsis, and tracheoesophageal fistula. It is important to examine infants in a well-lit room to assess for appearance and cyanosis.

The presentation of cyanotic CHD can be very similar to that of persistent pulmonary hypertension. Supplemental oxygenation with the "hyperoxia test" (discussed elsewhere in this article) fails to improve cyanosis in either condition. It is often difficult to recognize mild to moderate cyanosis, especially in infants with dark skin; therefore, a "pink" infant should not be reassuring. Pulse oximetry is an important vital sign for every neonate, because color change might not be evident on examination. Confounding the picture, the nadir of physiologic anemia of infancy typically occurs at 3 months of age in a term infant and sooner, at 4 to 6 weeks, for a preterm infant.[20] The timing of physiologic nadir coincides with the transition of shunting from right to left at birth, which progresses to left to right by 3 months of age as right ventricular compliance increases and pulmonary vascular resistance (PVR) decreases.[21] Differential cyanosis (ie, cyanosis of the lower extremities without accompanying cyanosis of the upper body) raises concern for persistent pulmonary hypertension of the newborn with right-to-left shunt, interrupted aortic arch, and coarctation of the aorta. In patients with these conditions, desaturated blood from the patent ductus arteriosus (PDA) supplies the postductal descending aorta and lower extremities and oxygenated blood from the preductal aortic arch supplies the upper extremities, creating a differential cyanosis. Reverse differential cyanosis is unique and requires a dextro-TGA (d-TGA) in combination with a PDA and severe coarctation of the aorta or interrupted aortic arch.[21] The upper extremities are supplied by deoxygenated blood from the transposed aortic arch. The lower extremities are supplied by oxygenated blood from the pulmonary artery shunting left to right distal to the coarctation through the PDA.

Cyanosis is part of the presentation of the following imminent emergencies: shock, cyanotic CHD, persistent pulmonary hypertension, and methemoglobinemia. Cyanotic CHD can be divided into right-sided obstructive ductal-dependent lesions, right outflow tract obstruction that diminishes blood flow to the pulmonary arteries, and mixing lesions (**Fig. 1**). Many children present to the ED without a known diagnosis of congenital cardiac disease, so management should be guided by considering the underlying physiology, as described elsewhere in this article.

Presentation

The diagnosis of CCHD might be missed during the birth hospitalization; therefore, clinicians should be aware of its clinical manifestations during the first week of life. Although there is no single test or historical feature that serves to differentiate CHD from other conditions in the differential for the ill-appearing infant, a compilation of red flags should alert the EP to the possibility of its presence. Few studies have examined the signs and symptoms that prompt parents to bring their children to the ED. Symptoms classically associated with CHD include irritability, sweating, and crying with feeding.[22] Other parental concerns include poor weight gain, cyanosis, respiratory difficulties, and decreased activity. The history alone is usually inadequate to differentiate between an inborn error of metabolism, sepsis, and a congenital cardiac lesion. The most sensitive and specific findings for serious congestive heart failure in infants is a history of less than 3 ounces of formula per feed or more than 40 minutes per breast feed, respiratory rate higher than 60 breaths per minute or irregular breathing, and the liver edge located more than 2.5 cm below the right costal margin.[23] Older children have symptoms similar to those of adults with congestive heart failure: dyspnea on exertion, exercise intolerance, syncope, facial or abdominal swelling, and abdominal pain. In addition to a thorough history of the chief complaint, a thorough family history must be obtained, because 20% of critical congenital cardiac defects have a genetic component.

In various studies, the common presenting signs documented as leading to the diagnosis of CHD are the presence of a murmur, cyanosis, respiratory distress, heart failure, and shock.[2,8,15] Two studies retrospectively examined pediatric ED presentations leading to a diagnosis of CHD.[2,8,15] A study from a US pediatric cardiology referral center found 8 new diagnoses of CHD among children admitted with decompensated CHD over a 5-year period.[2] Five children presented to the ED with pulmonary edema and 2 with cyanosis and circulatory collapse. Left obstructive lesions have the highest postdischarge mortality rate, and almost all infants with these lesions present by 3 weeks of age, the majority of them (68%) presenting with heart failure.[5]

DIAGNOSIS

The challenge for the EP is early identification of children with the potential for rapid decompensation. First and foremost, a neonate in distress should be presumed septic. Empiric antibiotics for sepsis should be initiated as soon as possible for every critically ill infant. Cefotaxime and ampicillin are recommended in neonates. For infants more than 1 month old, ceftriaxone and vancomycin can be used to cover for meningitis.[24] However, in the setting of cyanosis or hypotension, CCHD should also be

Pink Baby	Blue Baby	Blue Baby	Grey Baby
1-6 months	1-6 months	<2 weeks	<2 weeks
Too much pulmonary blood flow Qp>Qs	Obstruction of pulmonary blood return	Too little pulmonary blood flow Qp<Qs	Poor perfusion and oxygenation
Heart failure	Cyanosis + heart failure	Cyanosis	Circulatory collapse
Left-to-right shunt	Mixing right-to-left shunt	Right obstructive lesion	Left obstructive lesion
Toolkit clues: • CXR white lungs • Hepatomegaly • Murmur • BNP > 100 pg/mL • BLEEP: possible interventricular defect • ECG possible extreme superior axis or AV block	Toolkit clues: • Fail hyperoxia test • CXR white lungs • BNP >40-100 pg/mL • SpO$_2$ <80% • Hepatomegaly	Toolkit Clues: • Fail hyperoxia test • CXR black lungs • SpO$_2$ < 80% • ECG RVH	Toolkit clues: • CXR white lungs • Differential SpO$_2$ > 3%, BP > 10 mm Hg, pulse RUE vs RLE • Delayed capillary refill time • ECG LVH in >7 days of life, RVH in newborn • BLEEP possible single ventricle
Treatment goals • Increase PVR (decrease oxygen) • Decrease SVR • Increase Qs • Increase inotropy • Diuretics	Treatment goals: • Diuretics • Do not increase pulmonary blood flow • Restrict IV fluids • Increase right-to-left shunting and inotropy (milrinone)	Treatment goals: • Shunt left-to-right across ductus arteriosus (PGE) • Decrease PVR (add oxygen or iNO) • Increase Qp	Treatment goals: • Shunt right-to-left across ductus arteriosus (PGE) • Afterload reduction • Volume support • Minimize oxygen consumption • Initiate early antibiotics • May need pressors
Lesions: • PDA • VSD • AVM • AV canal defect	Lesions: • TAPVR • Truncus arteriosus • Double outlet right ventricle • d-TGA with a VSD (or PDA)	Lesions: • Tricuspid atresia • Pulmonary atresia • Pulmonary stenosis • Ebstein anomaly	Lesions: • Hypoplastic left heart syndrome • Coarctation of the aorta • Interrupted aortic arch • Aortic stenosis or atresia
		Exception: • d-TGA without a VSD • Tetralogy of Fallot	Exception: • Anomalous Left Coronary Artery from the Pulmonary Artery

Fig. 1. Diagnosis and management of the infant with undifferentiated critical congenital heart disease. [a] Goal oxygen saturations of greater than 80% are adequate for initial resuscitation, however Qp:Qs balance is obtained at different oxygen saturations for each critical congenital heart disease. Monitor resuscitation based on both the perfusion and respiratory examination. AV, atrioventricular; AVM, arteriovenous malformation; BLEEP, bedside limited echocardiography by the emergency physician; BNP, brain natriuretic peptide; CXR, chest x-ray; d-TGA, dextrotransposition of the great arteries; ECG, electrocardiograph; iNO, inhaled nitric oxide; PDA, patent ductus arteriosus; PGE, prostaglandin E; Qp, pulmonary blood flow; Qs, systemic blood flow; RLE, right lower extremity; RUE, right upper extremity; RVH, right ventricular hypertrophy; SVR, systemic vascular resistance; TAPVR, total anomalous pulmonary venous return; VSD, ventricular septal defect.

considered. Infants presenting at a younger age most likely have a ductal-dependent lesion; shunting lesions are more common during later infancy.[5,22] Several essential tests can aid in narrowing the differential diagnosis.

Hyperoxia Test

When a critically ill infant presents with cyanosis or respiratory distress, the "hyperoxia test" can be attempted to determine whether the symptoms are a result of a problem with the pulmonary or systemic circulation. The test is performed by measuring the infant's arterial blood gas while breathing room air, then remeasuring the arterial blood gas after providing 100% oxygen for 10 minutes. If the cause of the cyanosis is a primary pulmonary deficiency, then administration of 100% oxygen will augment the lungs' ability to saturate the blood with oxygen, and the partial pressure of oxygen in the arterial blood should increase to above 150 mm Hg. However, if the lungs are oxygenating fully, supplemental oxygen will have no significant effect, and the partial pressure of oxygen will usually remain below 100 mm Hg. In this circumstance, the cyanosis is most likely owing to a shunting lesion that bypasses the lung, such as a congenital heart lesion. Because of the difficulty in obtaining 1 arterial blood gas measurement, let alone 2, in a critically ill neonate, pulse oximetry can be used instead.[18] One should be wary of the pitfall that pulse oximetry is less accurate for saturations of less than 80%. Caution should be emphasized, because 100% oxygen is a pulmonary vasodilator and could worsen respiratory distress in a patient with ductal-dependent lesions by decreasing PVR and increasing pulmonary blood flow, leading to pulmonary overcirculation.

Physical Examination

Although the physical examination alone does not rule out cardiac disease, it can be helpful in the diagnosis or management of CHD. The routine examination should assess for cardiac murmur, tachypnea, adequate weight gain, presence and quality of LE pulses, capillary refill time, hepatomegaly, and lack of fever.

Vital signs should include preductal and postductal blood pressure and pulse oximetry measurements, respiratory rate, temperature, and weight. Tachypnea is commonly observed in infants with CCHD. An afebrile infant with respiratory distress should raise suspicion for CHD rather than infectious or primary pulmonary pathology. Poor weight gain (<30 g/d) or failure to regain birth weight by 2 weeks might be indicative of a progressively worsening process rather than an acute respiratory illness. Abnormally diminished or absent femoral pulses compared with brachial pulses could be indicative of aortic narrowing. Poor perfusion, evidenced by prolonged capillary refill time or peripheral pulses deficits, signifies profound hemodynamic collapse consistent with a left obstructive ductal-dependent lesion. In 1 study that involved almost 40,000 patients, the addition of pulse oximetry screening to the physical examination detected all cases of ductal-dependent lesions.[18] The term *preductal* refers to the RUE, because most ductus arteriosus attachments are distal to the subclavian artery. The term *postductal* refers to the right or the left LE. Any value less than 90% requires further investigation in a healthy neonate. A pulse oximetry differential of greater than 3% should raise concern because it might indicate a left obstructive lesion (see **Box 3**).[16–18] Ing and colleagues[25] observed that a murmur combined with a systolic blood pressure gradient of greater than 10 mm Hg between the arms and legs was the most consistent clinical finding in 50 patients with known coarctation of the aorta.

It is challenging to distinguish between pathologic murmurs caused by cardiac lesions and "innocent" physiologic murmurs. Six cardinal signs make a murmur more likely to be pathologic: pansystolic murmur, murmur intensity of 3/6 or greater grade intensity, point of maximal intensity at the upper left sternal border, harsh quality of the murmur, early midsystolic click, and abnormal second heart sound[26] (**Box 4**). In a series of 201 neonates without dysmorphic features or previous cardiology evaluation, the pediatric cardiologists to whom they were referred found murmur characteristic (harsh quality, location, and cardiac cycle timing) to be the most significant indication of a pathologic condition. Fifty-six percent of the study group had CHD. The pediatric cardiologists had a sensitivity of 81% and specificity of 91% for determining if the murmur was pathologic; those percentages were not changed by the addition of an electrocardiogram (ECG).[27] Farrer and Rennie[28] asked pediatric house officers to differentiate innocent from clinically significant murmurs in 112 neonates. They were accurate 76% of the time. Six percent of the murmurs they deemed innocent had echocardiographic evidence of structural heart disease.

In the ED, the lack of an audible murmur should not exclude CCHD. Similarly, the presence of a murmur does not mean a congenital cardiac lesion is present. Echocardiographic screening should be reserved for patients with a murmur. In a study of murmurs detected in newborns, which excluded children requiring neonatal intensive care or with risk factors for CHD, Lardhi[29] found that 43% had a structural defect, with ASD being the most common. When in doubt about a murmur, refer the patient to a cardiologist and prevent diagnostic delay.

Electrocardiography

An ECG can give valuable information regarding anatomy.[30–32] Similar to physiology, the ECG is also age dependent. Specific electrocardiographic abnormalities can be used to identify structural abnormalities, with special attention to axis deviation, atrioventricular (AV) prolongation, and atrial or ventricular enlargement. Intervals, axis, and criteria for ventricular hypertrophy are age dependent.[33,34] Although CHD physiology often results in electrical abnormalities, it is important to understand that a normal ECG does not rule out structural heart disease.

As the neonate transitions into infancy, the axis shifts from rightward to the normal adult leftward axis during the first 6 months of life. An extreme superior axis −90° to −180° suggests an AV canal defect or ostium primum ASD.[30] Right axis deviation suggests strong rightward forces, as noted in single ventricle physiology lacking leftward forces (eg, HLHS) and right outflow tract obstructive lesions causing right ventricular hypertrophy (RVH; eg, tricuspid atresia, pulmonary atresia, pulmonary stenosis, tetralogy of Fallot, and Ebstein's anomaly). Similarly, an AV block suggests either an AV canal defect or postoperative repair.

Box 4
Murmur characteristics that warrant echocardiography

- Pansystolic, continuous, diastolic
- Grade of 3/6 or greater murmur
- Point of maximal intensity at left upper sternal border
- Harsh quality
- Early midsystolic click
- Abnormal second heart sound

Data from McCrindle BW, Shaffer KM, Kan JS, et al. Cardinal clinical signs in the differentiation of heart murmurs in children. Arch Pediatr Adolesc Med 1996;150:169–74.

Voltage criteria for hypertrophy

The voltage criteria for both right and left ventricular hypertrophy (LVH) on ECG also vary with age, so close attention must be paid to age and relevant physiology to avoid confusion. Whereas right axis deviation is normal at birth, RVH is abnormal. Newborns have upright T waves in V1, which invert after the first week of life until adolescence, when they typically become upright again. Therefore, some important criteria for diagnosing RVH include a positive T wave in V1 after day of life 5 to 7, R in V1 of greater than the 98th percentile for age, or S in V6 of greater than the 98th percentile for age. The criteria for diagnosing LVH include the S wave in V1 of greater than the 98th percentile or the R wave in V6 of greater than the 98th percentile for age.

RVH in a newborn is likely a ductal-dependent left obstructive lesion, such as coarctation. LVH in a newborn, in combination with small right-sided forces, suggests an atretic right ventricle lesion, such as tricuspid or pulmonary atresia. In contrast, RVH in an infant suggests a ductal-dependent right obstructive lesion or right-to-left shunt. These infants typically present with cyanosis. LVH in an infant is typically a ductal-dependent left obstructive lesion, such as coarctation or a large hemodynamically significant left-to-right mixing lesion.

Laboratory analysis

Several laboratory studies can be helpful when considering causes in the differential diagnosis for the critically ill infant. Initial analysis should include a complete blood count for anemia, a complete metabolic panel for electrolyte derangements, methemoglobin level, lactic acid, pH, ammonia, blood culture, urine culture, urine organic acids, cortisol, thyroid-stimulating hormone, and free thyroxine.

Brain natriuretic peptide (BNP)/N-terminal pro-BNP (NT-proBNP) can be used as an adjunctive biomarker to differentiate a pulmonary process as a cause for respiratory distress from a cardiac disease in children. In contrast with the robust literature in the adult populations, there are fewer studies of BNP/NT-proBNP in the pediatric population.[35] Maher and associates[22] compared the results of laboratory tests for respiratory disease in children without a significant past medical history and with a new diagnosis of CCHD. The average BNP values were as follows: 3624 ± 1512 pg/mL among patients with congenital cardiac disease, 2837 ± 1681 pg/mL among those with acquired heart disease, and 17.4 pg/mL for those with respiratory illness. A cutoff BNP of less than 100 pg/mL for the identification of heart disease has a sensitivity of 100% and specificity of 98%.[22] In an evaluation of preterm infants with signs of CHD, Davlouros and associates[36] found that a BNP greater than 132.5 pg/mL had 93% sensitivity and 100% specificity for detecting hemodynamically significant left-to-right shunts. Koulouri and colleagues[37] calculated that a BNP concentration of greater than 40 pg/mL had 84% accuracy in differentiating cardiac from pulmonary causes of respiratory distress. In their series, the BNP value was observed to be significantly higher in patients with left ventricular systolic dysfunction than in those with left-to-right shunting lesions. Law and associates[38] studied the use of BNP as a diagnostic tool to differentiate hemodynamically significant cardiovascular disease from other disease processes with a similar presentation and found a cutoff of 170 pg/mL produced a sensitivity of 94% and specificity of 73% for neonates 0 to 7 days of age (n = 42). For the older age group (n = 58), a cutoff of 41 pg/mL produced a sensitivity of 87% and specificity of 70%.

Imaging

Chest radiography can reveal the causes of respiratory distress or shock as well as aid in the diagnosis of CCHD. Cardiomegaly, in which more than one-half of the chest cavity is consumed by the heart, can be an indicator of congenital cardiac disease. Some cardiac malformations are associated with classic appearances on radiographs. TGA has an "egg on a string" appearance owing to malrotation of the great vessels. TAPVR has a "snowman" or "**Fig. 1**" appearance owing to the input of pulmonary veins into the right atrium. Tetralogy of Fallot causes a "boot-shaped" heart on a chest radiograph. Radiography can also be used to evaluate other congenital causes of respiratory distress such as a diaphragmatic hernia or congenital cystic adenomatoid malformation.

The appearance of the radiograph can also guide management. A "white out" appearance suggests pulmonary vascular edema consistent with heart failure as seen in left-obstructive lesions and shunting lesions with left-to-right flow. These interstitial markings might be confused for infiltrates indicative of pneumonia. In contrast, right-obstructive lesions, right-to-left shunt lesions, and persistent pulmonary hypertension have a paucity of pulmonary vascular markings. This "black out" appearance is more suggestive of decreased pulmonary blood flow and cyanotic collapse as seen in right-obstructive lesions.

Echocardiography

Significant advances in the rapid diagnosis of life-threatening diseases have been made with the advent of bedside limited echocardiography by the emergency physician (BLEEP). The use of ultrasonography is becoming more prevalent in pediatric EDs owing to its ease of use, accessibility, and low radiation. With limited training, physicians can use this technology to obtain valuable information and provide evidence of CHD. Although no study has yet assessed the effectiveness of BLEEP for diagnosing CCHD in the ED, information about contractility and confirmation of the presence of 4 heart chambers has been obtained by using this modality to facilitate early diagnosis.[39–41]

EMERGENCY DEPARTMENT EVALUATION

Although congenital cardiac lesions can be differentiated broadly in 3 groups—left-sided obstructive ductal dependent, right-sided obstructive ductal dependent, and mixing—there is an even more simplified approach to categorize these disorders. Patients present in one of 3 ways: heart failure ("pink"), circulatory collapse ("gray"), or cyanotic ("blue"). The EP can identify which disorder is present by incorporating the age, history, physical examination, laboratory data, ECG, chest x-ray, and BLEEP (see **Fig. 1**).

Heart failure is a presentation of mixing lesions, typically in a "pink" well-perfused and oxygenated infant 1 to 6 months of age. The infant presents with tachypnea, poor feeding, inadequate weight gain, hepatomegaly, murmur, and "white out" on a chest radiograph. The ECG may show AV block or ventricular voltage criteria for hypertrophy, and BNP might be increased. BLEEP may show a septal defect.

Circulatory collapse is a presentation of a left-obstructive ductal-dependent lesion in a "gray" poorly perfused infant within the first few weeks of life. The neonate presents with hypotension, tachypnea, brachial–femoral pulse differential, systolic blood pressure differential greater than 10 mm Hg, and a pulse oximetry RUE and LE differential of greater than 3%. Poor perfusion evidenced by prolonged capillary refill time and peripheral pulse deficits signifies profound hemodynamic collapse consistent with a left obstructive ductal-dependent lesion. A chest radiograph shows "white out," the ECG varies based on age at presentation, and BNP is most likely increased. BLEEP may show a hypoplastic left ventricle or narrowing of the aorta.

Cyanosis, the "blue" baby, is a presentation of a right obstructive ductal-dependent or mixing lesion. An infant with a ductal-dependent lesion presents in the first weeks of life, "blue" with respiratory distress. After 1 month of age, the cyanotic mixing lesion presents with a combination of cyanosis and signs of heart failure. Examination reveals central cyanosis, murmur, and a "black" chest radiograph (unlike findings from a purely respiratory cause). The ECG might show either early dominant right forces or, after 1 week of life, dominant left forces. The BNP will not be increased. BLEEP may show hypoplastic right ventricular valves or septal defect. Once an infant with potential CHD has been identified and categorized by physiology, it is important to determine whether he or she would benefit from PGE1 and cardiology consultation.

It can be helpful to envision critical cardiac lesions in terms of a circuit in series with 2 systems: PVR and systemic vascular resistance (SVR). Managing the hemodynamics in these infants requires balancing the circulations like a teeter–totter. Pediatric cardiologists refer to the Qp:Qs ratio, in which Qp is the pulmonary blood flow and Qs is the systemic blood flow. Because each congenital cardiac disease has multiple variations, with each change altering the physiology, it might be simpler to consider the underlying physiology and balance the SVR and PVR instead of memorizing each defect. If PVR is decreased or SVR is increased, blood will flow to the lungs and become oxygenated. If SVR is decreased or PVR is increased, blood flows to the systemic vasculature but receives inadequate oxygenation in the lungs. The equation to guide the clinician is based on Fick's principle:

$$Qp:Qs = (SaO_2 - SvO_2):(SpvO_2 - SpaO_2),$$

where SaO_2 is the oxygen saturation, SvO_2 is the mixed venous oxygen saturation, $SpvO_2$ is the Pulmonary venous desaturation, and $SpaO_2$ is the pulmonary arterial oxygen saturation. The PVR and SVR must be manipulated to attain the goal Qp:Qs ratio of 1:1. If the child has had a surgical correction, the EP should ask the parents for the baseline oxygen saturation and target that goal. Increasing the oxygen saturation from 80% (Qp:Qs 25:20) to 100% for the hyperoxia test (Qp:Qs 25:0) increases the pulmonary vascular flow by 25 times. Oxygen is both a potent pulmonary vasodilator and vasoconstrictor of the ductus arteriosus. In fact, hypoxemia attained by blending nitrogen with oxygen can help to maintain the patency of the ductus arteriosus if prostaglandin is not available.[42] When considering an alteration of SVR, the goal mean arterial blood pressure is 40 mm Hg in neonates, which should be adjusted according to the normal mean arterial blood pressure for the child's age.

PVR can be manipulated by adding supplemental oxygen to vasodilate the pulmonary vasculature, thereby increasing pulmonary blood flow to assist with oxygenation in cyanosis. Alternatively, PVR can be increased to shunt blood toward the systemic circulation and decrease pulmonary edema or overload by mild hypoventilation, positive-pressure ventilation, and decreasing supplemental oxygen. SVR can be increased with medications such as phenylephrine, a purely α1-receptor agonist, and dopamine, a β1-agonist at low doses and β1-agonist with α1-agonist at higher doses. In a patient with a ductal-dependent right-obstructive lesion or a left-to-right shunting lesion, increased SVR will shunt blood from the systemic circulation to the pulmonary circulation, increasing oxygenation or pulmonary edema, respectively. In contrast, SVR can be decreased with medications such as milrinone, a phosphodiesterase III inhibitor, or nitroprusside. These vasodilators decrease SVR, promote right-to-left shunt, and increase systemic blood flow, decreasing pulmonary edema and oxygenation. Additionally, diuretics can be given for pulmonary edema.

As stated, infants with a hemodynamically significant cardiac lesion can be categorized by their appearance: pink, blue, or gray (see **Fig. 1**). A "pink" baby has too much pulmonary blood flow and too little systemic blood flow. A "pink" infant's oxygen saturation is greater than 85% to 90%; therefore, the Qp:Qs is 25:15 oxygen. To achieve a balanced Qp:Qs, the use of positive-pressure ventilation, hypoventilation, and vasodilators will increase the PVR, decrease the SVR, and increase systemic perfusion. Thus, the balance shifts from pulmonary overcirculation to balanced hemodynamics. A "blue" or cyanotic infant has too little pulmonary blood flow and too much systemic blood flow. The oxygen saturation for a "blue" infant is less than 75%, so the Qp:Qs is 25:25. Although this might seem to be balanced, recall that pulse oximetry is less reliable at oxygen saturations below 80%, so this would only be the best case scenario. Because the baby is "blue," the goal is to increase pulmonary blood flow. PGE1 can be initiated to increase flow to the lungs through the PDA, which typically improves oxygenation quickly. Furthermore, PVR can be decreased or SVR can be increased to increase pulmonary blood flow (Qp). PVR can be decreased with addition of supplemental oxygen, inhaled nitric oxide, and hyperventilation. SVR can be increased with intravenous fluids, phenylephrine, or knee-to-chest positioning. A "gray" baby is decompensated in circulatory collapse with hypoxemia and hypotension. The goal is to increase cardiac output globally and minimize oxygen consumption. It is critical to initiate PGE1 therapy to maintain patency of the ductus arteriosus. The addition of dopamine or epinephrine will augment systemic perfusion and improve inotropy. Intubation will increase oxygen saturation and provide positive-pressure ventilation to increase PVR. An exception is mixing "blue" lesions rather than right obstructive "blue" lesions, which have an obligatory shunt between the pulmonary and systemic circulations. The shunt is obligatory because, otherwise, the circulatory system would be a circuit in parallel, recycling blood within the same system instead of in series between the pulmonary and systemic circulation. Deoxygenated blood mixes with oxygenated blood. Eventually, this scenario creates pulmonary overcirculation and mixing of the deoxygenated and oxygenated blood, producing cyanosis and heart failure. Supplemental oxygen will decrease PVR and temporarily improve the clinical condition as less deoxygenated blood shunts to the systemic circulation. However, ultimately, the Qp:Qs balance needs to be obtained surgically.

Medical Management

After initiating the steps described to optimize the balance of pulmonary and systemic blood flow, consultation with a pediatric cardiologist is recommended to obtain diagnostic echocardiography and initiate transfer to the appropriate facility. As with any critically ill patient, the ABCs of resuscitation should be addressed sequentially. For intubation of children in respiratory distress or hypotension, ketamine is often chosen as an induction agent. However, caution is advised for its use the critically ill neonate, because it will increase SVR, further worsening left-to-right shunt. Hemodynamically neutral agents, such as etomidate, an α-agonist and a γ-aminobutyric acid receptor agonist, should be considered instead. Although sepsis is always on the differential diagnosis of a critically ill infant, the risks of adrenal suppression from etomidate are outweighed by the benefits of optimizing the hemodynamics of a decompensated cardiac lesion.[43–46] Rapid-sequence intubation should be induced with neuromuscular blockade using either rocuronium or vecuronium. After intubation, attention should be paid to hemodynamics, because positive-pressure ventilation increases PVR and decreases SVR and preload. This can affect shunting and the Qp:Qs flow, especially in a cyanotic baby. Children in respiratory distress should be intubated, especially those requiring PGE1 infusion. Prostaglandin has adverse effects, the most significant being apnea and hypotension. Thus, infants should be intubated empirically for transfer and given judicious use of intravenous fluids.

Vascular access and titrating hemodynamic medications is crucial to rapid-sequence intubation. In a neonate with circulatory collapse, rapid vascular access can be obtained by placement of a peripheral intravenous catheter, intraosseous catheter, or umbilical vein catheter. The umbilical stump is usually a viable vascular access option for up to 1 week after birth. The stump contains only 1 umbilical vein, which is larger and has less muscular walls than the arteries. An umbilical vein catheter has the advantage of providing central access and multiple ports for infusing medications. The emergent umbilical vein ("low lying") catheter should be advanced just beyond the point of initial blood flow within the catheter. Many umbilical lines are misplaced into the hepatic vein during cannulation, so low lying umbilical lines provide central vascular access without the risk of hepatic vein cannulation. The ideal depth of insertion of a nonemergent umbilical venous catheter can be estimated based on the infant's weight with the equation (weight in kilograms/2) + 9, and is confirmed radiographically by the location of the distal tip above the diaphragm between the seventh and ninth thoracic vertebrae. Alternatively, if peripheral intravenous access is not rapidly successful, intraosseous access should be established.[47–49]

PGE1 is a life-saving medication that stimulates ductal endothelium and maintains patency of the ductus arteriosus while awaiting definitive surgical management. PGE1 therapy should be implemented for any neonate with hemodynamic collapse or cyanosis in the first month of life.[50,51] The ductus arteriosus typically closes by 72 hours of life, but if flow depends on the ductus, it could take longer for the muscular walled conduit to become fibrotic. PGE1 is especially beneficial in neonates with coarctation of the aorta, hypoplastic left heart, critical aortic stenosis, interrupted aortic arch, transposition of the great vessels, tricuspid atresia/stenosis, pulmonary atresia/stenosis, and Ebstein's anomaly.[52] Because the diagnosis of CCHD is often unknown in the ED, infusion of PGE1 is critical for both "blue" babies with right-obstructive ductal-dependent physiology and "gray" babies with left-obstructive ductal-dependent physiology (see **Fig. 1**).

Further management is guided by the unique physiology of the type of CCHD. "Gray" shocklike infants with circulatory collapse require PGE1 to support systemic circulation. It may take hours for shock to resolve after PGE1 infusion and the patient will most likely remain undifferentiated until further diagnostic testing can be obtained in a tertiary pediatric intensive care unit. In addition to initiating a PGE1 infusion, additional therapeutic interventions include intubation to minimize oxygen consumption, inhaled nitric oxide, inotropic support, afterload reduction with milrinone, and hemodynamic support with dopamine or epinephrine. Oxygen administration should be adjusted to maintain the target Qp:Qs. Intravenous fluids boluses should be given to improve preload.

Neonates with cyanotic lesions causing circulatory collapse also require PGE1 to increase the pulmonary blood flow across the PDA. This should produce a prompt improvement. However, if the neonate is still cyanotic, consider the diagnosis of d-TGA without a VSD. Circulation in d-TGA flows in parallel, not in series like a normal heart, and would be immediately lethal without an intracardiac systemic to pulmonary connection. A PDA defect allows mixing until its closure, and a VSD or ASD could allow more permanent mixing by creating a circuit in series. d-TGA is a special scenario; it might require an emergent atrial septostomy to create a circuit in series.

Persistent pulmonary hypertension can also present in neonates as cyanosis with circulatory collapse. Persistent pulmonary hypertension can be differentiated from cyanotic CCHD after stabilization, and its initial management is similar to that of cyanotic CCHD with circulatory collapse. Patients with persistent pulmonary hypertension are difficult to ventilate after they are intubated, and their oxygen saturation will decrease episodically owing to vasospasm and ventilation/perfusion mismatch. Inhaled nitric oxide is beneficial for these patients and is usually instituted after echocardiography reveals the pulmonary hypertension and lack of cardiac defect at the tertiary care pediatric intensive care unit.

The "blue" infant with congestive heart failure is typically older than 1 month of age. These children do not need PGE1 and, in fact, might do worse if it is administered, because blood will be shunted left to right across the ductus, increasing the pulmonary blood flow. PGE1 will not alter the mixing of oxygenated and deoxygenated blood, which is the underlying cause of cyanotic congestive heart failure.

The "pink" infant with congestive heart failure is usually 1 to 6 months of age. The therapeutic goal is to increase PVR with low oxygen, positive-pressure ventilation, or intubation and to decrease SVR with a vasodilator such as milrinone. PGE1 is not necessary in these infants. Achieving an appropriate fluid balance is challenging in these infants because, although they have reduced preload, which may benefit from slow 10-mL/kg IV increments, they often need diuretics to prevent worsening of respiratory distress from volume overload.

Medications commonly used for the acutely decompensated infant with CCHD are listed in **Box 5**.[53]

SPECIAL CONSIDERATIONS

A child with anomalous left coronary artery from the pulmonary artery behaves similarly to the "pink" infant with heart failure or the "gray" neonate in shock. These babies typically present at 2 to 3 months of age. As the PVR decreases, decreased retrograde deoxygenated flow from the pulmonary artery to the left coronary artery causes myocardial ischemia in the left coronary distribution (anterolateral) and eventually heart failure. These babies typically have "white out" on chest radiography, caused by pulmonary edema, and a characteristic ECG, with Q waves laterally or ST elevation anterolaterally, from myocardial ischemia owing to persistent deoxygenated coronary perfusion. The ECG differentiates these infants from the "pink" CHF infant or the "gray" neonate in shock. Echocardiography or angiography should be obtained to diagnose the origin of the coronary arteries.

TAPVR is a problem of pulmonary overload returning to the right atrium. An infant with infradiaphragmatic or infracardiac obstructed TAPVR presents similarly to a cyanotic

Box 5 Emergency cardiac medications	
Medication	**Dose**
Dopamine	5–20 µg/kg/min
Epinephrine	0.01–0.1 µg/kg/min
Esmolol	500 µg/kg bolus, 50–300 µg/kg/min
Etomidate	0.3 mg/kg/dose
Fentanyl	1–3 µg/kg/min
Furosemide	0.5–2 mg/kg IV q6–12 h
IV fluid bolus	10 mL/kg/dose
Ketamine	1–2 mg/kg/dose
Milrinone	0.5 µg/kg load, 25–75 µg/kg/min
Morphine	0.1 mg/kg/dose
Nitroprusside	0.5–4 µg/kg/min
Phenylephrine	10–20 µg/kg bolus, 2–5 µg/kg/min
Prostaglandin E1	0.05–0.1 µg/kg/min titrating up q15–20 min

Data from Costello JM, Almodovar MC. Emergency care for infants and children with acute cardiac disease. Clin Pediatr Emerg Med 2007;8:145–55.

infant with congestive heart failure.[54] Infants with obstructed TAPVR typically present earlier than those with unobstructed forms of TAPVR. This is a unique scenario, in which prostaglandin can be detrimental. Opening the ductus arteriosus will increase left-to-right shunt and increase pulmonary blood flow, worsening heart failure.

Another scenario in which an infant with cyanosis might fail to improve or could worsen with prostaglandin infusion is a d-TGA with an intact ventricular septum or restrictive atrial or ventricular communication. Mixing in the heart via left-to-right shunt to oxygenate the systemic blood is required; thus, these infants need emergent atrial septostomy by a cardiologist.

Last, tetralogy of Fallot behaves differently with less ductal-dependent physiology. Its episodic presentation can occur earlier or later than the classic "blue" neonate. It can behave as a "blue tet" with right-obstructive ductal-dependent lesion early in life when PVR is still suprasystemic, owing to severe right ventricular outflow tract obstruction. The severe right ventricular outflow tract obstruction decreases pulmonary blood flow and will present as a cyanotic "blue" baby who is responsive to PGE1. If the obstruction is severe, left-to-right shunt at the ductus arteriosus might provide the much-needed pulmonary blood flow. In contrast, "pink tets" have enough mixing of blood at the VSD level that the preload can typically overcome a less severe obstruction. A classic "tet spell" can be seen in these babies awaiting surgical repair at 3 to 6 months of age. Decompensation, known as a "cyanotic tet spell," is caused by an acute decrease in pulmonary blood flow owing to either increased PVR (eg, from crying) or decreased preload from hypovolemia.[55] The agitation increases the heart rate and causes decreased diastolic filling time; therefore, the infundibulum does not fully relax, so the right ventricular outflow tract obstruction is worsened. The ductus arteriosus would subsequently shunt less blood left to right as the PVR nears the SVR. Tetralogy of Fallot spells are managed uniquely. The goal is to decrease PVR and increase SVR. If the first episode is presenting undiagnosed, PGE1 would not be detrimental and the infant can be treated like any other infant with a right-obstructive ductal-dependent lesion who is "blue." The chest radiograph will be black owing to decreased pulmonary blood flow. The ECG will show RVH. Hypercyanotic "tet spells" should be managed with calming. Child Life specialists and parents can be recruited for this endeavor. Morphine can be another adjunct. Bringing the child's knees to his or her chest will increase SVR, shunting more blood from left to right across a PDA or the VSD, and thus increasing preload in the right ventricle. A fluid bolus will also increase preload. Supplemental oxygen benefits by vasodilating the pulmonary vasculature, thereby decreasing PVR. Different modalities can be attempted to increase SVR and left-to-right shunt: manual external compression of the aorta, phenylephrine infusion, and ketamine.[55] Propranolol or esmolol can decrease the heart rate, thereby decreasing the infundibular overriding of the pulmonary artery and increasing time for diastolic filling.[56] If the child is still cyanotic after medical optimization and the Qp:Qs is balanced, then surgery may be the next best option.

SUMMARY

Any neonate with cyanosis or shock should be considered to have a ductal-dependent critical congenital cardiac disease until proven otherwise. Circulatory collapse and cyanosis caused by ductal-dependent lesions typically present within the first 2 weeks of life. Shunting lesions and those associated with heart failure present later during infancy. The crashing neonate certainly produces anxiety among ED providers, but following a clear and decisive algorithm can mitigate this stress. The essential elements discussed throughout this article provide a framework for the diagnosis of congenital cardiac disease. Cornerstones of this diagnosis include assessment of the neonate for cyanosis, hepatomegaly, murmur, and measurement of the proximal versus distal pulses and the blood pressure. Other vital tools include an ECG, chest x-ray, BNP, and BLEEP. Circulatory balance should be maintained with a Qp:Qs ratio of 1:1. Cyanotic infants require oxygen and most require PGE1 infusion. Infants with profound hemodynamic collapse can be harmed with oxygen and need circulatory support and PGE1 infusion. Owing to the complexity of CHD, in addition to age-dependent physiologic variability, a rapid compilation of data obtained from the history and physical (see **Box 2**) will guide the EP toward identifying and managing these infant. By using a simplified approach that categorizes the critically ill infant as "pink" (excessive pulmonary blood flow), "blue" (insufficient pulmonary blood flow), or "gray" (circulatory collapse; see **Fig. 1**), the EP will be able to provide life-saving stabilization until specialized care can be obtained.

REFERENCES

1. McCollough M, Sharieff GQ. Common complaints in the first 30 days of life. Emerg Med Clin North Am 2002;20:27–48.
2. Savitsky E, Alejos J, Votey S. Emergency department presentations of pediatric congenital heart disease. J Emerg Med 2003;24:239–45.
3. Hoffman JIE, Kaplan S. The incidence of congenital heart disease. J Am Coll Cardiol 2002;39:1890–900.
4. Wren C, Reinhardt Z, Khawaja K. Twenty-year trends in diagnosis of life-threatening neonatal cardiovascular malformations. Arch Dis Child Fetal Neonatal Ed 2008;93:F33–5.
5. Abu-Harb M, Wyllie J, Hey E, et al. Presentation of obstructive left heart malformations in infancy. Arch Dis Child 1994;71:F179–83.
6. Wren C, Richmond S, Donaldson L. Presentation of congenital heart disease in infancy: implications for routine examination. Arch Dis Child Fetal Neonatal Ed 1999;80:F49–53.
7. Liske MR, Greeley CS, Law DJ, et al. Report of the Tennessee Task Force on Screening Newborn Infants for Critical Congenital Heart Disease. Pediatrics 2006;118:e1250–6.
8. Dorfman AT, Marino BS, Wernovsky G, et al. Critical heart disease in the neonate: presentation and outcome at a tertiary care center. Pediatr Crit Care Med 2008;9:193–202.
9. Chang RR, Gurvitz M, Rodriguez S. Missed diagnosis of critical congenital heart disease. Arch Pediatr Adolesc Med 2008;162:969–74.
10. Chew C, Stone S, Donath SM, et al. Impact of antenatal screening on the presentation of infants with congenital heart disease to a cardiology unit. J Paediatr Child Health 2006;42:704–8.
11. Massin MM, Dessy H. Delayed recognition of congenital heart disease. Postgrad Med J 2006;82:468–70.
12. Mellander M, Sunnegardh J. Failure to diagnose critical heart malformations in newborns before discharge-an increasing problem? Acta Paediatr 2006;95:407–13.
13. Brown KL, Ridout DA, Hoskote A, et al. Delayed diagnosis of congenital heart disease worsens preoperative condition and outcome of surgery in neonates. Heart 2006;92:1298–302.
14. Abu-Harb M, Hey E, Wren C. Death in infancy from unrecognized congenital heart disease. Arch Dis Child 1994;71:3–7.

15. Lee YS, Baek JS, Kwon BS, et al. Pediatric emergency room presentation of congenital heart disease. Korean Circ J 2010;40:36–41.
16. Mahle WT, Newburger JW, Matherne GP, et al. Role of pulse oximetry in examining newborns for congenital heart disease. a scientific statement from the American Heart Association and American Academy of Pediatrics. Circulation 2009;120:447–58.
17. Frank LH, Bradshaw E, Beekman R, et al. Congenital heart disease screening using pulse oximetry. J Pediatr 2013;162:445–53.
18. Granelli AD, Mellander M, Sunnegårdh J, et al. Screening for duct-dependent congenital heart disease with pulse oximetry: a critical evaluation of strategies to maximize sensitivity. Acta Paediatr 2005;94:1590–6.
19. Mastropietro CW, Tourner SP, Sarnaik AP. Emergency presentation of congenital heart disease in children. Pediatr Emerg Med Pract 2008;5:1–30.
20. Custer JW, Rau RE. The Harriet Lane handbook. 19th edition. St Louis (MO): Mosby; 2012.
21. Lee JY. Clinical presentations of critical cardiac defects in the newborn: decision making and initial management. Korean J Pediatr 2010;53:669–79.
22. Maher KO, Reed H, Cuadrado A, et al. B-type natriuretic peptide in the emergency diagnosis of critical heart disease in children. Pediatrics 2008;121:e1484–8.
23. Ross RD, Bollinger RO, Pinsky WW. Grading the severity of congestive heart failure in infants. Pediatr Cardiol 1992;13:72–5.
24. Tunkel AR, Hartman BJ, Kaplan SL, et al. Practice guidelines for the management of bacterial meningitis. Clin Infect Dis 2004;39:1267–84.
25. Ing FF, Starc TJ, Griffiths SP, et al. Early diagnosis of coarctation of the aorta in children: a continuing dilemma. Pediatrics 1996;98:378–82.
26. McCrindle BW, Shaffer KM, Kan JS, et al. Cardinal clinical signs in the differentiation of heart murmurs in children. Arch Pediatr Adolesc Med 1996;150:169–74.
27. Mackie AS, Jutras LC, Dancea AB, et al. Can cardiologists distinguish innocent from pathologic murmurs in neonates? J Pediatr 2009;154:50–4.
28. Farrer KFM, Rennie JM. Neonatal murmurs: are senior house officers good enough? Arch Dis Child Fetal Neonatal Ed 2003;88:F147–51.
29. Lardhi AA. Prevalence and clinical significance of heart murmurs detected in routine neonatal exam. J Saudi Heart Assoc 2010;22:25–7.
30. O'Connor M, McDaniel N, Brady WJ. The pediatric electrocardiogram. Part I: age-related interpretation. Am J Emerg Med 2008;26:221–8.
31. O'Connor M, McDaniel N, Brady WJ. The pediatric electrocardiogram. Part II: dysrhythmias. Am J Emerg Med 2008;26:348–58.
32. O'Connor M, McDaniel N, Brady WJ. The pediatric electrocardiogram. Part III: congenital heart disease and other cardiac syndromes. Am J Emerg Med 2008;26:497–503.
33. Davignon A, Rautaharju P, Boisselle E, et al. Normal ECG standards for infants and children. Pediatr Cardiol 1980;1:123–31.
34. Rijnbeek PR, Witsenburg M, Schrama E, et al. New normal limits for the paediatric electrocardiogram. Eur Heart J 2001;22:702–11.
35. Cantinotti M, Law Y, Vittorini S, et al. The potential and limitations of plasma BNP measurement in the diagnosis, prognosis, and management of children with heart failure due to congenital cardiac disease: an update. Heart Fail Rev 2014;19:727–42.
36. Davlouros PA, Karatza AA, Xanthopoulou I, et al. Diagnostic role of plasma BNP levels in neonates with signs of congenital heart disease. Int J Cardiol 2011;147:42–6.

37. Koulouri S, Acherman RJ, Wong PC, et al. Utility of B-type natriuretic peptide in differentiating congestive heart failure from lung disease in pediatric patients with respiratory distress. Pediatr Cardiol 2004;25:341–6.
38. Law YM, Hoyer AW, Reller MD, et al. Accuracy of plasma B-type natriuretic peptide to diagnose significant cardiovascular disease in children: the better not pout children! Study. J Am Coll Cardiol 2009;54:1467–75.
39. Pershad J, Chin T. Early detection of cardiac disease masquerading as acute bronchospasm: the role of bedside limited echocardiography by the emergency physician. Pediatr Emerg Care 2003;19:e1–3.
40. Lambert M, Fox JC, Chhiv NB. Cyanotic congenital heart disease: emergency department diagnosis by limited bedside echocardiography. Adv Emerg Nurs J 2004;26:267–71.
41. Pershad J, Myers S, Plouman C, et al. Bedside limited echocardiography by the emergency physician is accurate during evaluation of the critically ill patient. Pediatrics 2004;114:e667–71.
42. Day RW, Barton AJ, Pysher TJ, et al. Pulmonary vascular resistance of children treated with nitrogen during early infancy. Ann Thorac Surg 1998;65:1400–4.
43. Guldner G, Schultz J, Sexton P, et al. Etomidate for rapid-sequence intubation in young children: hemodynamic effects and adverse events. Acad Emerg Med 2003;10:134–9.
44. Chan CM, Mitchell AL, Shorr AF. Etomidate is associated with mortality and adrenal insufficiency in sepsis: a meta-analysis. Crit Care Med 2012;40:2945–53.
45. McPhee LD, Badawi O, Fraser GL, et al. Single-dose etomidate is not associated with increased mortality in ICU patients with sepsis: analysis of a large electronic ICU database. Crit Care Med 2013;41:774–83.
46. Zuckerbraun NS, Pitetti RD, Herr SM, et al. Use of etomidate as an induction agent for rapid sequence intubation in a pediatric emergency department. Acad Emerg Med 2006;13:602–9.
47. Abe KK, Blum GT, Yamamoto LG. Intraosseous is faster and easier than umbilical venous catheterization in newborn emergency vascular access models. Am J Emerg Med 2000;18:126–9.
48. Rajani AK, Chitkara R, Oehlert J, et al. Comparison of umbilical venous and intraosseous access during simulated neonatal resuscitation. Pediatrics 2011;128:e954–8.
49. Haas NA. Clinical review: vascular access for fluid infusion in children. Crit Care 2004;8:478–84.
50. Olley PM, Coceani F, Bodach E. E-type prostaglandins: a new emergency therapy for certain cyanotic congenital heart malformations. Circulation 1976;53:728–31.
51. Danford DA, Gutgesell HP, McNamara DG. Application of information theory to decision analysis in potentially prostaglandin-responsive neonates. J Am Coll Cardiol 1986;8:1125–30.
52. Attenhofer Jost CH, Connolly HM, Dearani JA, et al. Ebstein's anomaly. Circulation 2007;115:277–85.
53. Costello JM, Almodovar MC. Emergency care for infants and children with acute cardiac disease. Clin Pediatr Emerg Med 2007;8:145–55.
54. Lawrence L, Lillis K. Identifying congenital heart disease in the emergency department: a case of total anomalous pulmonary venous return. Clin Pediatr Emerg Med 2005;6:273–7.
55. van Roekens CN, Zuckerberg AL. Emergency management of hypercyanotic crises in tetralogy of Fallot. Ann Emerg Med 1995;25:256–8.
56. Sun LS, Du F, Quaegebeur JM. Right ventricular infundibular β-adrenoreceptor complex in tetralogy of Fallot patients. Pediatr Res 1997;42:12–6.

Blunt Cardiac Injury

Evie G. Marcolini, MD[a,b,*], Joshua Keegan, MD[c]

KEYWORDS

- Blunt cardiac injury • Cardiac contusion • Cardiac concussion • Commotio cordis
- Contusio cordis

KEY POINTS

- Blunt cardiac injury encompasses multiple different injuries, including contusion, chamber rupture, and acute valvular disorders.
- Blunt cardiac injury is common and may cause significant morbidity and mortality; a high index of suspicion is needed for accurate diagnosis.
- Diagnostic work-up should always include electrocardiogram and cardiac enzymes, and may include echocardiography if specific disorders (ie, tamponade or valvular disorders) are suspected.
- Patients with myocardial contusion should be observed for 24 to 48 hours for arrhythmias.
- Many other significant forms of blunt cardiac injury require surgical intervention.

EPIDEMIOLOGY

"And always with a heart contusion arise both doubt and much confusion."[1]

Blunt cardiac injury (BCI) is not a straightforward entity. Because there is no widely accepted gold standard diagnostic test, it is difficult to quantify and there is little consensus on how to establish the diagnosis, even though the complications from BCI can range from asymptomatic ecchymosis to sudden death. A lack of consensus on the definition only limits research and understanding of the disease. The inconsistent nomenclature regarding this disease makes quantifying its incidence difficult at best. The diagnosis can be made clinically from complications, by diagnostic testing or laboratory evidence, or on postmortem examination. Given this lack of uniformity and specificity, well-validated diagnostic and treatment algorithms remain elusive.

Disclosures: None.
[a] Department of Emergency Medicine and Neurology, Division of Neurocritical Care and Emergency Neurology, Yale University School of Medicine, 464 Congress Street, Suite 260, New Haven, CT 06519, USA; [b] Division of Neurocritical Care and Emergency Neurology, Department of Neurology, Yale University School of Medicine, PO Box 208018, New Haven, CT 06520-8018, USA; [c] Department of Emergency Medicine, Yale University School of Medicine, New Haven, CT, USA
* Corresponding author. Department of Emergency Medicine and Neurology, Division of Neurocritical Care and Emergency Neurology, Yale University School of Medicine, 464 Congress Street, Suite 260, New Haven, CT 06519.
E-mail address: emarcolini@gmail.com

Emerg Med Clin N Am 33 (2015) 519–527
http://dx.doi.org/10.1016/j.emc.2015.04.003
0733-8627/15/$ – see front matter © 2015 Elsevier Inc. All rights reserved.
emed.theclinics.com

Mattox and colleagues[2] proposed eliminating the terms cardiac concussion and cardiac contusion, instead describing all cardiac conditions resulting from blunt trauma as BCI, with further delineation of specific injuries such as septal rupture, free wall rupture, coronary artery thrombosis, cardiac failure, minor electrocardiogram (ECG)/enzyme abnormality, or complex arrhythmia.

Motor vehicle crash (MVC) mechanisms account for most cases of BCI and approximately 20% of all MVC deaths involve blunt injury to the heart.[3] Some estimates place the incidence of cardiac trauma at slightly less than 1 million cases per year in the United States. Blunt thoracic trauma carries approximately a 20% risk of BCI, but with severe thoracic trauma or multisystem trauma the risk approaches 76%.[4]

In one study, significant chest wall trauma (multiple rib or sternal fractures, lung contusion, scapular fracture, hemopneumothorax, major intrathoracic vascular injury, or seat belt sign) predicted a 13% incidence of BCI.[5]

The clinical significance of this elusive diagnosis lies in its associated complications. The rationale of screening for BCI is to identify cases at high risk for complication that will benefit from intervention; a difficult proposition at best. In traumatic deaths, the cardiac injury is often overlooked, even in the setting of suggestive clinical features such as hypotension and jugular venous distention.[6,7] One autopsy series of 546 cases of nonpenetrating trauma to the heart found that 65% had a ruptured myocardium; in only 1 case was BCI clinically suspected in the medical documentation.[3] BCI is likely overlooked because patients at high risk for BCI commonly have multiple injured organ systems, which in turn overshadow the index of suspicion for BCI. In a series of 24 successfully treated blunt atrial injuries, 16 had a delay to treatment of more than an hour, and 15 had injury to other areas.[6,8] The same series found 2.3 to 3.4 total injured organ systems in patients with BCI.[6]

The picture is further clouded because manifestations of some cardiac injuries present in a delayed fashion. These injuries include intracardiac shunts or fistulae, valvular lesions, ventricular aneurysms, retained foreign bodies, tamponade from postpericardiotomy syndrome, hemopericardium or constrictive pericarditis, and coronary artery thrombosis. The clinical and diagnostic conundrum for emergency physicians is the differentiation between a benign cardiac insult and a significant episode with strongly associated morbidity and/or mortality. This article clarifies the available diagnostic and screening tools and presents a rational schema for their use. Practical classification schemes define BCI by its resulting complications: cardiac free wall rupture, septal rupture, coronary artery injury, cardiac failure, complex arrhythmias, and minor ECG or cardiac enzyme abnormalities.[2,9]

Note that there are limited data on BCI in the pediatric population. One registry of 1288 children with blunt thoracic trauma found a 4.6% incidence of BCI. However, most pediatric BCI is associated with nonaccidental trauma and concomitant head trauma.[6]

MECHANISMS AND INJURY PATTERNS

There are multiple potential mechanisms of injury for the blunt forces of BCI: direct, indirect, crush injury, bidirectional or compressive, decelerative, blast, concussive, and combined.[3] The most common site of injury is the right heart, because of its proximity to the chest wall, although more than half of patients with BCI experience injury to multiple cardiac chambers.[4]

Cardiac Concussion (Also Called Cardiac Contusion)

Cardiac concussion is histologically defined by myocardial hemorrhage, edema, and localized necrosis. In clinical practice, the term is loosely used to describe a spectrum of injuries from chest wall tenderness to wall motion abnormalities, decreased contractility, arrhythmia, or conduction abnormalities. The literature reports a wide-ranging incidence of myocardial contusion in patients with trauma, varying from 0% to 76% depending on the criteria used.[10]

A rare area of consensus is the lack of value in screening for myocardial contusion with biomarkers or echocardiography if there are no clinical sequellae.[11] These injuries typically resolve within 24 hours without intervention, and rarely manifest long-term effects. Any associated clinical features such as hypotension, pulmonary edema, malignant arrhythmia, or conduction disturbances should provoke suspicion for clinically significant contusion, and prompt further evaluation.

Commotio Cordis

Commotio cordis refers to sudden cardiac death from BCI where there is no evidence of morphologic injury or preexisting disease. This condition is differentiated from contusio cordis, which does have evidence of underlying morphologic injury. This differentiation requires autopsy evidence, and in practice does not have implications for treatment. Alcohol use, drug use, and preexisting cardiovascular disease increase the risk of commotio cordis.[12] Commotio cordis is the second most common cause of sudden cardiac death in young athletes and mostly occurs in boys less than 18 years old.[13] The prevailing pathophysiologic explanation for this is a high-velocity impact to the chest occurring during ventricular repolarization and inducing an R-on-T pheno-menon that manifests ventricular fibrillation.[14] Rapid recognition of dysrhythmia and prompt, high-quality bystander cardiopulmonary resuscitation have resulted in temporal trends toward improved outcomes for these patients.[15]

Cardiac Rupture

It is uncommon for direct BCI to result in serious complications, except in the setting of ruptured myocardium or fatal arrhythmia.[3] Cardiac wall rupture caused by blunt injury is possible and, in most cases, fatal. However, a pseudoaneurysm may develop if the myocardium is sealed off by an intact pericardium and development of thrombus. This defect is prone to spontaneous rupture after the patient has survived the acute trauma.[16]

Survival in patients with cardiac rupture with BCI is notably rare, but not nonexistent. Overall, ventricular rupture occurs more commonly than atrial rupture, but right atrial rupture is more common than left atrial rupture. These patients typically succumb rapidly to exsanguination, cardiac tamponade, or other concomitant injuries. However, patients with atrial rupture are more likely to survive the initial insult than those with ventricular rupture, so may live long enough to be considered for surgical intervention.

If discovered, septal injuries are also treatable. The presence of a murmur, thrill, arrhythmia, or conduction disturbance suggests this injury, and the severity of the signs typically portends the size of the injury. Severe injury typically results in overt cardiogenic shock. The natural history of septal injuries is contusion followed by necrosis and delayed rupture, which highlights the importance of early diagnosis.

Valvular Injury

Valvular injuries are typically either acutely severe, or insidious but amenable to repair if diagnosed. The morbidity and mortality of valvular injury in the context of BCI depend on the location and injury severity of the affected valve. Typically valvular injury associated with BCI is severe, hemodynamically consequential, and clinically manifests with cardiopulmonary sequelae. Minor valvular abnormalities detected during screening for BCI likely represent preexisting valvular disease.

Injury to atrioventricular valves is more common than injury to semilunar valves in the setting of chamber or septal injury.[15] Aortic valve injury is considered to be most common, and may result from sudden increase in intrathoracic pressure against a closed valve along with retrograde aortic pressure wave from a concomitant increase in intra-abdominal pressure.[15] Aortic valvular injury manifests as cardiovascular instability or cardiogenic shock, whereas acute mitral valve injury typically manifests as pulmonary edema and hypotension. These injuries are treated by afterload reduction as a bridge to definitive repair. Tricuspid injury may present more subacutely with long-term sequelae of right ventricular dysfunction manifesting over months to years.[6] In addition, injury to the papillary muscle or chordae tendineae injury is possible with BCI, and the left-sided structures are associated with higher morbidity and mortality than those on the right.[3]

Coronary Artery Injury

The possibility of coronary artery thrombosis as a direct result of BCI is controversial and lacking strong evidence. One case series of 546 patients with nonpenetrating trauma to the heart suggests that, even in the setting of significant surrounding injury, thrombosis does not occur.[3] Most coronary artery injuries take the form of laceration, dissection, aneurysm formation, and/or aneurysm rupture.[15]

Pericardial Injury

The pericardium is unlikely to rupture in the setting of BCI. Instead, pericardial injury typically results in pericarditis with subsequent effusion and tamponade. In rare cases, a pericardial laceration may result in myocardial herniation and strangulation.[16]

Dysrhythmias

Dysrhythmias are common in BCI, and most commonly manifest as sinus tachycardia, ventricular or atrial premature contractions, and atrial fibrillation. These dysrhythmias may represent benign sequelae, or be associated with catecholamine release, alcohol and drug use, or electrolyte abnormalities. In some cases, they can occur up to 48 hours postinjury. More sinister dysrhythmias, such as high-degree heart block, ventricular tachycardia, or fibrillation are described in severe trauma, but are associated with electrolyte disturbance, acidemia, and/or hypovolemia/hypotension.[16]

DIAGNOSIS

BCI is a difficult condition to diagnose, especially because it is a heterogeneous category of multiple specific injuries. The history and physical examination are often nonspecific. Patients may complain of chest pain or shortness of breath; in some cases, this even includes typical angina pain,[16] and patients may progress to myocardial infarction via an unknown mechanism.[17] However, because patients with clinically significant BCI are likely to have other traumatic injuries, the signs and symptoms may be nonspecific or masked by these other injuries.[4] The physical examination is often also nonspecific, although findings such as ecchymosis, chest tenderness, flail chest, and crepitus are markers for a high-risk mechanism of injury. Associated rib or sternal fractures also place patients at higher risk for BCI. More specific findings, such as friction rubs, distant heart sounds, and new murmurs, are more indicative of BCI, but are also less common and more difficult to appreciate in the acute care setting. The index of suspicion for BCI should be heightened in patients with dyspnea, distended jugular veins, chest wall ecchymosis, flail chest, sternal fracture, rib fracture, pneumothorax, hemothorax, great vessel injury, or hemodynamic instability not otherwise explained.

After the history and physical examination, the next step in evaluation for BCI is to obtain an ECG (**Fig. 1**). Given the poor sensitivity of the routine physical examination, a screening ECG should be performed on all patients with blunt chest injuries.[9] ECG should also be considered in patients without known blunt chest injuries, but whose traumatic mechanism places them at high risk for BCI. Electrocardiographic abnormalities may include sinus tachycardia, arrhythmias, and ST segment changes. Historically, most guidelines and supporting literature[18,19] concluded that a normal ECG was sufficient to exclude significant BCI. More recent series have described injuries despite a normal ECG,[5,20–22] including some that were clinically significant.[22] ECG abnormalities typically manifest within 48 hours of injury. The sensitivity of ECG is limited because, electrocardiographically, it represents mostly atrial and left ventricular conduction, which may overlook the (most frequently injured) right ventricle.[23] Consequently, the addition of a negative troponin I assay to an ECG is now required to exclude myocardial injury.[9] CK-MB is neither sensitive nor specific[21] for the detection of BCI, and is no longer recommended in the diagnostic evaluation.[9]

The sensitivity of troponin I varies considerably, from 23% to 100%,[24,25] and the optimal timing of its measurement is unclear. One series found that 1 out of 44 patients with clinically significant BCI developed a troponin level increase at 8 hours despite an initially normal level.[5] In addition, although the combination of a normal ECG and troponin I level excludes arrhythmias and cardiac contusion, acute valvular injury is still possible, even in the absence of cardiac contusion. However, the hemodynamic

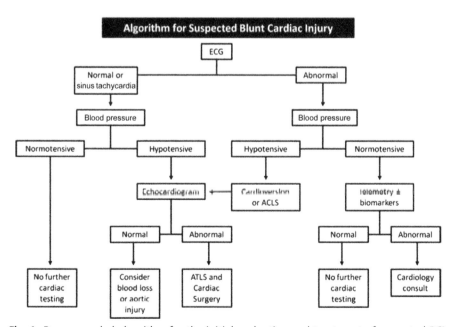

Fig. 1. Recommended algorithm for the initial evaluation and treatment of suspected BCI. Patients with blunt thoracic trauma who have a normal ECG and hemodynamics do well regardless of further laboratory or imaging studies. ACLS, advanced cardiac life support; ATLS, advanced trauma life support. (*From* Bock JS, Benitez RM. Blunt cardiac injury. Cardiol Clin 2012;30(4):550; with permission.)

derangements from acute valvular injuries are usually not subtle, often leading to the correct diagnosis so long as it is at least considered.

Although not routinely indicated, imaging may be a helpful adjunct in the diagnosis of BCI, usually in the form of transthoracic or transesophageal echocardiography. The combination of ECG and troponin I is adequate to exclude clinically significant injury. When these screening tests are abnormal, echocardiography should further characterize injuries that are present. This test includes quantifying the degree of left ventricular dysfunction resulting from contused or concussed myocardium (appearing as an area of thickened myocardium during end-diastole[21]) and identifying associated valvular disorders. Although the transesophageal approach is clearly superior to the transthoracic at image acquisition in BCI,[26] it is more time and resource intensive, and as ultrasonography technology improves, its relative advantage may diminish and it may not need to be routinely performed. Either modality also detects pericardial effusion caused by traumatic cardiac rupture, although this condition has a low prevalence (0.06% of patients with blunt trauma) and high mortality despite operative intervention. One series estimated the need for approximately 4800 echocardiograms in patients with blunt chest trauma to diagnose 1 survivor.[27] Other modalities, such as computed tomography (CT), MRI, and magnetic resonance coronary angiography have been used to evaluate BCI, but all have significant limitations and should be considered only on a case-by-case basis in consultation with a trauma surgeon and/or radiologist. Nuclear scintigraphy is not useful in the evaluation of BCI.[10]

TREATMENT

At a minimum, all patients with abnormal ECG or positive troponin level should be admitted for observation to monitor for dysrhythmias. Dysrhythmias and hypokinesis from myocardial contusion frequently resolve within 24 hours, but some experts recommend observation for at least 48 hours.[16] Admission location (telemetry vs intensive care unit) should depend on concomitant injuries, the type of ECG abnormality, and the degree of hemodynamic derangement.[28] Patients who develop significant heart failure or cardiogenic shock should be treated with inotropic agents and/or mechanical support.

There is no evidence to support or refute the use of specific antidysrhythmics in this population; consequently, providers should follow the standard approach to dysrhythmia management, including electrolyte repletion, avoidance of hypoxia and acidosis, antidysrhythmic medications, and defibrillation if necessary. The most common dysrhythmia is sinus tachycardia, which is addressed by treating the underlying cause (eg, volume resuscitation, analgesia, or transfusion). Atrial fibrillation is the second most common dysrhythmia, with the most common causes being alcohol or drug use, fluid shifts, electrolyte abnormalities, and/or catecholamine surge. Although uncommon, persistent complete heart block requiring permanent pacemaker placement has been described.[29,30] Such cases may necessitate temporary pacemaker placement in the acute care setting.

Patients with ST segment elevations on ECG represent a management dilemma, because these elevations may be caused by either traumatic myocardial infarction (from coronary rupture, dissection, or thrombosis) or myocardial contusion. Consequently, some experts recommend coronary angiography for patients with BCI when myocardial infarction is suspected (ie, ST segment elevation is observed),[31] although there is no clear standardized approach or guideline recommendation to differentiate infarction from contusion.

Most structural injuries, including myocardial rupture, pericardial rupture, hemopericardium, and traumatic valvular injuries, require operative repair and warrant immediate surgical evaluation.[32] A variety of temporizing measures may be performed depending on the specific structure injured. Mitral valve injuries with significant regurgitation may require vasodilators to reduce afterload and improve the forward stroke volume and ejection fraction. In such cases, mechanical support with an intra-aortic balloon pump may also be beneficial before valve repair or replacement.[33] Aortic valvular injuries are typically not amenable to stabilizing measures and require emergent surgery. Pericardiocentesis or emergent thoracotomy may be indicated for hemopericardium, depending on the degree of hemodynamic instability and the acuity of decompensation. In these cases, injuries caused by pulmonary vein or vena caval lacerations carry a much better prognosis than those caused by blunt cardiac rupture.

There is a paucity of literature addressing long-term functional outcomes of patients with BCI, especially given the lack of standardization in diagnostic terminology. Lindstaedt and colleagues[11] found normalization of echocardiographic findings and no cardiac limitations in 12-month follow-up of 118 patients with cardiac contusion.

SUMMARY

In spite of its elusive nature, BCI offers the opportunity for emergency physicians to discover disorders that can lead to timely treatment. The key to excellence in care is maintenance of suspicion, especially in patients with multiple injured organ systems, and use of readily available diagnostic tests to screen for further investigation and determine the need for treatment. The literature on BCI is wide and varied, inasmuch as the term encompasses multiple injury patterns within the realm of blunt trauma to the heart. The most important diagnostic pearls are (1) using ECG and troponin assays as screening tools, (2) obtaining echocardiography in cases with abnormalities screening, and (3) recognizing that signs of cardiac contusion can take up to 48 hours to manifest. Patients with abnormal ECG or biomarkers should be admitted for observation.

REFERENCES

1. Burchell HB. Unusual forms of heart disease. Circulation 1954;10(4):574–9.
2. Mattox KL, Flint LM, Carrico CJ, et al. Blunt cardiac injury. J Trauma 1992;33(5): 649–50.
3. Parmley LF, Manion WC, Mattingly TW. Nonpenetrating traumatic injury of the heart. Circulation 1958;18(3):371–96.
4. Schultz JM, Trunkey DD. Blunt cardiac injury. Crit Care Clin 2004;20(1):57–70.
5. Velmahos GC, Karaiskakis M, Salim A, et al. Normal electrocardiography and serum troponin I levels preclude the presence of clinically significant blunt cardiac injury. J Trauma 2003;54(1):45–50 [discussion: 50–1].
6. Baum VC. The patient with cardiac trauma. J Cardiothorac Vasc Anesth 2000; 14(1):71–81.
7. Liedtke AJ, DeMuth WE Jr. Nonpenetrating cardiac injuries: a collective review. Am Heart J 1973;86(5):687–97.
8. Patton AS, Guyton SW, Lawson DW, et al. Treatment os severe atrial injuries. Am J Surg 1981;141(4):465–71.
9. Clancy K, Velopulos C, Bilaniuk JW, et al. Screening for blunt cardiac injury: an Eastern Association for the Surgery of Trauma practice management guideline. J Trauma Acute Care Surg 2012;73(5 Suppl 4):S301–6.

10. Maenza RL, Seaberg D, D'Amico F. A meta-analysis of blunt cardiac trauma: ending myocardial confusion. Am J Emerg Med 1996;14(3):237–41.
11. Lindstaedt M, Germing A, Lawo T, et al. Acute and long-term clinical significance of myocardial contusion following blunt thoracic trauma: results of a prospective study. J Trauma 2002;52(3):479–85.
12. Marshall DT, Gilbert JD, Byard RW. The spectrum of findings in cases of sudden death due to blunt cardiac trauma–'commotio cordis'. Am J Forensic Med Pathol 2008;29(1):1–4.
13. Maron BJ, Doerer JJ, Haas TS, et al. Sudden deaths in young competitive athletes: analysis of 1866 deaths in the United States, 1980–2006. Circulation 2009;119(8):1085–92.
14. Link MS, Maron BJ, Wang PJ, et al. Upper and lower limits of vulnerability to sudden arrhythmic death with chest-wall impact (commotio cordis). J Am Coll Cardiol 2003;41(1):99–104.
15. Bock JS, Benitez RM. Blunt cardiac injury. Cardiol Clin 2012;30(4):545–55.
16. El-Chami MF, Nicholson W, Helmy T. Blunt cardiac trauma. J Emerg Med 2008; 35(2):127–33.
17. McGillicuddy D, Rosen P. Diagnostic dilemmas and current controversies in blunt chest trauma. Emerg Med Clin North Am 2007;25(3):695–711, viii–ix.
18. Collins JN, Cole FJ, Weireter LJ, et al. The usefulness of serum troponin levels in evaluating cardiac injury. Am Surg 2001;67(9):821–5 [discussion: 825–6].
19. Pasquale M, Fabian TC. Practice management guidelines for trauma from the Eastern Association for the Surgery of Trauma. J Trauma 1998;44(6):941–56 [discussion: 956–7].
20. Fulda GJ, Giberson F, Hailstone D, et al. An evaluation of serum troponin T and signal-averaged electrocardiography in predicting electrocardiographic abnormalities after blunt chest trauma. J Trauma 1997;43(2):304–10 [discussion: 310–2].
21. Garcia-Fernandez MA, Lopez-Perez JM, Perez-Castellano N, et al. Role of trans-esophageal echocardiography in the assessment of patients with blunt chest trauma: correlation of echocardiographic findings with the electrocardiogram and creatine kinase monoclonal antibody measurements. Am Heart J 1998; 135(3):476–81.
22. Gibel W, Schramm T. Passive smoking in controversy. Z Arztl Fortbild (Jena) 1988;82(5):213–6 [in German].
23. Kaye P, O'Sullivan I. Myocardial contusion: emergency investigation and diagnosis. Emerg Med J 2002;19(1):8–10.
24. Adams JE 3rd, Davila-Roman VG, Bessey PQ, et al. Improved detection of cardiac contusion with cardiac troponin I. Am Heart J 1996;131(2):308–12.
25. Bertinchant JP, Polge A, Mohty D, et al. Evaluation of incidence, clinical significance, and prognostic value of circulating cardiac troponin I and T elevation in hemodynamically stable patients with suspected myocardial contusion after blunt chest trauma. J Trauma 2000;48(5):924–31.
26. Chirillo F, Totis O, Cavarzerani A, et al. Usefulness of transthoracic and transoesophageal echocardiography in recognition and management of cardiovascular injuries after blunt chest trauma. Heart 1996;75(3):301–6.
27. Press GM, Miller S. Utility of the cardiac component of FAST in blunt trauma. J Emerg Med 2013;44(1):9–16.
28. Tenzer ML. The spectrum of myocardial contusion: a review. J Trauma 1985; 25(7):620–7.
29. Benitez RM, Gold MR. Immediate and persistent complete heart block following a horse kick. Pacing Clin Electrophysiol 1999;22(5):816–8.

30. Lazaros GA, Ralli DG, Moundaki VS, et al. Delayed development of complete heart block after a blunt chest trauma. Injury 2004;35(12):1300–2.
31. Plautz CU, Perron AD, Brady WJ. Electrocardiographic ST-segment elevation in the trauma patient: acute myocardial infarction vs myocardial contusion. Am J Emerg Med 2005;23(4):510–6.
32. El-Menyar A, Al Thani H, Zarour A, et al. Understanding traumatic blunt cardiac injury. Ann Card Anaesth 2012;15(4):287–95.
33. Wolfson AB, Harwood-Nuss A. Harwood-Nuss' clinical practice of emergency medicine. 4th edition. Philadelphia: Lippincott Williams & Wilkins; 2005.

Chameleons

Electrocardiogram Imitators of ST-Segment Elevation Myocardial Infarction

Jose V. Nable, MD, NRP[a],*, Benjamin J. Lawner, DO, EMT-P[b]

KEYWORDS

- Electrocardiography • STEMI • Myocardial infarction • Electrocardiogram

KEY POINTS

- Rapid recognition of ST-segment elevation myocardial infarction (STEMI) is imperative; however, the characteristic electrocardiographic (ECG) pattern of ST-segment elevation may be seen in other diagnoses.
- An understanding of these other diagnoses, and an awareness of how to distinguish them from STEMI, often requires obtaining a satisfactory history, comparing with previous ECGs, assessing serial tests, and uncovering subtle clues in the ECG pattern.
- The morphology of ST-segment elevation may provide a valuable clue at determining if the evaluated pattern is concerning for either STEMI or one of its imitators.
- Specifically, ST-segment elevation may be seen in patients with left ventricular hypertrophy, early repolarization, left bundle branch block, myopericarditis, Brugada syndrome, hyperkalemia, Takotsubo cardiomyopathy, and ventricular aneurysm.

INTRODUCTION

The need for timely reperfusion is critical to improving outcomes following ST-segment elevation myocardial infarction (STEMI). Indeed, the most recent iteration of the guideline from the American College of Cardiology Foundation (ACCF) and American Heart Association (AHA) continues to emphasize rapid recognition and reperfusion for patients with STEMI.[1] Clinicians must recognize electrocardiographic (ECG) patterns diagnostic of STEMI and rapidly coordinate the delivery of definitive care in the form of percutaneous coronary intervention or fibrinolysis. Importantly,

Disclosures: The authors have no commercial associations or sources of support that might pose a conflict of interest.
[a] Department of Emergency Medicine, MedStar Georgetown University Hospital, Georgetown University School of Medicine, 3800 Reservoir Rd NW, G-CCC, Washington, DC 20007, USA;
[b] Department of Emergency Medicine, University of Maryland School of Medicine, 6th floor, Suite 200110 South Pace Street, Baltimore, MD 21201, USA
* Corresponding author.
E-mail address: JoseVictor.L.Nable@medstar.net

Emerg Med Clin N Am 33 (2015) 529–537
http://dx.doi.org/10.1016/j.emc.2015.04.004   emed.theclinics.com

the 2013 ACCF/AHA guideline clarified the definition of STEMI to include elevations, as measured from the J point, of at least 1 mm in two or more anatomically contiguous leads (with allowance of up to 1.5 mm in leads V_2–V_3 for women and 2 mm in the same leads in men).[1]

Unfortunately, ECG features seen in association with STEMI also appear in other benign, nonischemic presentations. Although a certain amount of overtriage is accepted, it is desirable to minimize patient risk. Patients with evidence of left ventricular hypertrophy (LVH) without actual acute infarction, for example, will likely not benefit from emergent reperfusion. Risks associated with inappropriate coronary revascularization include radiation exposure, dye administration, and medication-induced bleeding. A thorough understanding of conditions that have the potential to mimic or confound the diagnosis of STEMI is essential to the provision of timely and safe patient care. This article focuses on ECG findings, specifically ST-segment elevation, occurring in the absence of ischemia.

LEFT VENTRICULAR HYPERTROPHY

Chronic and uncontrolled hypertension results in remodeling of the heart's left ventricle. The increase in muscle mass also alters the manner in which cardiac repolarization occurs. Characteristic ECG changes associated with LVH may mimic the ST-segment elevation seen in the setting of acute myocardial infarction (AMI).[2] Other changes attributed to LVH include prominent septal q waves, T-wave inversion, and ST-segment depression.[3] Several features unique to LVH assist the emergency clinician in differentiating it from the STEMI-related ECG changes. First, ECG changes in the setting of LVH are static. Unlike an evolving ischemic event, the ST-segment morphology of the ECG in LVH remains constant. Serial ECGs are therefore of value when considering the diagnosis of LVH. The ST-segment changes are appropriately discordant with respect to hypertrophy (**Figs. 1–3**). Deep QS waves appear in the septal precordial leads. The resultant repolarization is upright and occurs on the opposite side of the baseline.

Similarly, high-amplitude R waves occur in the lateral precordial leads. ST-segment changes, including strain-associated ST-segment depression, occur below the isoelectric line.[3] ECG "strain" seen in LVH does not typically manifest as ST-segment elevation. A characteristic strain pattern reveals a downsloping ST segment ending

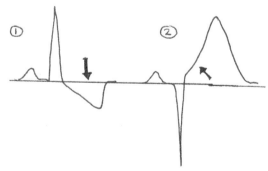

Fig. 1. Left ventricular hypertrophy appropriate discordance. Appropriately discordant ST segment changes in the setting of left ventricular hypertrophy. The ST segment is below baseline when the QRS complex is positively deflected (*1*), whereas the ST segment is above baseline when the QRS complex is negatively deflected (*2*).

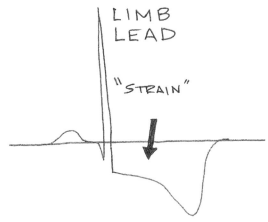

Fig. 2. Strain pattern. A characteristic strain pattern reveals a downsloping ST segment ending in a terminally negative, and asymmetric T wave.

in a terminally negative and asymmetric T wave. Finally, the ECG usually reveals a rapid return to the baseline. Strain patterns are thought to result from hypertensive heart disease.

The emergency physician should be keenly aware of the possibility of LVH confounding the ability to recognize true STEMI. The presence of LVH, and its concomitant perturbing of the ST segment, has been demonstrated as a risk factor for false-positive STEMI diagnosis, not uncommonly leading to unnecessary reperfusion therapy.[4,5]

EARLY REPOLARIZATION

Early repolarization occurs in approximately 1% of the population.[6] Patients with early repolarization may present to the emergency department complaining of chest pain with an ECG potentially mimicking STEMI. There are several clues, however, that may assist the physician in correctly distinguishing early repolarization from an AMI.

The ST-segment elevation typically found in early repolarization is less than 2 mm in the precordial leads and less than 0.5 mm in the limb leads.[7] Additionally, the morphology of the ST segment in early repolarization is generally upsloping in concavity (**Fig. 4**)[7,8] Although a nonconcave morphology is often worrisome for MI,[9] morphology is not completely sensitive for detecting ongoing infarction.[7] Other clues, such as notching of the terminal QRS complex, prominent T waves that are concordant with the ST segment, and the persistent nature of early repolarization, should also be

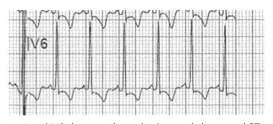

Fig. 3. Strain pattern. Lead V6 shows a downsloping and depressed ST segment.

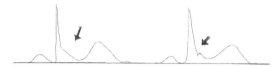

Fig. 4. Early repolarization. Typical early repolarization pattern with ST-segment elevation, prominent T waves that are concordant with the ST segment, and not uncommonly a notched terminal QRS complex.

considered.[7] The importance of assessing for dynamic ECGs to assist in differentiating early repolarization from STEMI underscores the necessity of frequently obtaining serial tests.

LEFT BUNDLE BRANCH BLOCK

The left bundle branch block (LBBB) pattern complicates the physician's ability to assess for STEMI because the pattern by definition includes ST-segment elevation.[10] Additionally, the presence of LBBB during an AMI has previously been associated with increased risk for mortality.[11] For many years, it was recommended that patients with new or presumably new LBBB in the setting of chest pain or other ischemic symptoms should undergo emergent reperfusion therapy.[12]

More recent literature, however, has caused a dramatic shift in the approach to management of patients with LBBB. Although LBBB may identify a high-risk population, only a small proportion of these patients are ultimately diagnosed with AMI.[13] The presence of LBBB also has been shown to be a poor predictor for infarction.[14] The most recent ACCF/AHA guideline on STEMI management notes that LBBB may interfere with the ability to detect STEMI and should not be used in isolation to diagnose AMI.[1] Because patients with LBBB, however, not uncommonly do present with acute coronary syndrome, the clinician must remain vigilant.

Criteria developed by Sgarbossa and colleagues[15] may potentially be useful in identifying those with LBBB who require emergent reperfusion.[16] This score-based criteria system includes the presence of (1) ST-segment elevation of at least 1 mm concordant with the QRS complex in any lead (5 points); (2) ST-segment depression of at least 1 mm in leads V_1, V_2, or V_3 (3 points); or (3) ST-segment elevation of at least 5 mm discordant with the QRS complex in any lead (2 points).[15] A composite score of 3 or greater has been shown to have an estimated sensitivity of 20% and specificity of 98% to predict AMI.[17] A score of 0, however, does not reliably exclude MI.[17] In light of the recent ACCF/AHA guideline changes regarding LBBB, and the relatively low sensitivity of Sgarbossa's criteria, the development of more versatile clinical criteria may be necessary.[15]

MYOPERICARDITIS

Myopericarditis is classically associated with diffuse elevations of the ST segment, usually with upward concavity, along with PR-segment depressions.[18] These elevations may be confused with STEMI. Furthermore, similar to MI, patients may present with chest pain radiating to the arms or neck.[18] Cardiac biomarkers are generally elevated in patients with myocarditis[10] and in up to 50% of patients with pericarditis.[18]

Inflammation of the pericardium and heart muscle is typically idiopathic, although most often presumed to be caused by a viral infection.[19] It is believed that PR-segment depressions are a manifestation of inflammation of the pericardial sac.[20] PR-segment changes, however, are dynamic in the course of acute myoperi-carditis, typically seen in the early phases of the disease process.[20]

Myopericarditis is an example of the importance of obtaining serial ECGs to help the clinician distinguish STEMI from other ECG-mimicking processes. As opposed to myopericarditis, the evolution of STEMI is typically much more rapid, with changes to the ST-segment and T-wave morphology often occurring over the course of only several minutes.[10] Furthermore, although patients with multiple coronary artery occlusions may present with diffuse ST-segment elevations, such patients tend to have a much sicker and more dramatic presentation than those with myopericarditis, often in cardiogenic shock.[21] A sicker patient presentation may thus be more worrisome for the need for rapid reperfusion therapy.

BRUGADA SYNDROME

Brugada syndrome is described as a right bundle branch block with ST-segment elevation in leads V_1 through V_3.[22] Three types of this pattern have been described (**Fig. 5**). In type 1, a coved-appearing ST-segment elevation of at least 2 mm is proceeded by a negative T wave; type 2 contains an ST segment that remains above baseline followed by an upright or biphasic T wave, giving rise to a "saddle-back" appearance; type 3 is typified by ST-segment elevation of less than 1 mm, with either a coved or "saddle-back" appearance.[23]

Patients with this particular ECG pattern have been observed to be at risk for sudden ventricular arrhythmias leading to death.[24] A genetic mutation linked to a sodium channelopathy has been attributed to this process.[25] Although some patients with the Brugada pattern may have significant ST-segment elevation, chest pain is not considered part of the syndrome.[10] These patients are, however, at risk for sudden death.

PROMINENT T WAVES

Hyperacute T waves, as manifested by increased T-wave amplitudes, is considered to be one of the earliest ECG signs of AMI.[26] Indeed, the early temporal nature of large T waves in the evolution of ST-segment elevation has been described since the early half of the twentieth century.[27] The astute clinician, however, should note that large T waves may be found in a variety of other conditions.

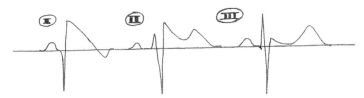

Fig. 5. Brugada syndrome. Type I demonstrates a coved-appearing ST segment with elevation of at least 2 mm followed by a negatively deflected T wave. Type II contains an ST segment that remains above baseline followed by an upright or biphasic T wave with a "saddle-back" appearance. Type III has ST-segment elevation of less than 1 mm with either a coved or "saddle-back" appearance. (*Data from* Wilde AA, Antzelevitch C, Borggrefe M, et al. Proposed diagnostic criteria for the Brugada syndrome: consensus report. Circulation 2002;106:2514–9.)

Hyperkalemia

Elevated serum potassium is known to cause a variety of ECG changes, including increasing amplitudes of the T wave. Hyperkalemic T waves, however, tend to maintain a narrow base with a symmetric morphology.[26] In contrast, hyperacute T waves associated with AMI tend to be broad-based and asymmetric. Although ST-segment elevation may also be seen in hyperkalemia,[28] such elevations are typically diffuse. Additional historical factors, such as the presence of kidney failure, may also provide valuable insight.

Finally, the evolution of ECG changes may provide some clues. The typical pattern of progressing hyperkalemia includes (1) peaked T waves, (2) prolonging PR interval, (3) widening QRS complex, and (4) sinusoidal pattern (**Figs. 6** and **7**).

Early Repolarization

Early repolarization can be confused with STEMI. In particular, the large T waves not uncommonly found with early repolarization may mimic the early stages of AMI. These enlarged T waves, however, tend to be symmetric and concordant with the ST segment.[10]

TAKOTSUBO OR STRESS-RELATED ST-SEGMENT ELEVATION

Takotsubo cardiomyopathy (TTCM) was first recognized in 1990 at Hiroshima City Hospital. Dr Sato detailed a syndrome of apical wall motion abnormality and ECG changes occurring in the absence of coronary artery disease.[29] TTCM presents with signs and symptoms similar to those seen in acute coronary syndromes. Patients may report chest discomfort and shortness of breath. The accompanying ECG may show ST-segment abnormalities including ST-segment elevation.

A recent review documented the prevalence of ST-segment elevation in cases of TTCM as high as 90%.[30] The magnitude of ST-segment deviation in TTCM tends to be less than the elevation occurring with STEMI, and TTCM is less likely to present with reciprocal changes.[29,31] Because the left ventricle is most commonly affected in TTCM, ECG changes may be more likely to occur in the lateral, septal, and anterior leads.[30] History may offer additional diagnostic clues because patients often report a stressful or precipitating event in these cases. Currently, the ECG is not useful as a stand-alone tool to set TTCM apart from STEMI. Both conditions produce ST-segment elevation and elevated cardiac biomarkers. If available, emergent transthoracic echocardiography may identify typical wall motion abnormalities that accompany TTCM. The literature is not clear about the underlying physiology. Catecholamine release and an upregulation of myocardial β-receptor activity have been implicated in the disease process.[29]

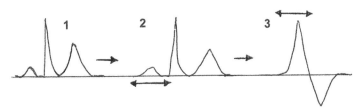

Fig. 6. Early hyperkalemia. The typical pattern of progressing hyperkalemia includes (*1*) peaked T waves, (*2*) prolonging PR interval, and (*3*) widening QRS complex.

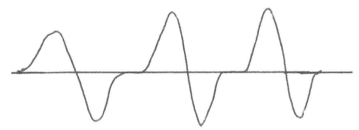

Fig. 7. Severe hyperkalemia. Sinusoidal pattern not uncommonly seen in severe hyperkalemia.

VENTRICULAR ANEURYSM

The finding of persistent ST-segment elevation following a recent MI has long been recognized as a possible sign of the development of a ventricular aneurysm.[32,33] Although the exact mechanism for its persistence has yet to be elucidated, at least one study has shown that continued ST-segment elevation may be a further marker of extensive transmural necrosis and microvascular damage.[34] Because of the typical location of ventricular aneurysm postinfarction, ST-segment elevation in this setting is most commonly in the anterior leads.[35]

Historical factors, such as known recent AMI, should help provide the emergency physician some clues in distinguishing an acute STEMI from ventricular aneurysm. Additionally, comparison with prior ECGs may be helpful.

SUMMARY

The time-sensitive diagnosis of STEMI demands that emergency clinicians maintain proficiency in the interpretation of the ECG. In addition to the recognition of potentially life-threatening ECG patterns, emergency clinicians must separate STEMI patterns from mimics, confounders, and other conditions that produce similar changes. Fortunately, close scrutiny of the ECG in combination with a focused clinical history assists practitioners with sorting out conditions that likely do not benefit from urgent percutaneous coronary intervention. ST-segment morphology yields valuable diagnostic clues and represents another tool useful for the triage of patients with ECG findings.

REFERENCES

1. O'Gara PT, Kushner FG, Ascheim DD, et al. 2013 ACCF/AHA guideline for the management of ST-elevation myocardial infarction. J Am Coll Cardiol 2013;61: e78–140.
2. Brady WJ, Perron AD, Martin ML, et al. Cause of ST segment abnormality in ED chest pain patients. Am J Emerg Med 2001;19:25–8.
3. Brady WJ. Electrocardiographic left ventricular hypertrophy in chest pain patients: differentiation from acute coronary ischemic events. Am J Emerg Med 1998;16:692–6.
4. McCabe JM, Armstrong EJ, Kulkarni A, et al. Prevalence and factors associated with false-positive ST-segment elevation myocardial infarction diagnoses at primary percutaneous coronary intervention–capable centers: a report from the activate-SF registry. Arch Intern Med 2012;172:864–71.

5. Khoury NE, Borzak S, Gokli A, et al. "Inadvertent" thrombolytic administration in patients without myocardial infarction: clinical features and outcome. Ann Emerg Med 1996;28:289–93.

6. Mehta MC, Jain AC. Early repolarization on scalar electrocardiogram. Am J Med Sci 1995;309:305–11.

7. Brady WJ, Chan TC. Electrocardiographic manifestations: benign early repolarization. J Emerg Med 1999;17:473–8.

8. Wasserburger RM, Alt WJ, Lloyd C. The normal RS-T segment elevation variant. Am J Cardiol 1961;8:184–92.

9. Brady WJ, Syverud SA, Beagle C, et al. Electrocardiographic ST-segment elevation: the diagnosis of acute myocardial infarction by morphologic analysis of the ST segment. Acad Emerg Med 2001;8(10):961–7.

10. Pollak PM, Brady WJ. Patterns mimicking ST segment elevation myocardial infarction. Cardiol Clin 2012;30:601–15.

11. Fibrinolytic Therapy Trialists' (FTT) Collaborative Group. Indications for fibrinolytic therapy in suspected acute myocardial infarction: collaborative overview of early mortality and major morbidity results from all randomized trials of more than 1000 patients. Lancet 1994;343:311–22.

12. Antman EM, Anbe DT, Armstrong PW, et al. ACC/AHA guidelines for the management of patients with ST-elevation myocardial infarction: a report of the American College of Cardiology/American Heart Association task force on practice guidelines. J Am Coll Cardiol 2004;44:E1–211.

13. Jain S, Ting HT, Bell M, et al. Utility of left bundle branch block as a diagnostic criterion for acute myocardial infarction. Am J Cardiol 2011;107:1111–6.

14. Chang AM, Shofer FS, Tabas JA, et al. Lack of association between left bundle-branch block and acute myocardial infarction in symptomatic ED patients. Am J Emerg Med 2009;27:916–21.

15. Sgarbossa EB, Pinski SL, Barbagelata A, et al. Electrocardiographic diagnosis of evolving acute myocardial infarction in the presence of left bundle-branch block. N Engl J Med 1996;334:481–7.

16. Cai Q, Mehta N, Sgarbossa EB, et al. The left bundle-branch block puzzle in the 2013 ST-elevation myocardial infarction guidelines: from falsely declaring emergency to denying reperfusion in a high-risk population. Are the Sgarbossa criteria ready for prime time? Am Heart J 2013;166:409–13.

17. Tabas JA, Rodriguez RM, Seligman HK, et al. Electrocardiographic criteria for detecting acute myocardial infarction in patients with left bundle branch block: a meta-analysis. Ann Emerg Med 2008;42:329–36.

18. Lange RA, Hillis LD. Clinical practice. Acute pericarditis. N Engl J Med 2004;351:2195–202.

19. Zayas R, Anguita M, Torres F, et al. Incidence of specific etiology and role of methods for specific etiologic diagnosis of primary acute pericarditis. Am J Cardiol 1995;75:378–82.

20. Porela P, Kytö V, Nikus K, et al. PR depression is useful in the differential diagnosis of myopericarditis and ST elevation myocardial infarction. Ann Noninvasive Electrocardiol 2012;17:141–5.

21. Pollak PM, Parikh SV, Kizilgul M, et al. Multiple culprit arteries in patients with ST segment elevation myocardial infarction referred for primary percutaneous coronary intervention. Am J Cardiol 2009;104:619–23.

22. Brugada J, Brugada R, Brugada P. Right bundle-branch block and ST-segment elevation in leads V1 through V3: a marker for sudden death in patients without demonstrable structural heart disease. Circulation 1998;97:457–60.

23. Wilde AA, Antzelevitch C, Borggrefe M, et al. Proposed diagnostic criteria for the Brugada syndrome: consensus report. Circulation 2002;106:2514–9.
24. Brugada P, Brugada J. Right bundle branch block, persistent ST segment elevation and sudden cardiac death: a distinct clinical and electrocardiographic syndrome: a multicenter report. J Am Coll Cardiol 1992;20:1391–6.
25. Veerakul G, Nademanee K. Brugada syndrome: two decades of progress. Circ J 2012;76:2713–22.
26. Somers MP, Brady WJ, Perron AD, et al. The prominent T wave: electrocardiographic differential diagnosis. Am J Emerg Med 2002;20:243–51.
27. Dressler W, Hugo R. High T waves in the earliest stage of myocardial infarction. Am Heart J 1947;45:627–45.
28. Simon BC. Pseudomyocardial infarction and hyperkalemia: a case report and subject review. J Emerg Med 1988;6:511–5.
29. Kurisu S, Kihara Y. Tako-tsubo cardiomyopathy: clinical presentation and underlying mechanism. J Cardiol 2012;60:429–37.
30. Sanchez-Jimenez EF. Initial clinical presentation of Takotsubo cardiomyopathy with-a focus on electrocardiographic changes: a literature review of cases. World J Cardiol 2013;5:228–41.
31. Prasad A, Lerman A, Rihal CS. Apical ballooning syndrome (Tako-Tsubo or stress cardiomyopathy): a mimic of acute myocardial infarction. Am Heart J 2008;155:408–17.
32. Arvan S, Varat MA. Persistent ST-segment elevation and left ventricular wall abnormalities: a 2-dimensional echocardiographic study. Am J Cardiol 1984;53:1542–6.
33. Cohn K, Dymnicka S, Forlini FJ. Use of the electrocardiogram as an aid in screening for left ventricular aneurysm. J Electrocardiol 1976;9:53–8.
34. Napodano M, Tarantini G, Ramondo A, et al. Myocardial abnormalities underlying persistent ST-segment elevation after anterior myocardial infarction. J Cardiovasc Med (Hagerstown) 2009;10:44–50.
35. Engel J, Brady WJ, Mattu A, et al. Electrocardiographic ST segment elevation: left ventricular aneurysm. Am J Emerg Med 2002;20:238–42.

Hypertensive Emergencies in the Emergency Department

 CrossMark

Omoyemi Adebayo, MD*, Robert L. Rogers, MD

KEYWORDS

• Hypertension • Hypertensive emergency • Hypertensive crisis

KEY POINTS

- Hypertensive emergency cannot be diagnosed based only on the combination of severely increased blood pressure with symptoms such as headache, shortness of breath, and blurred vision.
- Hypertensive urgency is defined as severe hypertension in a patient with comorbidities that place the patient at higher risk of end-organ dysfunction. Hypertensive emergency is defined as objective findings of end-organ damage.
- Asymptomatic and otherwise healthy patients with severe essential hypertension should be referred to a primary care doctor within a week for nonurgent blood pressure control; treatment of this group with aggressive intravenous medications can precipitate hypotension and subsequent end-organ damage.
- Select a therapeutic agent that has rapid and reliable pharmacodynamics that can be turned on and off easily.
- The goal in treating most hypertensive emergencies is to reduce the blood pressure 25% within the first 24 hours after diagnosis. An exception is in patients with aortic dissection, which calls for much more rapid blood pressure reduction.

INTRODUCTION

In 2014, the American Heart Association (AHA) estimated that 77.9 million Americans older than 20 years of age have hypertension (HTN).[1] That is approximately 1 in every 3 adults, which is a staggering figure compared with other common diseases such as diabetes and hyperlipidemia. In 2009, the AHA reported that almost a third of the population with HTN was unaware of their underlying diagnosis[2]; this percentage has decreased to 19% according to recent figures from the National Health and Nutrition

Disclosures: The authors have no relevant financial relationships to disclose.
Department of Emergency Medicine, University of Maryland School of Medicine, 110 South Paca Street, 6th Floor, Suite 200, Baltimore, MD 21201, USA
* Corresponding author.
E-mail address: yadebayo@umem.org

Emerg Med Clin N Am 33 (2015) 539–551
http://dx.doi.org/10.1016/j.emc.2015.04.005   emed.theclinics.com

Examination Survey.[1] Nearly 70% of all patients with a first-time myocardial infarction, stroke, or congestive heart failure have poorly controlled blood pressure.[1] However, the 2014 Joint National Committee (JNC) guidelines for blood pressure management recommend a less aggressive treatment approach for older hypertensive patients than that proposed in the JNC 7 guidelines,[3] which could increase the number of patients found to be in a hypertensive crisis in the emergency department (ED).[4]

HTN is associated with significant short-term and long-term morbidity and mortality. The effects of HTN often build to hypertensive crises that can affect numerous organ systems either individually or simultaneously. The JNC 7 recommendations laid the groundwork for the identification and treatment of hypertensive crisis, but they did not clearly distinguish hypertensive urgency from hypertensive emergency. This distinction is important because their treatment approaches for blood pressure control are different. Despite the lack of large randomized controlled trials designed to establish evidence-based guidelines for the management of hypertensive emergencies, general consensus exists regarding the need for a timely response to prevent adverse outcomes.

This article discusses essential concepts in the evaluation and treatment of hypertensive emergencies that are encountered commonly in the ED. These emergencies include encephalopathy, pulmonary edema, myocardial ischemia, aortic dissection, nephropathy, and eclampsia (**Box 1**).

DEFINITION

Hypertension is defined as a systolic blood pressure greater than 140 mm Hg or a diastolic pressure greater than 90 mm Hg.[4] Hypertensive crises are separated into 2 broad categories of urgency and emergency. They are both defined by a systolic blood pressure greater than 180 mm Hg and a diastolic pressure greater than 120 mm Hg but are differentiated by the absence or presence, respectively, of end-organ damage.[4] End-organ damage is typically manifested by dysfunction in the cerebrovascular, cardiovascular, pulmonary, or renovascular systems. Organ dysfunction is the sole element that dictates the rapidity and modality of treatment required in a hypertensive crisis.

Hypertensive urgency is characterized by an acute increase of blood pressure that is not associated with end-organ damage. Recognition of hypertensive urgency can generate anxiety in emergency physicians (EPs), leading to the decision to administer intravenous (IV) medications. This therapeutic approach could inadvertently cause hypotension and organ hypoperfusion. In its definition of hypertensive urgency, the JNC includes symptoms such as headache, shortness of breath, and epistaxis. Many EPs are opposed to the term hypertensive urgency, citing its lack of meaningful definition. They prefer to refer to this entity as severe HTN.

Patients with hypertensive urgency are typically either noncompliant with prescribed medications or have been lost to follow-up and therefore lack proper titration of their medication dosages. Optimal treatment in this population is close outpatient follow-up with a gradual move toward oral antihypertensive medications.[5] No validated studies have shown that acutely reducing blood pressure in ED patients who present with severe HTN has any benefits in short-term risk reduction. In its 2013 clinical policy, the American College of Emergency Physicians discouraged initiation of blood pressure medication in the ED for asymptomatic patients with HTN.[6]

In contrast, hypertensive emergencies are associated with significant short-term and long-term morbidity and mortality: 5-year mortality approaches 100%.[7] Hypertensive emergencies represent up to one-fourth of all ED visits.[4] The JNC recommends

| Box 1 |
| Causes of hypertensive crises |

Essential hypertension

Endocrine

    Pheochromocytoma

    Cushing syndrome

    Renin-secreting tumor

    Primary hyperaldosteronism

Renovascular disease

    Renal artery stenosis

    Polyarteritis nodosa

    Takayasu arteritis

Drugs

    Cocaine

    Phencyclidine

    Sympathomimetics

    Antihypertensive medication withdrawal

    Amphetamines

    Lead intoxication

    Tyramine reaction with use of monoamine oxidase inhibitors

    Serotonin syndrome from selective serotonin reuptake inhibitor use

Central nervous system

    Cerebral edema

    Cerebral hemorrhage

    Brain tumor

    Spinal cord injury

Coarctation of the aorta

Pain

Burns

the following therapeutic approach after a hypertensive emergency has been diagnosed: (1) mean arterial pressure reduction by ~25% in the first 1 hour of treatment, and (2) avoidance of precipitously reducing blood pressure (except in patients with aortic dissection) to preclude organ hypoperfusion.[4]

EVALUATION
History

Hypertensive emergencies can be identified based on the patient's past and present history, results of the physical examination, laboratory analysis, and imaging. Any patient who presents to the ED with severely increased blood pressure should have a thorough evaluation. The EP's evaluation and treatment algorithms are different for an acutely increased blood pressure in a patient with no history of HTN compared with another patient with known chronic HTN. For example, a previously normotensive woman who comes to the ED after her twentieth week of gestation with a severely increased blood pressure and headache raises concern for preeclampsia requiring emergent management; however, if the same gravid woman presents to the ED with chronic pregestational HTN and a headache, the level of concern and management approach are different than for the patient described earlier.

The EP should obtain the patient's current complete medication list: drug names, doses, any recent changes in their administration, and sudden discontinuations from previously taken prescriptions. Sympatholytic medications such as clonidine are notorious for causing severe rebound HTN. Another pertinent piece of information to obtain from the patient is the use of illicit substances. Cocaine and phencyclidine are sympathomimetics that cause severe increases in blood pressure, as well as other symptoms. A family history of sudden death, premature cardiac disease, or endocrine disorders should prompt the EP to consider pheochromocytoma, multiple endocrine neoplasm, and hyperthyroidism as possible causes of episodic blood pressure increase and tachycardia in a young healthy patient. The most vital part of the history is assessment of signs and symptoms associated with the patient's chief complaint (eg, chest pain, shortness of breath, urine output, weakness, or sensory loss) and targeted evaluation of end organs. The presence of symptoms alone does not confirm a hypertensive emergency, but it suggests that an organ might be affected, requiring further assessment.

Physical Examination

If high blood pressure is detected during the triage process, the measurement must be repeated in the examination room after the patient has rested for 5 minutes without perturbation. The one-size-fits-all approach to blood pressure cuffs can produce falsely high or low blood pressure readings; a cuff of appropriate size for each patient is required for accurate measurements.[8]

When examining a patient with suspected hypertensive emergency, several crucial parts of the examination indicate whether further testing is needed. Assessment of mental status is one of the first steps in a thorough neurologic examination. Confusion, delirium, or seizure without other cause or reason suggests hypertensive encephalopathy. Other telltale signs of neurologic impairment are motor or sensory deficits and papilledema on funduscopic evaluation. A complete ocular examination is vital; if not performed by the EP, ophthalmologic consultation is warranted to guard against permanent vision damage. The pulmonary examination should focus on evidence of rales, hypoxia, or tachypnea, which imply flash pulmonary edema. Murmurs heard on cardiac examination (specifically, a diastolic decrescendo murmur of aortic regurgitation that was not previously known to exist in the patient) could signify a type A aortic dissection. A careful vascular assessment of proximal and distal pulses and blood pressures allows stratification of the likelihood of this rare, and potentially deadly, diagnosis. Auscultation of an abdominal bruit should raise concern for renal artery stenosis. An often-overlooked part of the examination of a hypertensive patient is evaluation of volume status. An acute increase in blood pressure results in natriuresis, a physiologic response that decreases the blood volume in an effort to reduce the blood pressure. This response becomes extremely important when IV medications are administered to treat a hypertensive emergency; the combination of natriuresis and the effects of a potent antihypertensive agent could induce a dangerously fast reduction in blood pressure.

Diagnostic Testing

Laboratory analysis should be based on which organ system the EP thinks could be damaged. Any patient thought to have had a stroke, seizure, or any neurologic derangement secondary to hypertensive emergency should undergo computed tomography of the head as a priority. Based on a small study, Roque and colleagues[9] concluded that measurements of optic nerve sheath diameter by bedside ultrasonography can accurately predict which patients have increased intracranial pressure. Every patient presenting with chest pain should have an electrocardiogram (ECG) to assess for signs of cardiac ischemia or infarct. If the patient's history of present illness suggests acute coronary syndrome (ACS) (exertional chest pain, dyspnea, diaphoresis, fatigue, jaw/arm pain, and nausea with epigastric pain), cardiac biomarker measurements should also be obtained. Dyspnea has a myriad of causes (eg, an anginal equivalent, pulmonary edema, renal failure, and anemia), all of which could stem from a hypertensive emergency. Obtaining both a screening ECG and chest radiograph (CXR) in dyspneic patients is recommended. If renal dysfunction is suspected, urinalysis and a basic metabolic panel should be requested. Abnormalities that suggest hypertensive nephropathy include proteinuria, muddy casts, and an increased blood urea nitrogen or creatinine level. A complete blood count with manual differentiation showing schistocytes suggests microangiopathic hemolytic anemia, which is another sign of end-organ damage. Diagnostic testing should be tailored to focus on patient complaints and the end organ in question to both maximize ED efficiency and minimize costly unnecessary work-ups.[10]

MANAGEMENT OF HYPERTENSIVE EMERGENCIES

Definitive treatment of any hypertensive emergency is the acute reduction of blood pressure to prevent ongoing organ damage. The JNC 7 guidelines recommend that this be done within the first hour.[4] Therapy decisions should be considered carefully, weighing risks and benefits and taking into account which end organ is compromised as well as the patient's comorbidities. A patient in a hypertensive emergency should be admitted to an intensive or intermediate care unit for meticulous IV titration of antihypertensive medications and close cardiopulmonary monitoring. With the number of critically ill patients increasing and hospital overcrowding, EPs are likely to be responsible for managing patients with hypertensive emergencies for longer periods of time, including adjusting the therapeutic approach if the patient's condition improves or deteriorates in the ED. For patients who improve, it is important for the EP to institute oral antihypertensive agents for long-acting therapy before discontinuation of IV agents. If the patient was already on an oral antihypertensive at home, restarting that medication is appropriate, keeping in mind its side effect profile, onset of action, and half-life, because iatrogenic hypotension is common in this population.

Hypertensive Encephalopathy

The brain, like other organs, possesses an autoregulatory system to maintain a certain cerebral perfusion pressure. The autoregulatory system of a normotensive patient maintains a steady state, adequate for perfusion, by maintaining a mean arterial pressure (MAP) of 60 to 120 mm Hg. In normotensive patients who suddenly become hypertensive, the regulator system quickly becomes overwhelmed and can no longer maintain autoregulation through vasoconstriction and dilation. In contrast, in patients with long-standing hypertension, the autoregulatory system gradually adapts to severely increased blood pressures and accommodates a higher set-point and thus decreases the likelihood of a hypertensive emergency at moderately increased pressures. When the cerebral regulatory system becomes overwhelmed, the patient is at risk for cerebral edema. The subsequent syndrome is known as hypertensive encephalopathy. It can manifest in many ways, including acute delirium, lethargy, confusion, severe headache, or seizure. In addition, it is important to consider other equally dangerous causes of altered mental status (eg, infection and cerebrovascular accidents), because they have entirely different management strategies. In patients experiencing ischemic stroke, the blood pressure should not be reduced by more than 10% to 15% over the first 24 hours, because it is thought that HTN protects the ischemic penumbra of the brain.[11–14]

The treatment of hypertensive encephalopathy begins with symptom control. Expert opinion suggests that medications such as benzodiazepines, fosphenytoin, phenytoin, or barbiturates should be given for delirium and seizure control; they provide the added benefit of further blood pressure reduction.[15] For blood pressure management of hypertensive encephalopathy not complicated by cerebral vascular accident, the MAP should be reduced by about 20% to 25% in the first 1 hour of treatment. Traditionally used medications include IV nitroprusside, labetalol, nicardipine, and enalapril (**Table 1**). Centrally acting medications such as clonidine should be avoided for the acute management of hypertensive emergencies because their sedative side effects can make it difficult to appreciate the resolution of encephalopathic symptoms.[15]

Pulmonary Edema

One of the most harrowing hypertensive emergencies is hypoxic respiratory failure with acute flash pulmonary edema. Certain patient populations (ie, those with congestive heart failure and end-stage renal disease) are unable to tolerate fluctuations in their blood pressure easily, resulting in volume overload and pulmonary edema. In recent years, attention has centered on the use of noninvasive ventilation therapy, such as bilevel positive airway pressure ventilation, to circumvent the likelihood of these patients progressing to intubation. Treatment of the underlying cause, along with blood pressure reduction, is key to clinical improvement.

For patients with flash pulmonary edema, preload and afterload reduction remains the goal of treatment. One or more medications that work either alone or in conjunction with each other have been the traditional treatment. Nitrates such as nitroglycerin are effective in reducing preload because of their venodilatory effects. Afterload reducers, such as angiotensin-converting enzyme inhibitors, are also used as key treatment of flash pulmonary edema. Loop diuretics such as furosemide are often used to treat symptomatic dyspnea secondary to pulmonary edema. In a recent randomized, double-blind prospective study, Holzer-Richling and colleagues[16] found that administration of furosemide versus placebo to a cohort of patients did not improve outcomes. Study participants who received furosemide required lower doses of antihypertensive agents, suggesting a role for loop diuretics in reducing blood pressure.[16] Caution is needed when giving a diuretic during a hypertensive crisis, because more than half of patients with pulmonary edema are euvolemic or hypovolemic, not overloaded in terms of total body volume; in contrast, patients with renal or hepatic failure tend to be overloaded, so diuretics have benefit in the acute phase to excrete the excess fluid and off-load the lungs.

Nitroprusside, one of the fastest acting agents in the treatment armamentarium, is considered ideal for patients with flash pulmonary edema.[17] It has the profile benefit of being rapid in onset as well as a venous and arterial dilator. Its use carries a small risk of thiocyanate and cyanide toxicity, but that side effect is seen more commonly with excessive dosing and refractory blood pressure response. Clevedipine, one of the newest IV antihypertensive medications (approved by the US Food and Drug

Administration in 2008) has shown great promise in clinical trials for treatment of severe hypertension, particularly for pulmonary edema and postoperative hypertension.[18] Clevedipine is a dihydropyridine calcium channel blocker that has the added benefit of not being metabolized by the kidney or liver.[19–21]

Myocardial Ischemia

Classically, ACS develops as the result of an acute coronary thrombus. Cardiac ischemia can also be the result of other uncommon causes, such as hypertensive emergency. Patients with cardiac ischemia typically present with chest pain, dyspnea, diaphoresis, vomiting, and, especially in the elderly, generalized fatigue. Severe hypertension is usually associated with increased myocardial work and oxygen demand. Patients with previously diseased hearts are at increased risk of further myocardial ischemia. Electrocardiographic abnormalities and increased cardiac biomarkers indicate hypertension-induced cardiac ischemia or infarction. Treatment of ischemic chest pain is 3-fold: (1) reduction in myocardial work, (2) reduction in myocardial oxygen consumption, and (3) improvement in coronary artery perfusion.

The first intervention that should be performed in a patient with suspected ACS is administration of aspirin.[22] Severely hypertensive patients with suspected ACS should be given an IV β-blocker (class IIa recommendation by the AHA).[23] Other commonly recommended agents are nitroglycerin and labetalol. Nitroglycerin is often titrated to resolution of chest pain or hypotension, whichever occurs first. Nitroglycerin has the added effect of coronary vasodilation, which improves cardiac tissue perfusion. No specific recommendations exist on which β-blocker is preferred, but it is best to use a medication with a quick pharmacokinetic profile so that it can be titrated easily. Care should be used with medications such as hydralazine and nitroprusside. Hydralazine causes reflex tachycardia, which increases myocardial work and oxygen consumption. It also has an extremely variable dose response curve from patient to patient, which can cause a precarious situation for EPs when the blood pressure decreases precipitously. Nitroprusside has the potential to cause coronary steal syndrome, which worsens ischemia and could increase risk of death if it is given after acute myocardial infarction (AMI).[24,25] Similarly, β-blockers should not be administered after AMI because of the risk that they could worsen underlying congestive heart failure and cause cardiogenic shock.

Aortic Dissection

When a patient describes the sudden-onset chest pain that radiates to the back, the EP should put aortic dissection (AD) at the top of the differential diagnosis. However, more subtle presentations should not be overlooked. chest pain accompanied by pain in any extremity, neurologic symptoms, abdominal or back pain, or gastrointestinal bleeding should raise concern for AD. The mortality for AD increases 1% to 2% every hour during the first 24 hours after the onset of symptoms. The Stanford classification distinguishes dissections as either type A or type B. Type A involves the aortic arch only; type B involves the descending aorta. Most type B dissections and some type A dissections can be managed with medical therapy but that determination should be made by the vascular surgeon. All type A dissections should be referred to a vascular surgeon for likely surgical repair.

Whenever AD is suspected, it is important to measure the blood pressure in both arms and to assess the pulses in all 4 extremities. It is critical not to rely on classic findings: ~19% of patients with type A dissections and ~9% of those with type B dissections have no identifiable pulse deficits.[26] More reliable is identification of a new diastolic murmur suggestive of aortic regurgitation, which is seen in up to 44% of type A

Table 1
Pharmacologic agents for hypertensive emergencies

Drug	Dose	Onset of Action (min)	Duration of Action	Adverse Effects	Indications
Vasodilators					
Nitroglycerin	5–100 µg/min as IV infusion	2–5	5–30 min	Headache, vomiting, methemoglobinemia; caution in right ventricular infarct	Cardiac ischemia; flash pulmonary edema; caution with recent use of phosphodiesterase inhibitors
Sodium nitroprusside	0.25–10 µg/kg/min as IV infusion	Immediate	1–2 min	Nausea, vomiting, muscle twitching, sweats, thiocyanate and cyanide toxicity	Most hypertensive emergencies; caution with high intracranial pressure or azotemia
Nicardipine hydrochloride	5–15 mg/h IV	5–10	15–30 min, may last several hours	Tachycardia, headache, flushing, local phlebitis	Most hypertensive emergencies; caution of coronary steal with cardiac ischemia
Fenoldopam mesylate	0.1–0.3 µg/kg per min IV fusion	<5	30 min	Tachycardia, headache, nausea, flushing	Best for hypertensive nephropathy emergencies
Enalaprilat	1.25–5 mg every 6 h IV	15–30	6–12 h	Significant reductions in blood pressure in high-renin states	Acute left ventricular failure and flash pulmonary edema; avoid in AMI
Hydralazine hydrochloride	10–20 mg IV 10–40 mg IM	10–20 IV 20–30 IM	1–4 h IV 4–6 h IM	Tachycardia, flushing, headache, vomiting, worsening angina	Eclampsia; caution given erratic response

Drug	Dose			Adverse Effects	Special Indications
Clevidipine	Initial infusion of 1–2 mg/h, titrate every 5–10 min	2–4	5–15 min	Headache, nausea, vomiting, hypotension, rebound hypertension, reflex tachycardia	Postoperative hypertension, hypertensive emergency in renal dysfunction or acute heart failure
Adrenergic Antagonists					
Esmolol hydrochloride	250–500 μg/kg/min IV bolus, then 50–100 μg/kg/min by infusion; repeat bolus after 5 min if needed or increase infusion to 300 μg/min	1–2	10–30 min	Hypotension, nausea, asthma exacerbation, first-degree heart block, heart failure	Aortic dissection, perioperative
Labetalol hydrochloride	20–80 mg IV bolus every 10 min; alternatively, 0.5–2 mg/min IV infusion	5–10	3–6 h	Vomiting, scalp tingling, bronchoconstriction, dizziness, nausea, heart block, orthostatic hypotension	Most hypertensive emergencies except acute heart failure; ideal for preeclampsia
Phentolamine	5-mg to 15-mg IV bolus	1–2	10–30 min	Tachycardia, flushing, headache	Pheochromocytoma and other catecholamine excess states

Abbreviations: AMI, acute myocardial infarction; IM, intramuscular.

Adapted from Chobanian AV, Bakris GL, Black HR, et al. Seventh report of the Joint National Committee on Prevention, Detection, Evaluation, and Treatment of High Blood Pressure. Hypertension 2003;42:1206–52.

dissections.[26] A CXR obtained as part of the work-up might show a widened medias-tinum, but as many as 15% of patients with AD have normal chest radiographs.[27]

The goal of medical therapy for AD is rapid and large reduction of vascular sheer stress and blood pressure. The initial medication should be able to reduce the sheer-ing force; a β-blocker is typically used for this purpose, because this drug group both decreases the heart rate (HR) and prevents reflex tachycardia when arteriodilators are introduced. Esmolol is an ideal agent for this purpose because of its rapid on/off qual-ities and its ability to reduce the HR to less than 60 beats per minute. A medication is also needed to reduce the systolic blood pressure to less than 120 mm Hg. Nitroprus-side has long been used for this purpose and is a reasonable option for fast and reli-able blood pressure control.[27]

Acute Renal Failure

Acute renal failure (ARF) can be either the direct cause or an observed effect of a hy-pertensive emergency. A patient's history, specifically renal transplant and renal func-tion, can help differentiate cause from effect. Assessment of the patient's volume status is also important to determine the need for adjunctive therapies, such as positive-pressure ventilation or diuretics for patients who present with dyspnea from fluid overload. Calcium channel blockers (eg, nicardipine) are typically preferred in ARF because they do not affect renal perfusion or clearance. Nitroprusside and fenol-dopam are also commonly used. Nitroprusside is effective in reducing blood pressure, but it places the patient at risk of cyanide toxicity because it decreases renal clearance and thus causes a buildup of metabolites. Fenoldopam is a more desirable second-line medication. An arterial vasodilator, it not only decreases blood pressure but also promotes renal excretion via its specific effects on the dopamine receptors in the nephron. It produces no toxic metabolites and has been shown to be as effective in blood pressure reduction as nitroprusside.[28,29] In the special case of scleroderma renal crisis, angiotensin-converting enzyme inhibitors (eg, captopril and enalapril) are first-line agents for effect management.[30]

Sympathomimetic Crisis

This category encompasses severe increases in blood pressure secondary to many causes: cocaine, phencyclidine, or amphetamine abuse; pheochromocytoma; interac-tion of monoamine oxidase inhibitor drugs with selective serotonin reuptake inhibitors or with wine and cheese (tyramine reaction); abrupt cessation of sympatholytic medi-cations such as clonidine; and alcohol withdrawal. The treatment of all these crises is similar. The sole use of β-blockers is not recommended because of the reflex tachy-cardia that it induces, which could precipitate a rapid increase in blood pressure and cardiovascular collapse.[31,32] Phenoxybenzamine, phentolamine, nitroprusside, and labetalol are good first-line medications.[33,34] In cocaine-induced crisis, benzodiaze-pines should be used in conjunction with antihypertensive drugs. In a study involving 378 patients with cocaine-induced chest pain, Ibrahim and colleagues[35] found no dif-ference in the troponin levels of patients who received β-blockers and those who did not. This observation challenges convention, which has created a culture of fear around using such drugs in these patients. More studies are needed to validate or challenge these controversial findings. In the treatment of a hypertensive emergency in patients with clonidine withdrawal, the first step is to administer clonidine.

Hypertensive Emergency in Pregnancy

Pregnancy causes many deviations from women's pregravid physiology. Blood pres-sure decreases in the second trimester of pregnancy before increasing back to baseline values in the third trimester. Preeclampsia is a poorly understood disorder of hypertension that occurs for unknown reasons in 2% to 6% of pregnancies after the 20th week of gestation. It can be a serious disorder, with consequences for both mother and fetus. The dramatic increase in maternal blood pressure affects the placenta, which is the end organ that is vital to fetal development. Preeclampsia has mild and severe forms. Mild preeclampsia and severe preeclampsia are essentially distinguished by the degree of hypertension that persists and not the degree of proteinuria because both forms can exist without proteinuria. The treatment of severe preeclampsia is 2-fold: (1) delivering the fetus as soon as possible (ideally after the administration of steroids for fetal lung maturity in viable fetuses), and (2) reducing the blood pressure and reversing end-organ damage. Preeclampsia can also lead to other end-organ dysfunction such as the HELLP (hemolysis, elevated liver enzymes, and low platelet count) syndrome. Failure to achieve rapid control of the blood pressure can lead to the potentially fatal progression to eclampsia, characterized by seizures, strokes, and death.

The approach to blood pressure management in a preeclamptic patient is a balancing act. When the fetus is viable and delivery is not imminent, antihypertensive therapy must be chosen so that precipitous decreases in blood pressure do not cause placental hypoperfusion and compromise fetal blood flow. Labetalol, nifedipine, nicardipine, and hydralazine have been common choices for this condition for years. However, the safety of hydralazine and nifedipine in gravid patients has been questioned. Those medications, particularly hydralazine, should be considered second-line or third-line choices because of their unpredictability in duration of action and degree of hypotension. Labetalol and nicardipine are more predictable.[36] Another hallmark in the treatment of severe preeclampsia and eclampsia is the use of magnesium sulfate, which is given as a bolus followed by an infusion. Patients should be monitored closely for the development of magnesium toxicity. Magnesium is thought to be neuroprotective to the mother, preventing the onset of eclampsia (or terminating seizures once eclampsia has set in), and possibly to the fetus.[37]

SUMMARY

Hypertension is a multifaceted disease process that affects the US and global populations in massive proportions. The most accurate indicator of hypertensive emergency is the presence of end-organ damage. The EP's role is pivotal in rapidly identifying and differentiating hypertensive emergency from hypertensive urgency and providing the appropriate intervention. Actions that are fundamental to identifying individuals at risk include obtaining a targeted history, performing a careful physical examination, and requesting the appropriate laboratory and diagnostic screening. Many medications are available to treat hypertensive emergencies but none is universally recognized as being superior to the others. Important considerations in drug selection include an understanding of the underlying physiology of the crisis, the patient's comorbid conditions, and associated risk factors. Once a drug is chosen, it should be given quickly because "time is tissue" in hypertensive emergency. Patients should be managed in an intensive care unit because critical care monitoring is required. With appropriate identification and management, hypertensive crises can be halted and reversed.

REFERENCES

1. Go AS, Mozaffarian D, Roger VL, et al. Heart disease and stroke statistics—2014 update: a report from the American Heart Association. Circulation 2014;129:e28–292.

2. Lloyd-Jones D, Adams R, Carnethon M, et al. Heart disease and stroke statistics—2009 update: a report from the American Heart Association Statistics Committee and Stroke Statistics Subcommittee. Circulation 2009;119:e21–181.
3. James PA, Oparil S, Carter BL, et al. 2014 evidence-based guideline for the management of high blood pressure in adults: report from the panel members appointed to the eighth Joint National Committee (JNC 8). JAMA 2014;311:507–20.
4. Chobanian AV, Bakris GL, Black HR, et al. Seventh report of the Joint National Committee on Prevention, Detection, Evaluation, and Treatment of High Blood Pressure. Hypertension 2003;42:1206–52.
5. Vaidya CK, Ouellette JR. Hypertensive urgency and emergency. Hosp Physician 2007;43:43–50.
6. Wolf SJ, Lo B, Shih RD, et al. Clinical policy: critical issues in the evaluation and management of adult patients in the emergency department with asymptomatic elevated blood pressure. Ann Emerg Med 2013;62:59–68.
7. Webster J, Petrie JC, Jeffers TA, et al. Accelerated hypertension—patterns of mortality and clinical factors affecting outcome in treated patients. Q J Med 1993;86:485–9.
8. Graves JW. Prevalence of blood pressure cuff sizes in a referral practice of 430 consecutive adult hypertensives. Blood Press Monit 2001;6:17–20.
9. Roque PJ, Wu TS, Barth L, et al. Optic nerve ultrasound for the detection of elevated intracranial pressure in the hypertensive patient. Am J Emerg Med 2012;30:1357–63.
10. Dedic A, ten Kate G, Nieman K, et al. Coronary CT angiography outperforms calcium imaging in the triage of acute coronary syndrome. Int J Cardiol 2013;167:1597–602.
11. Papadopoulos DP, Votteas V. Role of perindopril in the prevention of stroke. Recent Pat Cardiovasc Drug Discov 2006;1:283–9.
12. Lavin P. Management of hypertension in patients with acute stroke. Arch Intern Med 1986;146:66–8.
13. Adams HP Jr, del Zoppo G, Alberts MJ, et al. Guidelines for the early management of adults with ischemic stroke: a guideline from the American Heart Association/American Stroke Association Stroke Council, Clinical Cardiology Council, Cardiovascular Radiology and Intervention Council, and the Atherosclerotic Peripheral Vascular Disease and Quality of Care Outcomes in Research Interdisciplinary Working Groups: the American Academy of Neurology affirms the value of this guideline as an educational tool for neurologists. Stroke 2007;38:1655–711.
14. O'Connell JE, Gray CS. Treatment of post-stroke hypertension: a practical guide. Drugs Aging 1996;8:408–15.
15. Vaughan CJ, Delanty N. Hypertensive emergencies. Lancet 2000;356:411–7.
16. Holzer-Richling N, Holzer M, Kerkner H, et al. Randomized placebo controlled trial of furosemide on subjective perception of dyspnea in patients with pulmonary edema because of hypertensive crisis. Eur J Clin Invest 2011;41:627–34.
17. Aggarwal M, Khan I. Hypertensive crisis: hypertensive emergencies and urgencies. Cardiol Clin 2006;24:135–46.
18. Aronson S, Dyke SM, Stierer KA, et al. The ECLIPSE trials: comparative studies of clevidipine to nitroglycerin, sodium nitroprusside, and nicardipine for acute hypertension treatment in cardiac surgery patients. Anesth Analg 2008;107:1110–21.
19. Pollack CV, Varon J, Garrison NA, et al. Clevidipine, an intravenous dihydropyridine calcium channel blocker, is safe and effective for the treatment of patients with acute severe hypertension. Ann Emerg Med 2009;53:329–38.

20. Cleviprex (clevidipine butyrate) [package insert]. Clayton, NC: Hospira; 2008.
21. Marik P, Rivera R. Hypertensive emergencies: an update. Curr Opin Crit Care 2011;17:569–80.
22. Randomized trial of intravenous streptokinase, oral aspirin, both, or neither among 17187 cases of suspected acute myocardial infarction. Lancet 1988; 2(8607):349–60.
23. O'Gara PT, Kushner FG, Ascheim DD, et al. 2013 ACCF/AHA guideline for the management of ST-elevation myocardial infarction: a report of the American College of Cardiology Foundation/American Heart Association Task Force on Practice Guidelines. J Am Coll Cardiol 2013;61:e78–140.
24. Mann T, Cohn PF, Holman LB, et al. Effect of nitroprusside on regional myocardial blood flow in coronary artery disease: results in 25 patients and comparison with nitroglycerin. Circulation 1978;57:732–8.
25. Cohn JN, Franciosa JA, Francis GS, et al. Effect of short-term infusion of sodium nitroprusside on mortality rate in acute myocardial infarction complicated by left ventricular failure: results of a Veterans Administration cooperative study. N Engl J Med 1982;306:1129–35.
26. Hagan PG, Nienaber CA, Isselbacher EM, et al. International Registry of Acute Aortic Dissection (IRAD): new insights from an old disease. JAMA 2000;283: 897–903.
27. Braverman AC. Acute aortic dissection: clinician update. Circulation 2010;122: 184–8.
28. Elliott WJ, Weber RR, Nelson KS, et al. Renal and hemodynamic effects of intravenous fenoldopam versus nitroprusside in severe hypertension. Circulation 1990;81:970–7.
29. Reisin E, Huth MM, Nguyen BP, et al. Intravenous fenoldopam versus sodium nitroprusside in patients with severe hypertension. Hypertension 1990;15:I59–62.
30. Mouthon L, Bérezné A, Bussone G, et al. Scleroderma renal crisis: a rare but severe complication of systemic sclerosis. Clin Rev Allergy Immunol 2011;40: 84–91.
31. Lange RA, Cigarroa RG, Flores ED, et al. Potentiation of cocaine-induced coronary vasoconstriction by beta-adrenergic blockade. Ann Intern Med 1990;112: 897–903.
32. Pitts WR, Lange RA, Cigarroa JE, et al. Cocaine-induced myocardial ischemia and infarction: pathophysiology, recognition, and management. Prog Cardiovasc Dis 1997;40:65–76.
33. Kitiyakara C, Guzman NJ. Malignant hypertension and hypertensive emergencies. J Am Soc Nephrol 1998;9:133–42.
34. Rhoney D, Peacock W. Intravenous therapy for hypertensive emergencies, part 1. Am J Health Syst Pharm 2009;66:1343–52.
35. Ibrahim M, Maselli D, Hasan R, et al. Safety of β-blockers in the acute management of cocaine-associated chest pain. Am J Emerg Med 2013;31:613–6.
36. Magee LA, Cham C, Waterman EJ, et al. Hydralazine for treatment of severe hypertension in pregnancy: meta-analysis. BMJ 2003;327:955–60.
37. Doyle LW, Crowther CA, Middleton P, et al. Magnesium sulfate for women at risk of preterm birth for neuroprotection of the fetus. Cochrane Database Syst Rev 2009;(1):CD004661.

Congestive Heart Failure

Michael C. Scott, MD[a,b], Michael E. Winters, MD[a,*]

KEYWORDS

- Congestive heart failure • Acute decompensated heart failure
- Noninvasive positive pressure ventilation • Nitrates
- Angiotensin converting enzyme inhibitors • Diuretics • Inotropes

KEY POINTS

- Many patients with acute decompensated heart failure do not have intravascular volume overload.
- The foundation of emergency department management of acute decompensated heart failure is the use of noninvasive positive pressure ventilation and nitrate medications.
- Diuretics should not be used until optimal preload and afterload reduction has been achieved.
- Morphine, nesiritide, β-blockers, and intraaortic balloon pump should not routinely be used in the management of patients with acute heart failure in the emergency department.

INTRODUCTION

Congestive heart failure (CHF) remains the most common reason for hospitalization in the United States for people aged 65 years and older, with more than 1 million patients admitted for this condition each year.[1,2] Despite improvements in diagnosis and treatment, approximately 300,000 deaths each year can be attributed to CHF. Furthermore, the in-hospital mortality rate can be as high as 12% for patients admitted with an acute exacerbation of CHF.[2] Patients with acute decompensated heart failure (ADHF) frequently present to the emergency department (ED) for evaluation; many of

Disclosure: The authors have no relevant financial relationships to disclose.

The article was copyedited by L.J. Kesselring, MS, ELS, the technical writer/editor in the Department of Emergency Medicine at the University of Maryland School of Medicine.

[a] Emergency Medicine/Internal Medicine/Critical Care Program, Department of Emergency Medicine, University of Maryland Medical Center, 110 South Paca Street, 6th Floor, Suite 200, Baltimore, MD 21201, USA; [b] Department of Medicine, University of Maryland Medical Center, 22 South Greene Street, Baltimore, MD 21201, USA

* Corresponding author. Department of Emergency Medicine, University of Maryland Medical Center, 110 South Paca Street, 6th Floor, Suite 200, Baltimore, MD 21201.

E-mail address: mwinters@umem.org

them are critically ill, requiring immediate treatment. In 2007, CHF accounted for 6.3% of ED patients requiring hospital admission.[3] It is imperative that the emergency physician be expert in the rapid assessment and treatment of patients with ADHF. The article focuses on the management of the ED patient with ADHF, with attention to therapies that improve patient symptoms, morbidity, and mortality.

PATHOPHYSIOLOGY

Recent reports have improved our understanding of the pathophysiology of ADHF. Although some patients present with the textbook description of preexisting systolic dysfunction and progressive volume overload, most ED patients with ADHF have preserved systolic function and are not overloaded in terms of total body volume. In fact, most acutely ill ED patients with ADHF harbor processes much more complex than an excess of intravascular volume. These processes can be divided into 2 categories: cardiac failure and vascular failure.[4,5]

Patients with cardiac failure represent the textbook description of ADHF, that is, a patient with chronic heart failure who develops intravascular volume overload through a variety of mechanisms (eg, medication noncompliance, dietary noncompliance, acute kidney injury). Quite simply, their damaged heart cannot tolerate increases in intravascular volume, so edema develops in the lungs and peripheral tissues. In general, symptoms develop gradually in the patient with this type of ADHF.

Patients with vascular failure have an abrupt increase in vasoconstriction and afterload, resulting in acute decompensation. This sharp increase in afterload is believed to occur through neurohumoral pathways involving the sympathetic and renin–angiotensin–aldosterone axes.[4,5] Patients with vascular failure typically present with an acute onset of symptoms, often lack the classic signs of peripheral edema, and generally have preserved cardiac function. In addition, these patients are frequently hypertensive upon ED presentation and can be either euvolemic or hypovolemic.

CLASSIFICATION

The European Society of Cardiology has classified acute heart failure into distinct clinical syndromes (**Box 1**).[6,7] Some patients present with overlapping features, but their appropriate classification is important, because each requires a specific therapeutic approach.

Box 1
Classification of acute heart failure

- Acute decompensated heart failure
- Hypertensive acute heart failure
- Pulmonary edema
- Cardiogenic shock
- Right heart failure
- Acute coronary syndrome complicated by acute heart failure

Adapted from Dickstein K, Cohen-Solal A, Filippatos G, et al. ESC guidelines for the diagnosis and treatment of acute heart failure 2008. Eur J Heart Fail 2008;10:968.

CAUSES

Common precipitants of ADHF are listed in **Box 2**.

SYMPTOMS AND SIGNS

Regardless of the underlying pathophysiology, the most common complaint of ED patients with ADHF is dyspnea. Additional symptoms can include orthopnea, paroxysmal nocturnal dyspnea, decreased exercise tolerance, peripheral edema, weakness, and fatigue. Depending on the classification and cause, patients with ADHF can present with either hypertension or hypotension. Although most patients are tachycardic, bradycardia can be seen in the setting of medication toxicity (eg, β-blocker, digoxin) or high-degree atrioventricular block. Physical examination findings in patients with ADHF include pulmonary edema, peripheral edema, jugular venous distention, hepatomegaly, hepatojugular reflux, and a third heart sound.

DIAGNOSTIC TESTING

The diagnostic evaluation of the patient with suspected ADHF generally includes electrocardiogram, chest radiography (CXR), bedside echocardiogram, and laboratory analysis.

Electrocardiogram

After an evaluation and stabilization of airway, breathing, and circulation, it is crucial that an electrocardiogram be obtained as soon as possible in patients with suspected ADHF to evaluate for signs of acute myocardial ischemia or infarction. For patients with electrocardiographic signs of acute myocardial ischemia or infarction, emergent cardiac catheterization should be performed, because restoring perfusion by percutaneous coronary intervention is the most successful therapy for ADHF in this setting. Additional electrocardiographic findings that might be seen in ADHF include atrial or ventricular hypertrophy, arrhythmias, or conduction abnormalities.

Chest Radiography

A CXR should also be obtained as soon as possible to evaluate for findings consistent with ADHF. Typical CXR findings of ADHF include pulmonary edema, hilar fullness,

---

Box 2
Precipitants of acute decompensated heart failure

- Medication noncompliance[a]
- Dietary noncompliance[a]
- Acute coronary syndrome
- Arrhythmias
- Acute valvular dysfunction
- Hypertensive crisis
- Infection
- Anemia

[a] Most common causes.
Adapted from Kosowsky JM. Congestive heart failure. In: James GA, editor. Emergency medicine: clinical essentials. Philadelphia: Elsevier; 2013. p. 477.

increased vascularization, pleural effusions, and cardiomegaly. **Fig. 1** illustrates classic CXR finding of ADHF.

Echocardiography

As with other critical illnesses, the use of bedside ultrasonography and echocardiography has become a keystone in the diagnosis and management of ADHF in the ED. The portability and rapidity of ultrasound as a diagnostic modality lends itself quite well to this setting. The finding of diffuse b-lines (**Fig. 2**), although not truly specific to ADHF, helps the emergency physician to refine the differential diagnosis in the setting of undifferentiated dyspnea. Furthermore, the ability to evaluate ejection fraction, exclude other causes of dyspnea such as pleural or pericardial effusion, and evaluate for diastolic or valvular dysfunction makes bedside echocardiography an enormously valuable tool in the evaluation of the ED patient with ADHF.

Laboratory Testing

In the patient with suspected ADHF, a complete blood count should be obtained to exclude anemia, along with a basic metabolic panel to evaluate for renal dysfunction. Cardiac biomarkers (eg, troponin I) are commonly obtained and increased in many patients with ADHF.[8] Although increases in troponin might simply reflect the severity of heart failure and not myocardial necrosis, elevated values are associated with increased short-term mortality.[8]

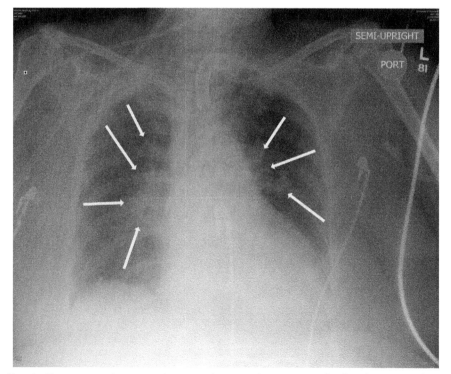

Fig. 1. Chest x-ray demonstrating vascular prominence typical of pulmonary edema (*arrows*).

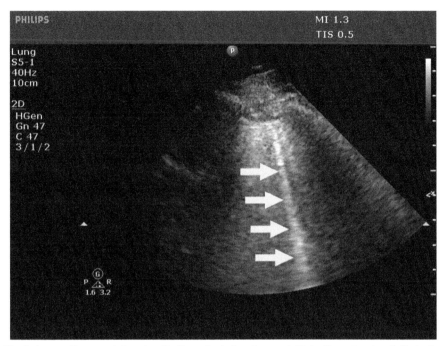

Fig. 2. Lung ultrasound showing finding of a b-line (*arrows*). Note the extension fully to the end of the field. Multiple, diffuse b-lines suggests the presence of fluid in the lung fields, as in pulmonary edema.

A common laboratory test obtained in the patient with ADHF is the measurement of B-type natriuretic peptide (BNP) or the N-terminal proBNP (NT-proBNP).[9] BNP is released from cardiac myocytes in response to volume overload and has been used in the evaluation of ED patients with undifferentiated dyspnea. In general, BNP values of less than 100 pg/mL indicate that ADHF is an unlikely cause of dyspnea, whereas values of greater than 400 pg/mL strongly suggest the presence of ADHF.[9] Although NT-proBNP has a different half-life and different cutoff values for ADHF than BNP, both are degradation products of a common precursor and are clinically interchangeable. Importantly, ADHF is not the only cause of increases in BNP or NT-proBNP. Any condition that increases the stretch of the left or right ventricle (eg, pulmonary embolism) can result in elevated BNP and NT-proBNP levels. In addition, elevated BNP and NT-proBNP levels can also be seen in older patients and those with renal dysfunction. In contrast, obese patients often have lower values of BNP and NT-proBNP. Optimal cutoff values for both BNP and NT-proBNP in these patient populations remain controversial; therefore, values must be interpreted within the clinical context of the patient's history, the clinical presentation, and prior BNP or NT-proBNP values. Regardless of the cause, increases in BNP and NT-proBNP are associated with increased in-hospital mortality and therefore have prognostic importance.[10]

EMERGENCY DEPARTMENT TREATMENT

Patients with ADHF often present to the ED in extremis and require rapid treatment. Similar to other critical conditions, patients with suspected ADHF should be placed on a cardiac monitor and continuous pulse oximetry and should be given supplemental oxygen. Adequate intravenous access should be obtained and blood sent for the laboratory studies previously described. Rapid initiation of noninvasive ventilation and appropriate pharmacologic therapy form the foundation of ED therapy for patients with ADHF.

Noninvasive Positive-Pressure Ventilation

Noninvasive positive-pressure ventilation (NPPV), whether it is continuous positive airway pressure (CPAP) or bilevel positive airway pressure (BiPAP), provides numerous benefits to the patient with ADHF. NPPV reduces afterload by reducing the transmural pressure across the left ventricle.[11] In addition, NPPV increases intrathoracic pressure, thereby reducing venous return and preload. Decreases in both afterload and preload significantly benefit the acutely failing left heart. Through these mechanisms, NPPV reduces the work of breathing and improves oxygenation. A recent Cochrane review found that, compared with standard medical therapy alone, the addition of NPPV resulted in significant reductions in the rates of in-hospital mortality and endotracheal intubation in patients with ADHF.[12] Neither CPAP nor BiPAP has been shown to be superior. A recent metaanalysis found no difference in in-hospital mortality, need for intubation and mechanical ventilation, or rate of acute myocardial infarction between CPAP and BiPAP for patients with ADHF.[13] It is more important to initiate NPPV early in the course of ED treatment than to deliberate over which modality to use. A typical initial setting for CPAP ranges from 5 to 10 mm Hg, whereas initial settings for BiPAP are an inspiratory positive airway pressure of 10 mm Hg and an expiratory positive airway pressure of 5 mm Hg.

Pharmacologic Therapy

The primary objective of pharmacologic therapy in the patient with ADHF is to decrease preload and afterload. Decreases in preload decrease myocardial wall tension and, ultimately, myocardial oxygen demand. Decreases in afterload decrease the myocardial work of the left ventricle, resulting in increased cardiac output and tissue perfusion. Common classes of medications used to treat the ED patient with ADHF are nitrates, angiotensin-converting enzyme (ACE) inhibitors, diuretics, and inotropes.

Nitrates, namely nitroglycerin, are the initial medications of choice for patients with ADHF. At low doses, nitroglycerin reduces preload primarily through its dilatory effects on the venous system. At higher doses, nitroglycerin causes arterial dilation, thereby also reducing afterload.[14] Initially, nitroglycerin can be given via the sublingual route (400 μg every 5 minutes) while adequate intravenous access is being secured. Once that access is established, a nitroglycerin infusion should be started. The infusion often begins at 20 μg/min, depending on institutional guidelines. It is critically important for the emergency physician to titrate the infusion rapidly to clinical improvement.[15] In general, the dose of nitroglycerin can be increased by 40 μg/min every 5 minutes to a maximum of 200 μg/min. Recent studies involving small numbers of patients demonstrated lower intubation rates, without the adverse effect of hypotension, when nitroglycerin infusions were started at doses higher than the traditional 20 μg/min.[16–18] Larger studies are required to validate the safety and efficacy of this approach.

For patients unresponsive to nitroglycerin and for those with severe hypertension, sodium nitroprusside can be considered for additional afterload reduction. Nitroprusside is given intravenously at a starting dose of 0.100 to 0.125 μg/kg per minute. The infusion can be increased by 0.1 μg/kg per minute every 5 minutes until a maximum dose of 400 μg/min is reached. Importantly, nitroprusside is metabolized to cyanide, which can accumulate rapidly in patients with renal dysfunction. In addition, nitroprusside might increase the mortality rate among patients with acute myocardial infarction.[19]

ACE inhibitors are effective at reducing afterload and have been used in the ED treatment of patients with ADHF. Several small studies on ACE inhibitors in patients with ADHF demonstrated improvement in hemodynamic markers.[20,21] In addition, a single-center study demonstrated reduced rates of intubation and intensive care unit admission for patients who received sublingual captopril as a component of their ED treatment.[22] Importantly, current guidelines from the American College of Emergency Physicians include ACE inhibitors in the treatment options for ED patients with ADHF.[23] The most commonly used ACE inhibitors in studies of patients with ADHF are enalaprilat and captopril. Enalaprilat can be given intravenously at a dose of 1.25 mg over 5 minutes, whereas captopril can be administered via intravenous or sublingual routes.

Traditionally, diuretic medications have been considered the mainstay of pharmacologic therapy for patients with ADHF. Because the majority of acutely ill ED patients with ADHF are not volume overloaded, indiscriminate administration of diuretics could be harmful.[5] Adequate renal perfusion is necessary for these medications to be effective. As a result, the role of diuretics in the ED management of patients with ADHF is limited.[19] The administration of a diuretic should not supersede known effective therapies, namely NPPV and nitrates. When a diuretic is deemed appropriate, furosemide is used most commonly. For patients not routinely taking furosemide as an outpatient, an initial dose of 20 to 40 mg can be given. For patients already prescribed furosemide, an initial intravenous dose equivalent to their oral outpatient dose can be given. Studies comparing high- and low-dose diuretic therapy, as well as those comparing intermittent bolus dosing with continuous infusions, have not demonstrated superior outcomes with any dose or method.

Inotropic medications should be considered in patients with ADHF who manifest signs of cardiogenic shock. Bedside echocardiography performed by the emergency physician can be immensely helpful in identifying patients who might benefit from inotropic support. Current guidelines generally recommend initiating inotropic medications after optimizing administration of nitrates and diuretics.[24,25] Dobutamine and milrinone are the most common inotropic medications used in these patients. A dobutamine infusion can be initiated at 2.5 μg/kg per minutes and titrated by 2.5 μg/kg per minute every 10 minutes to a maximum dose of 20 μg/kg per minute. These 2 agents have important differences in mechanism and duration of action. Although dobutamine stimulates adrenergic receptors, resulting in increased contractility and reduced afterload milrinone inhibits phosphodiesterase, the resultant increase in cyclic adenosine monophosphate causes increased contractility and diastolic relaxation, as well as vasodilation and, therefore, decreased afterload. Because it does not rely on sympathetic receptors, it may be preferred in patients on chronic β-blocker therapy. Furthermore, milrinone has more potent vasodilatory effects, making it more attractive than dobutamine in patients with severe pulmonary hypertension. Finally, it is important to note that milrinone's half-life is 2 to 4 hours, whereas dobutamine has a half-life of just 2 minutes.[26] If the patient's blood pressure remains inadequate despite inotropic therapy, a vasopressor medication (ie, norepinephrine, epinephrine) can be initiated. It is important to recall that inotropic medications can have the significant adverse effects of hypotension and tachydysrhythmias. As a result, they should not be used routinely for all patients with ADHF. In fact, several studies suggested an increase in mortality rate when these agents were used liberally.[27,28]

The use of morphine in the treatment of ADHF has long been considered standard care, even though no well-designed, randomized trials have established its efficacy for these purposes. Over the past 10 to 15 years, evidence has been mounting to suggest that morphine is actually not helpful in the treatment of ADHF and very likely could carry significant harm. Sacchetti and colleagues[22] reported an increased rate of mechanical ventilation and admission to the intensive care unit for ADHF patients treated with morphine and Peacock and associates[29] found an increased likelihood of mortality. These studies are based on retrospective reviews and are, therefore, subject to the flaws inherent in such research, but they are far from unique in suggesting that morphine might very well worsen the effects of ADHF.[30] Given these unsettling findings, we recommend against the use of morphine in the management of ED patients with ADHF.

Nesiritide, a recombinant form of BNP with vasodilatory and diuretic properties, received initial positive reviews as well as approval for use by the US Food and Drug Administration, but controversy arose when 2 metaanalyses indicated a significant increase in kidney injury and a trend toward increased mortality among ADHF patients receiving this drug.[31,32] The ASCEND-HF trial failed to demonstrate a reduction in the 30-day mortality rate and the rate of rehospitalization for patients with ADHF receiving nesiritide.[33] The same trial also demonstrated significantly higher rates of hypotension in patients randomized to the nesiritide group compared with patients in the control group. As a result, nesiritide should not be used commonly in the treatment of ED patients with ADHF.

β-Blocker medications are an integral component of the outpatient management of patients with chronic heart failure. In general, these medications are not used in patients with ADHF, because of their negative inotropic effects. For patients who take these medications routinely, it is common to withhold them during an acute exacerbation of chronic heart failure. However, recent guidelines indicate that withholding β-blocker therapy from patients with chronic heart failure is not beneficial and recommend continuing the medication at its previously prescribed doses during an episode of ADHF.[25] The decision to continue β-blocker therapy for ED patients with ADHF is best left to the inpatient team in consultation with the patient's cardiologist.

Mechanical Assistance

Traditionally, placement of an intraaortic balloon pump (IABP) was recommended as a bridge to surgery for patients with refractory cardiogenic shock that is complicating acute myocardial infarction. An IABP inflates during diastole, improving coronary artery perfusion, and deflates during systole, decreasing afterload. The recently completed IABP-SHOCK II trial failed to demonstrate improvement in the 30-day mortality rate for patients randomized to receive an IABP compared with patients in the control group.[34] As a result of that trial, routine placement of an IABP can no longer be recommended.

SUMMARY

Patients with ADHF who come to the ED are usually critically ill and require immediate treatment. In contrast with traditional teaching, many of them are not volume overloaded. The foundation of ED management of patients with ADHF is rapid initiation of NPPV along with aggressive titration of nitrates. For patients who do not respond to escalating doses of nitrates, afterload reduction with an ACE inhibitor can be considered. A diuretic should not be administered before these critical interventions have been completed, but can be given after optimal preload and afterload reduction has been achieved. Short-term inotropic therapy can be considered in select patients with cardiogenic shock and ADHF who fail to respond to standard therapy. Morphine, nesiritide, β-blockers, and placement of an IABP are not recommended for routine use in the ED management of patients with ADHF.

REFERENCES

1. Roger VL. Epidemiology of heart failure. Circ Res 2013;113:646–59.
2. Bui AL, Horwich TB, Fonarow GC. Epidemiology and risk profile of heart failure. Nat Rev Cardiol 2011;8:30–41.
3. Niska R, Bhuiya F, Xu J. National hospital ambulatory medical care survey: 2007 emergency department summary. Natl Health Stat Report 2010;6:1–31.
4. Gheorghiade M, De Luca L, Fonarow GC, et al. Pathophysiologic targets in the early phase of acute heart failure syndromes. Am J Cardiol 2005;19:11G–7G.
5. Cotter G, Felker GM, Adams KF, et al. The pathophysiology of acute heart failure – is it all about fluid accumulation? Am Heart J 2008;155:9–18.
6. Nieminen MS, Bohm M, Cowie MR, et al. Executive summary of the guidelines on the diagnosis and treatment of acute heart failure: the task force on acute heart failure of the European society of cardiology. Eur Heart J 2005;26: 384–416.
7. Dickstein K, Cohen-Solal A, Filippatos G, et al. ESC guidelines for the diagnosis and treatment of acute heart failure 2008: the task force for the diagnosis and treatment of acute and chronic heart failure 2008 of the European society of cardiology. Eur J Heart Fail 2008;10:933–89.
8. Peacock WF, De Marco T, Fonarow GC, et al. Cardiac troponin and outcome in acute heart failure. N Engl J Med 2008;358:2117–26.
9. Maisel A, Mueller C, Adams K Jr, et al. State of the art: using natriuretic peptides levels in clinical practice. Eur J Heart Fail 2008;10:824–39.
10. Fonarow GC, Peacock WF, Phillips CO, et al. Admission B-type natriuretic peptide levels and in-hospital mortality in acute decompensated heart failure. J Am Coll Cardiol 2007;49:1943–50.
11. Bellone A, Barbieri A, Bursi F, et al. Management of acute pulmonary edema in the emergency department. Curr Heart Fail Rep 2006;3:129–35.
12. Vital FM, Ladeira MT, Atallah AN. Non-invasive positive pressure ventilation (CPAP or bilevel NPPV) for cardiogenic pulmonary oedema. Cochrane Database Syst Rev 2013;(5):CD005351.
13. Li H, Hu C, Xia J, et al. A comparison of bilevel and continuous positive airway pressure noninvasive ventilation in acute cardiogenic pulmonary edema. Am J Emerg Med 2013;31:1322–7.
14. Moazemi K, Chana JS, Willard AM, et al. Intravenous vasodilator therapy in congestive heart failure. Drugs Aging 2003;20:485–508.
15. Mattu A, Martinez JP, Kelly BS. Modern management of cardiogenic pulmonary edema. Emerg Med Clin North Am 2005;23:1105–25.
16. Cotter G, Metzkor E, Kaluski E, et al. Randomized trial of high-dose iso-sorbide dinitrate plus low-dose furosemide versus high-dose furosemide plus low-dose isosorbide dinitrate in severe pulmonary oedema. Lancet 1998;351:389–93.
17. Sharon A, Shpirer I, Kaluski E, et al. High-dose intravenous isosorbide-dinitrate is safer and better than Bi-PAP ventilation combined with conventional treatment for severe pulmonary edema. J Am Coll Cardiol 2000;36:832–7.
18. Levy P, Compton S, Welch R, et al. Treatment of severe decompensated heart failure with high-dose intravenous nitroglycerin: a feasibility and outcome analysis. Ann Emerg Med 2007;50:144–52.

19. Mebazaa A, Gheorghiade M, Pina IL, et al. Practical recommendations for prehospital and early in-hospital management of patients presenting with acute heart failure syndromes. Crit Care Med 2008;36:S129–39.
20. Varriale P, David W, Chryssos BE. Hemodynamic response to intravenous enalaprilat in patients with severe congestive heart failure and mitral regurgitation. Clin Cardiol 1993;16:235–8.
21. Podbregar M, Voga G, Horvat M, et al. Bolus versus continuous dose of enalaprilat in congestive heart failure with acute refractory decompensation. Cardiology 1999;91:41–9.
22. Sacchetti A, Ramoska E, Moakes ME, et al. Effect of ED management on ICU use in acute pulmonary edema. Am J Emerg Med 1999;17:571–4.
23. Silvers SM, Howell JM, Kosowsky JM, et al. Clinical policy: critical issues in the evaluation and management of adult patients presenting to the emergency department with acute heart failure syndromes. Ann Emerg Med 2007;49:627–69.
24. Yancy CW, Jessup M, Bozkurt B, et al. 2013 ACCF/AHA guideline for the management of heart failure: a report of the American college of cardiology foundation/American heart association task force on practice guidelines. J Am Coll Cardiol 2013;62:147–239.
25. McMurray JJ, Adamopoulos S, Anker SD, et al. ESC guidelines for the diagnosis and treatment of acute and chronic heart failure 2012: the Task Force for the Diagnosis and Treatment of Acute and Chronic Heart Failure 2012 of the European Society of Cardiology. Developed in collaboration with the heart failure association (HFA) of the ESC. Eur Heart J 2012;33:1787–847.
26. Overgaard CB, Dzavik V. Inotropes and vasopressors: review of physiology and clinical use in cardiovascular disease. Circulation 2008;118:1047–56.
27. Abraham WT, Adams KF, Fonarow GC, et al. In-hospital mortality in patients with acute decompensated heart failure requiring intravenous vasoactive medications: an analysis form the acute decompensated heart failure national registry (ADHERE). J Am Coll Cardiol 2005;46:57–64.
28. Arnold LM, Crouch MA, Carroll NV, et al. Outcomes associated with vasoactive therapy in patients with acute decompensated heart failure. Pharmacotherapy 2006;26:1078–85.
29. Peacock WF, Hollander JE, Diercks DB, et al. Morphine and outcomes in acute decompensated heart failure: an ADHERE analysis. Emerg Med J 2008;25:205–9.
30. Sosnowski MA. Review article: lack of effect of opiates in the treatment of acute cardiogenic pulmonary oedema. Emerg Med Australas 2008;20:384–90.
31. Sackner-Bernstein JD, Kowalski M, Fox M, et al. Short-term risk of death after treatment with nesiritide for decompensated heart failure: a pooled analysis of randomized controlled trials. JAMA 2005;293:1900–5.
32. Sackner-Bernstein JD, Skopicki HA, Aaronson KD. Risk of worsening renal function with nesiritide in patients with acutely decompensated heart failure. Circulation 2005;111:1487–91.
33. O'Connor CM, Starling RC, Hernandez AF, et al. Effect of nesiritide in patients with acute decompensated heart failure. N Engl J Med 2011;365:32–43.
34. Thiele H, Zeymer U, Neumann FJ, et al. Intraaortic balloon support for myocardial infarction with cardiogenic shock. N Engl J Med 2012;367:1287–96.

Cardiotoxicodynamics
Toxicity of Cardiovascular Xenobiotics

Nathan B. Menke, MD, PhD[a],*, Steven J. Walsh, MD[b], Andrew M. King, MD[c]

KEYWORDS

- Cardiac electrophysiology • Antidysrhythmics • β-blockers
- Calcium channel blockers • Cardioactive steroids • β-agonists • Methylxanthines
- Central α_2-agonists

KEY POINTS

- Mechanistic knowledge of the physiological derangements caused by cardiovascular xenobiotics helps with the diagnosis and management of the poisoned patient.
- Management of most drug-induced cardiotoxicity includes close monitoring and aggressive supportive care.
- Treatment of drug-induced dysrhythmias are unique in that they may require the use of uncommon interventions such as serum alkalinization or antidotal therapy.
- Extracorporeal support (eg, intra-arterial balloon pump, cardiac bypass, etc) should be considered in cases of severe toxicity refractory to medical therapy.

BASIC CARDIAC ELECTROPHYSIOLOGY
Ion Channels and the Myocardial Cell Action Potential

Cardiac contractility requires the rhythmic generation of a myocardial action potential conducted through the heart to coordinate myocardial contractions. Molecular studies have identified the major ion channels critical for cardiac conduction. Voltage-gated sodium channels are responsible for initiating myocardial membrane depolarization and rapid electrical impulse transmission throughout the myocardium (via rapidly conducting Purkinje fibers). Potassium channels maintain resting potential and are the main

Disclosures: None.
Funding Sources: None.
Conflict of Interest: None.
[a] Division of Medical Toxicology, Department of Emergency Medicine, University of Pittsburgh Medical Center, 3600 Forbes Avenue, Iroquois Building, Suite 402, Pittsburgh, PA 15213, USA;
[b] Division of Medical Toxicology, Department of Emergency Medicine, Einstein Medical Center, Korman Research Building, Suite B9, 5501 Old York Road, Philadelphia, PA 19141, USA;
[c] Department of Emergency Medicine, Detroit Medical Center, Children's Hospital of Michigan Regional Poison Control Center, Detroit Receiving Hospital, Wayne State University School of Medicine, 4201 St Antoine Street, Suite 3R, Detroit, MI 48201, USA
* Corresponding author.
E-mail address: menkenb@upmc.edu

determinants of repolarization. Transmembrane calcium channel conductivity is critical for appropriate duration of cell membrane depolarization and mechanical activity.

The myocardial action potential is divided into 5 phases: phase 0 (depolarization), phase 1 (overshoot), phase 2 (plateau), phase 3 (repolarization), and phase 4 (resting) (**Figs. 1** and **2**). During phases 0, 1, and 2, the cell cannot be depolarized again by a stimulus of any magnitude—the cell is absolutely refractory. As calcium channels convert from inactivated to resting state during phase 3, a sufficient stimulus may cause another depolarization (the cell is relatively refractory). During phase 4, any appropriate stimulus that reaches threshold may initiate another depolarization.

Cardiac Dysrhythmia Initiation and Propagation

Dysrhythmias refer to any disruption in the usual coordinated conduction and contraction of the heart. A general discussion of cardiac dysrhythmias is a considerable undertaking and is beyond the scope of this article, thus this discussion is limited to xenobiotic-induced dysrhythmias.

Xenobiotics often directly or indirectly cause metabolic derangements that are detrimental to the cardiac conduction system. Abnormalities such as hypotension, tachycardia, bradycardia, acidemia, and electrolyte disorders, whether directly drug induced or not, often exacerbate a xenobiotic's direct cardiac effects. Similar to any other critical illness, the terminal phase of any poisoning may include dysrhythmia and associated cardiovascular (CV) collapse; therefore, correction of these processes is of paramount importance.

Xenobiotics that directly cause dysrhythmia typically affect the cardiac action potential via direct actions on the cell membrane. Cardiac myocyte ion channel characteristics vary (ie, epicardial cells have a shorter action potential duration than does the subendocardium, a phenomenon known as dispersion), allowing the heart to function as a synchronous unit despite the fact that the action potential requires time to propagate through the full thickness of the myocardial wall.

Dysrhythmias are typically related to 3 mechanisms: abnormal spontaneous depolarization (increased automaticity), afterdepolarizations (triggered automaticity), and reentrant rhythms. In the absence of metabolic derangements that predispose to

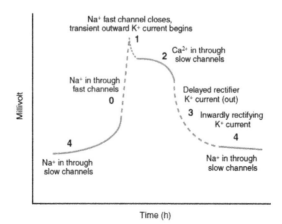

Time (h)

Fig. 1. Ion flow during Purkinje cell action potential. (*From* Shannon MW, Borron SW, Burns MJ, editors. Haddad and Winchester's clinical management of poisoning and drug overdose. Philadelphia: Saunders/Elsevier; 2007; with permission.)

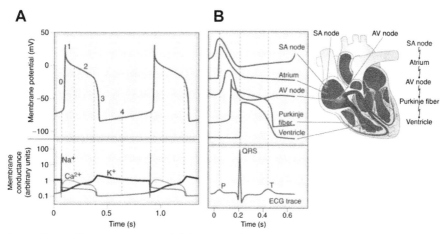

Fig. 2. The cardiac action potential. (*A*) Phases of the action potential: 0, rapid depolarization; 1, partial repolarization; 2, plateau; 3, repolarization; 4, pacemaker depolarization. The lower panel shows the accompanying changes in membrane conductance for Na^+, K^+, and Ca^{2+}. (*B*) Conduction of the impulse through the heart, with the corresponding electrocardiogram (ECG) trace. Note that the longest delay occurs at the atrioventricular (AV) node, where the action potential has a characteristically slow waveform. SA, sinoatrial. (*From* Dale MM, Rang HP, Dale MM. Rang & Dale's pharmacology. Edinburgh (United Kingdom): Churchill Livingstone; 2007; with permission.)

dysrhythmia, most xenobiotic-associated dysrhythmias are likely attributable to reentry[1] (**Fig. 3**).

Under normal circumstances, spontaneous depolarization (phase 4) occurs most rapidly in the heart's normal pacemaker, the sinus node. Increases or decreases in the rate of phase 4 depolarization in the sinus node result in sinus tachycardia or bradycardia, respectively. Xenobiotics may affect the depolarization rates in myocytes that have pacemaker potential, allowing these cells to overtake the sinus node as the primary cardiac pacemaker. These abnormal spontaneous depolarizations are one example of xenobiotic-associated dysrhythmia initiation.

Afterdepolarizations are spontaneous oscillations in the membrane potential because of inward calcium currents (primarily through L-type calcium channels) and occur during phase 3 or 4 (**Fig. 4**). If the magnitude of these variations is large enough, fast sodium channels open and trigger an action potential. Early afterdepolarizations occur during phase 2 plateau or phase 3 repolarization, while variations in membrane potential that occur during phase 4 resting are termed delayed afterdepolarizations.

Early afterdepolarizations commonly take place in situations in which the cardiac action potential is prolonged by potassium rectifying channels (I_{Kr}) blockade and subsequent prolongation of outward potassium flux. Delayed afterdepolarizations occur mostly secondary to increased intracellular calcium concentration (as in the case of cardiac steroid exposure).

Most early and late afterdepolarizations generate an ectopic beat (a premature atrial or ventricular contraction) and are otherwise benign. However, when xenobiotics have altered normal dispersion, these ectopic beats may spread within the myocardium resulting in a dysrhythmia. The mechanism is as follows. (1) An impulse arrives at a region of the heart that is relatively refractory (ie, the cell is in phase 3). (2) The impulse spreads locally and reaches the distal end of the previously refractory region. (3)This

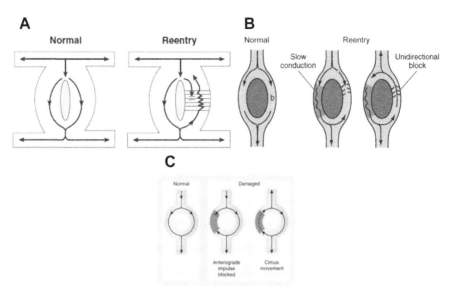

Fig. 3. (*A*) Drug-induced reentry: Schema of Purkinje tissue or ventricular muscle through which impulse transmission occurs. (*Left*) Normal depolarization of a muscle segment. Impulses spread simultaneously down various conduction pathways to depolarize distal areas. Depolarization and repolarization proceed homogeneously. (*Right*) Reentry. The hatched area represents a local area with depressed conduction, which might be produced by a membrane-depressant drug. An impulse traveling in an anterograde direction in an area of depressed conduction is blocked (*dark horizontal lines*); impulses traveling in adjacent pathways, however, can pass through the area of conduction delay in a retrograde manner. If tissue proximal to the depressed area is repolarized already and is now excitable, restimulation (reentry) occurs. (*B*) Normal reentry. Ring model reentry. (*C*) Reentrant rhythm. Generation of a reentrant rhythm by a damaged area of myocardium. (*From* [*A*] Shannon MW, Borron SW, Burns MJ, editors. Haddad and Winchester's clinical management of poisoning and drug overdose. Philadelphia: Saunders/Elsevier; 2007; and [*B*] Vincent JL, Abraham E, Moore FA, et al, editors. Textbook of Critical Care. 6th edition. Philadelphia: Elsevier; 2011; and [*C*] Dale MM, Rang HP, Maureen MD, editors. Rang & Dale's pharmacology. Edinburgh (United Kingdom): Churchill Livingstone; 2007, with permission.)

area then conducts the action potential in a retrograde manner, creating a continuous circuit that depolarizes repeatedly resulting in a malignant dysrhythmia (see **Fig. 4**).

ANTIDYSRHYTHMICS
Introduction

Antidysrhythmics are drugs intended to prevent life-threatening dysrhythmias and maintain sinus rhythm; however, because of their narrow therapeutic index, these agents have been found to promote dysrhythmias and increase mortality in many large studies (CAST [Cardiac Arrhythmia Suppression Trial] I and II[2];). Owing to their potent modulation of cardiac electrical activity, as little as twice the daily therapeutic dose can be lethal.

The Vaughan-Williams classification system categorizes antidysrhythmics by their ion channel interactions (**Box 1**). Class I drugs alter sodium conductance through cardiac fast inward voltage-gated sodium channels and are further divided into subtypes IA, IB, and IC based on each drug's effect on the action potential, conduction, and

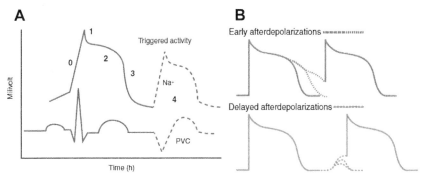

Fig. 4. (*A*) Afterdepolarization. If the inhibition of the Na^+/K^+-ATPase pump leads to Ca^{2+} overload of the cell, sarcoplasmic reticulum is unable to compensate by sequestration and the internal charge begins to increase, leading to delayed afterdepolarization formation. (*B*) Afterdepolarizations (*dotted lines*). Early afterdepolarizations are retardations in repolarization with prolongation in action potential duration (*top*). Delayed afterdepolarizations represent spontaneous depolarizations that occur after repolarization is over (*bottom*). Afterdepolarizations that reach threshold trigger an action potential. (*From [A]* Shannon MW, Borron SW, Burns MJ, editors. Haddad and Winchester's clinical management of poisoning and drug overdose. Philadelphia: Saunders/Elsevier; 2007; and [*B*] Vincent JL, Abraham E, Moore FA, et al, editors. Textbook of critical care. 6th edition. Philadelphia: Elsevier; 2011, with permission.)

refractory period. Class II and IV antidysrhythmics are β-adrenergic and calcium channel antagonists, respectively. Class III antidysrhythmics block potassium channels responsible for action potential duration and repolarization.

Pathophysiology

Class I (sodium channel blockers) are thought to exhibit their antidysrhythmic effect by reducing the number of sodium channels available to participate in impulse conduction and lessening myocardial excitability. With fewer sodium channels available for impulse conduction, the probability of an abnormal impulse being generated decreases. However, excessive sodium channel inhibition can depress physiologic electrical conduction and contractility, and ultimately, cardiac output. Clinically, this can result in a widened QRS interval, bradycardia, ventricular dysrhythmias, sinus arrest, and asystole.

Class III (potassium channel blockers) drugs increase the duration of both the action potential and the refractory period of the myocardium. With more tissue refractory to depolarization, reentrant dysrhythmias are prevented. Thus, class III agents are primarily used to treat ventricular tachydysrhythmias. Potassium channel blockade increases both the absolute and the relative refractory periods, producing QTc prolongation. Dysrhythmogenesis begins with an area of myocardial tissue in a heterogeneously relative refractory state. This area is then exposed to an early afterdepolarization (often termed the R-on-T phenomenon) and results in a characteristic reentrant dysrhythmia known as polymorphic ventricular tachycardia or torsades de pointes (TdP) (**Fig. 5**).

Class III antidysrhythmics are not the only medications that have potassium channel blocking properties; other therapeutic medication classes (antipsychotics, antiemetics, antihistamines, etc.) share this property. Potassium channel blockade and its subsequent risk of TdP and sudden death has resulted in the US Food and Drug

---

Box 1
Vaughan-William antidysrhythmics and primary mechanism of action

1A. Na and K blockade

- Disopyramide, most anticholinergic
- Procainamide
- Quinidine/quinine
- Others (cyclic antidepressants, antihistamines)
- Prolonged QRS and QTc

1B. Na blockade

- Lidocaine
- Phenytoin
- Decreased QT

1C. Na and K blockade

- Encainide
- Flecainide
- Morizicine
- Propafenone
- Prolonged PR, QRS, and QTc

2. β-blockers

3. K blockade

- Amiodarone
- Azimilide
- Bretylium
- Dofetilide
- Dronedarone
- Ibutilide
- Sotalol
- Prolonged PR and QT

4. Calcium channel blockers

Administration assigning such drugs a black box warning or withdrawing them from the market. Prominent examples include astemizole, terfenidine, droperidol, and cisapride.

Clinical Effects

Sodium channel blockers

The key clinical findings that should prompt the emergency department physician to consider sodium channel toxicity are the electrographic changes described earlier (QRS widening, ventricular dysrhythmias, etc). Transient ventricular dysrhythmias may manifest clinically as syncopal events (eg, quinidine syncope). All class I agents may cause significant CV toxicity including atrioventricular (AV) block, bradydysrhythmias, ventricular dysrhythmias, hypotension, and asystole. In addition, sodium channel blockers may also have extracardiac effects, predominantly in nervous tissue. The most common extracardiac manifestations include paresthesias, dizziness, ataxia, tremor, sedation, confusion, seizures, coma, and respiratory arrest. Central nervous system (CNS) toxicity may precede CV toxicity and should warrant immediate evaluation of the CV system.

Sodium channel blockers interact with a myriad of other receptors, causing additional toxicity. Diphenhydramine, disopyramide, and cyclic antidepressants strongly antagonize muscarinic receptors, leading to the usual manifestations of antimuscarinic toxicity (tachycardia, mydriasis, delirium, hyperthermia, anhydrosis, erythema, urinary retention, and ileus). Quinine and quinidine can cause cinchonism, which, in addition to many of the above-mentioned effects, includes the loss of vision, vertigo, and disturbances in hearing from direct retina and inner ear hair cell toxicity.[3] Members of both the IA and IC group block potassium channels, affecting not only the heart but also pancreatic β-islet cells leading to insulin release and hypoglycemia. Finally, many of these agents are associated with immune-related phenomena. Hypersensitivity reactions, symptoms of which include fever, rash, hepatitis, and blood dyscrasias, have been described.[3] Procainamide, quinidine, and tocainide have been associated with drug-induced lupus.[4]

Potassium channel blockers
Therapeutic use or overdose of potassium channel blockers should be anticipated to increase the duration of the QTc intervals, thus placing the patient at risk for TdP. Episodes may resolve spontaneously, causing syncope, or may persist and degenerate to ventricular fibrillation and sudden death. **Table 1** elucidates the toxicity associated with individual potassium channel blockers.

Management
General management includes meticulous attention to airway, breathing, and circulation. All patients with suspected antidysrhythmic toxicity should be placed on a continuous cardiopulmonary monitor, and vital signs should be obtained frequently. An electrocardiogram (ECG) should be obtained as soon as possible. Management of antidysrhythmic toxicity is summarized in **Table 2**.

Sodium bicarbonate should be administered to any patient with evidence of severe sodium channel blockade (defined as QRS duration >120 ms), hypotension, or bradydysrhythmia. Sodium bicarbonate infusion should be titrated to a goal serum pH of 7.5 to 7.55. Potassium should be replaced liberally; sodium bicarbonate therapy causes kaliuresis and hypokalemia, and appropriate serum alkalinization is difficult (if not impossible) to maintain in the setting of hypokalemia. Furthermore, hypokalemia may also contribute to toxicity by increasing the QTc interval. Alkalinization should continue for a minimum of 24 hours. Placement of an arterial catheter is recommended for continuous hemodynamic monitoring and frequent blood draws.

Seizures should be treated aggressively because the resultant acidosis potentiates further cardiotoxicity. Benzodiazepines, propofol, and barbiturates are appropriate anticonvulsants. Other antiepileptic medications are discouraged.

Direct-acting vasopressors should be administered to any hypotensive patient not responsive to crystalloid administration and sodium bicarbonate therapy. Dopamine, especially in the setting of cyclic antidepressant overdose, is discouraged. Although dopamine exhibits direct α-adrenergic agonism at high doses, lower to moderate doses may cause vasodilation and hypotension because of inhibition of its uptake at the nerve terminal by cyclic antidepressants with concomitant stimulation of dopamine receptors.

A

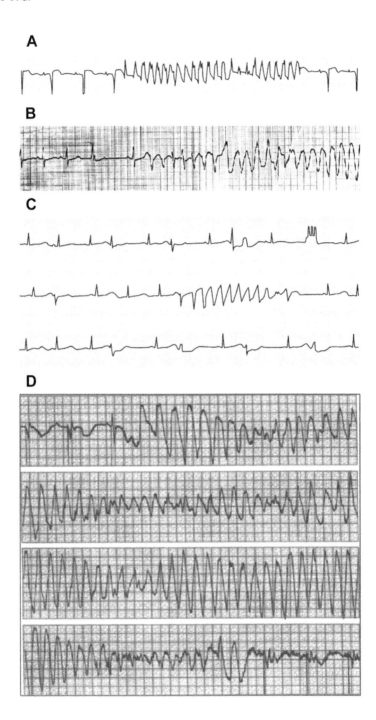

B

C

D

Table 1
Potassium channel blocker toxicity

Agent	Clinical Effects
Amiodarone	Decrease inotropy with IV dosing
	Pulmonary fibrosis
	Skin discoloration
	Corneal deposits
	Peripheral neuropathy
	Thyroid dysfunction
	Hepatitis
Bretylium	Initial sympathomimetic effect followed by hypotension
Dofetilide	TdP
Ibutilide	Available in IV form only
	TdP
	AV block

Abbreviation: IV, intravenous.

Recurrent polymorphic ventricular tachycardia should be treated as per advanced cardiovascular life support (ACLS) protocols, with cardioversion, intravenous magnesium sulfate, electrolyte optimization, and overdrive pacing as indicated.

Administration of intravenous fat emulsion (IFE, trade name Intralipid) therapy should be considered in any patient with local anesthetic toxicity (eg, lidocaine, bupivacaine) having seizures or severe cardiotoxicity (ie, malignant dysrhythmia and/or hypotension). IFE consists of a 30% mixture of multiple types of fats. IFE can also be considered in patients with severe toxicity from other fat-soluble medications; however, the supporting literature consists mainly of case reports and animal models and is associated with complications such as pancreatitis, laboratory interference, and death[5,6] (see **Table 2**).

Fig. 5. (*A*) Tdp. Rhythm strip showing polymorphous ventricular tachycardia occurring abruptly and without warning. This particular arrhythmia often is referred to as TdP, reflecting a twisting of the QRS complexes around the electrocardiographic baseline; it occurs in association with prolongation of the QT interval due to any cause (including idiopathic) and may also be seen in acute ischemic heart disease. In this tracing, the QT interval, measured from other leads, was 0.56 seconds. (*B*) TdP. Rhythm strip of a patient with TdP having chronic procainamide toxicity. Procainamide level was 27.5 µg/mL, and N-acetylprocainamide (NAPA) level was 62.4 µg/mL. (*C*) TdP. The patient is a 64-year-old woman who was given oral quinidine therapy for frequent premature ventricular beats associated with palpitations. These continuous lead II rhythm strips were recorded after the third 200-mg dose and show a markedly prolonged QT interval, frequent multiform ventricular ectopic beats, and a self-terminating burst of polymorphous ventricular tachycardia. The serum level of quinidine obtained after the recording of these tracings was 3.6 mg/mL. Quinidine was withdrawn and oral procainamide substituted without further complications. (*D*) TdP. A patient with a demand ventricular pacemaker developed QT prolongation ($\approx$ 640 ms, seen during paced rhythm) after treatment with amiodarone for recurrent ventricular tachycardia (VT). An episode of TdP developed that spontaneously terminated with resumption of a paced ventricular rhythm. (*From* [*C*] Shannon MW, Borron SW, Burns MJ, editors. Haddad and Winchester's clinical management of poisoning and drug overdose. Philadelphia: Saunders/Elsevier; 2007; and [*D*] Braunwald E, Zipes D, Libby P, editors. Heart disease: a textbook of cardiovascular medicine. 6th edition. Philadelphia: Saunders; 2001. p. 868, with permission.)

Table 2
Treatment recommendations for toxicity due to class I and III antidysrhythmics

Abnormality	Treatment	Treatment Goal
Prolonged QRS (>120 ms)	1- to 2-mEq/kg (2–4 vials) NaHCO$_3$ bolus, followed by a continuous infusion of 150 mEq/L NaHCO$_3$ + 40 mEq KCL at 200 mL/h	QRS <120 ms pH 7.5–7.55
Prolonged QRS (>120 ms) with hypotension despite bicarbonate therapy	Hypertonic saline (3%) 100-mL bolus Lidocaine 1-mg/kg bolus; followed by continuous infusion at 50 μg/kg/min Direct-acting vasopressor (epinephrine)	QRS <120 ms Hemodynamic stability
Prolonged QTc (>500 ms)	Magnesium sulfate 2- to 4-g bolus Optimize electrolytes	Prevent development of TdP Has no effect on QTc
TdP	Magnesium sulfate bolus Overdrive pacing Electrical cardioversion	Resolution of TdP
Refractory hypotension	Intralipid bolus 1.5 mL/kg, followed by continuous infusion at 0.25 mL/kg/min Extracorporeal cardiopulmonary support	Hemodynamic stability
Seizure	Benzodiazepine Barbiturates Propofol	Resolution of seizure

- General management includes meticulous attention to airway, breathing, and circulation. The patient should be placed on a continuous cardiac monitor, and an ECG should be obtained as soon as possible.
- Sodium bicarbonate should be started in any patient with exposure to any medications with sodium channel blocking activity and a QRS greater than 120 ms.
- Blood gases should be obtained every 1 to 2 hours, and bicarbonate infusion should be titrated for a goal pH between 7.5 and 7.55.
- Electrolytes, especially potassium and magnesium, should be replaced aggressively.
- Hypotension should be treated with volume resuscitation and direct-acting vasopressors.
- Seizures should be treated aggressively with benzodiazepines, barbiturates, or propofol.
- IFE therapy should be administered for local anesthetic toxicity or as salvage therapy, although optimal timing is controversial.
- Polymorphic ventricular tachycardia should be treated with cardioversion, magnesium sulfate, or overdrive pacing (mechanical or pharmacologic) as per ACLS protocols.
- Cardiac dysrhythmias that result from antidysrhythmics should not be treated with antidysrhythmics.
- Extracorporeal mechanical support should be strongly considered in any patient with cardiac collapse not responsive to medical therapy.

β-BLOCKERS AND CALCIUM CHANNEL BLOCKERS
Background

β-Adrenergic blockers (BBs) and calcium channel blockers (CCBs) are both widely used and the source of significant morbidity and mortality. In overdose, BBs and

CCBs have similar presentations and similar treatment strategies and are often refractory to standard supportive care. Both BBs and CCBs inhibit calcium entry into cells and, with toxicity, share the common clinical presentation of bradycardia and hypotension[7–9] **(Fig. 6)**.

Pathophysiology

β-blockers

β-Adrenergic receptors (ARs) are G protein receptors with 3 known subtypes. β_1-Receptors primarily regulate myocardial tissue and affect the rate of contraction via impulse conduction. β_2-Receptors regulate smooth muscle tone and influence vascular and bronchiolar relaxation. β_3-Receptors effect lipolysis and may increase cardiac inotropy. Each BB has relative specificity for different β-subreceptors; some agents may antagonize α-receptors (eg, labetalol), whereas others block potassium channels (eg, sotalol). BBs may have mixed agonist and antagonist activity; this agonist property is commonly referred to as intrinsic sympathomimetic activity (eg, pindolol, carteolol, and penbutolol). In overdose, β-receptor antagonists lose selectivity for their usual subreceptors. In addition, BBs may antagonize cardiac sodium channels, producing toxicity similar to class IA sodium channel blockers, potentiating cardiac toxicity in overdose. Finally, an important determinant of adverse effects with BBs is lipid solubility. Highly lipophilic drugs (such as propranolol) cross the blood-brain barrier (BBB) and can result in CNS depression and seizures. In contrast, hydrophilic β-blockers (such as atenolol) have low CNS toxicity **(Table 3)**.

Calcium channel blockers

Voltage-gated calcium channels are found in myocardial cells, smooth muscle cells, and β-islet cells of the pancreas. CCBs prevent the opening of these voltage-gated

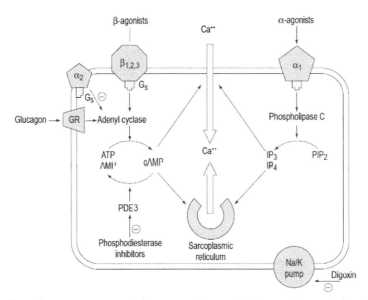

Fig. 6. Schematic representation of the action of inotropic drugs on intracellular calcium in myocytes. cAMP, cyclic AMP; GR, glucagon receptor; G_s, G protein complex; IP_3, inositol triphosphate; PDE3, phosphodiesterase 3; PIP_2, phosphoinositol diphosphate. (*From* Myburgh JA. Inotropes and vasopressors. In: Bersten AD, Soni N, editors. Oh's Intensive Care Manual. 5th edition. Edinburgh (United Kingdom): Butterworth-Heinemann; 2003. p. 13; with permission.)

Table 3
Properties of individual BB

	Receptor Antagonist	Intrinsic Sympathomimetic Activity	Sodium Channel Blockade	Lipophilicity
Atenolol	β_1	No	No	Hydrophilic
Carvedilol	β_1,β_2,α_1	No	Yes	Lipophilic
Esmolol	β_1	No	No	Hydrophilic
Labetalol	β_1,β_2,α_1	β_2	Yes	Lipophilic
Metoprolol	β_1	No	Yes	Lipophilic
Pindolol	β_1,β_2	Yes	Yes	Lipophilic
Propranolol	β_1, β_2	No	Yes	Lipophilic
Sotalol	β_1, β_2	No	No	Hydrophilic

calcium channels and reduce calcium entry into cells during phase 2 of the action potential. Lack of intracellular calcium within the cardiomyocyte reduces inotropy, and calcium channel blockade of vascular smooth muscle results in vasodilation. Differential selectivity exists with respect to cardiac and vascular smooth muscle channels, based on the CCB class (**Table 4**). Dihydropyridines such as amlodipine and nifedipine act predominantly on peripheral vasculature. The nondihydropyridines such as verapamil and diltiazem are not only more cardioselective but also have peripheral vascular activity. Physiologically, this translates to decreased sinoatrial (SA) and AV nodal conduction, myocardial contractility, and peripheral vascular resistance (PVR). Impaired impulse generation can range from sinus bradycardia to complete AV dissociation and sinus node arrest. Decreased PVR reduces afterload and systemic blood pressure. Because dihydropyridine-type CCBs preferentially act in the peripheral vascular system, initial vasodilation with reflex tachycardia may result. Of note, in large overdoses, receptor selectivity is lost and the toxicity of each class is indistinguishable. Finally, voltage-gated calcium channel inhibition of pancreatic β-islet cells results in decreased insulin release.

Clinical Effects

Cardiovascular
Cardiotoxicity characterized by hypotension and bradycardia (sinus pauses/arrest, junctional escape rhythms, idioventricular rhythm, and AV blockade) is common to both BBs and CCBs. Widened QRS due to sodium channel blockade is typically associated with BB toxicity. BBs may have compensatory peripheral vasoconstriction as opposed to vasodilation. Finally, noncardiogenic pulmonary edema is more commonly observed in CCB poisoning.[10–12]

Table 4
CCB classes

Class	Examples
Benzothiazepines	Diltiazem
Dihydropyridine	Pines (amlodipine, felodipine, nicardipine, nifedipine, nimodipine, etc...)
Phenylalkylamines	Verapamil, fendiline, and gallapamil

Central nervous system

Lipophilic BBs (eg, propranolol) are likely to cause CNS depression, whereas hydrophilic BBs (eg, atenolol) generally do not produce the same degree of sedation. Although BB themselves may cause CNS depression, an inadequately perfused brain also manifests clinically with an altered mental status. Other CNS manifestations may include confusion, agitation, and seizures.

Endocrine

CCB toxicity is likely to result in hyperglycemia. In fact, the degree of hyperglycemia correlates with the degree of CCB cardiotoxicity.[13] Conversely, in BB toxicity, hypoglycemia may be observed (especially in children). BB toxicity may also lead to hyperkalemia.

Owing to their common cardiac effects, BBs and CCBs often have similar clinical manifestations, and it may be difficult to determine the causative agent. Peripheral vasoconstriction and cool extremities, hypoglycemia or euglycemia, sodium channel blockade, as well as CNS depression would favor the diagnosis of β-blocker toxicity, whereas peripheral vasodilation, hyperglycemia, noncardiogenic pulmonary edema, and a normal sensorium would suggest CCB toxicity (**Table 5**).

Final common pathway

In patients who are severely poisoned and underresuscitated, tissue hypoperfusion results in lactate-associated acidosis and resultant acidemia. Similarly, CNS effects, including drowsiness, confusion, agitation, and seizures may be observed secondary to CNS hypoperfusion. Acute lung injury, acute renal failure, and gastrointestinal (GI) ischemia may develop secondary to hypoperfusion and portend a grim prognosis.

Management

There is insufficient evidence that GI decontamination improves outcome. Therefore, airway, ventilation, and CV resuscitation take precedence over GI decontamination after overdose. The exception is a patient who is awake, alert, and oriented with normal vital signs. In this setting, potential morbidity and mortality from these CV drugs may warrant decontamination if the clinician has a high index of suspicion that the patient has consumed a life-threatening amount of BB and/or CCBs.

Immediate and reliable intravenous access is critical, and all poisoned patients should be placed on a continuous cardiopulmonary monitor. An ECG should be obtained as early as possible. Placement of a central venous catheter is required in any hypotensive patient in anticipation of treatment with direct vasopressors. An

Table 5		
Clinical characteristics of BB and CCB toxicity		
	CCB	**BB**
Glucose	Hyperglycemia	Normoglycemia or hypoglycemia
Potassium	Normal	Hyperkalemia
Mental status	Normal	AMS
HR	Bradycardia	Bradycardia
BP	Hypotension	Hypotension
Pulmonary edema	Yes	No
Tachycardia	Yes (dihydropyridines)	No
PVR	Decreased	Normal or increased

Abbreviations: AMS, altered mental status; BP, blood pressure; HR, heart rate.

arterial catheter allows for close monitoring of the blood pressure and to obtain frequent blood samples.

For cases of BB poisoning, therapies include judicious use of intravenous crystalloids, calcium, glucagon, direct-acting vasopressors, high-dose insulin, and extracorporeal cardiopulmonary support. In BB poisoning where symptomatic bradycardia and hypotension are present, high-dose glucagon (0.1 mg/kg) is considered the first-line therapy. Glucagon is able to bypass the β-AR and activate adenylate cyclase (see **Fig. 6**). After the initial bolus of glucagon, hemodynamic improvement should occur within 5 minutes. If the bolus improves hemodynamic parameters, a continuous infusion should be initiated. Administration of the bolus dose and waiting more than 5 minutes to obtain another set of vital signs to assess efficacy is a common error. For cases of CCB poisoning in which cardiotoxicity is evident, first-line therapy is a combination of high-dose insulin, judicious use of intravenous crystalloids, calcium, and direct-acting vasopressors.

Unlike other hypotensive patients, most patients with overdose are not volume depleted. Thus, using resuscitation strategies geared toward sepsis may lead to volume overload and pulmonary edema. Pulmonary edema in a patient with a poisoned myocardium presents significant difficulties in management and should be avoided.

Given the mechanism of action of both BB and CCB, there is no maximum dose of epinephrine. The ischemic complications that are seen with high-dose epinephrine in other disease states are only seen in the context of profound hypoperfusion in the context of BB or CCB toxicity. Levine and colleagues published a series of 48 patients who were treated with vasopressors alone (maximum dose of epinephrine was 150 μg/min) with recovery in all but 1 patient.

High-dose insulin with euglycemia was traditionally reserved for refractory cases but has become the first-line therapy in many centers for severe BB and CCB toxicity. In addition to its critical role with respect to its effects on metabolism and glucose homeostasis, insulin also possesses inotropic properties, improving myocardial function in depressed hearts because of ischemic and nonischemic causes.[14,15] However, direct comparison with appropriate vasopressor administration has not been performed in humans.

Extracorporeal cardiopulmonary support of BB- and CCB-poisoned patients is a treatment modality reserved for patients refractory to medical management. Intraaortic balloon pump counterpulsation may be successfully deployed but requires placement by an interventional cardiologist. Severely poisoned patients have also been supported for days using extracorporeal membrane oxygenation and/or cardiopulmonary bypass allowing metabolism and subsequent elimination of the xenobiotic, with associated clinical improvement. Transthoracic or transvenous pacing may be attempted, but it is unlikely to be beneficial in a profoundly poisoned myocardium.

Regardless of the treatment modality, the goal in BB and CCB overdose is to maintain adequate perfusion to vital organs. A reasonable goal and surrogate for adequate endorgan perfusion is to maintain mean arterial pressure (MAP) of 65 mm Hg or more. The previously mentioned therapies should be titrated to maintaining adequate urine output, improvement of metabolic acidosis, and improvement of lactate levels (**Table 6**).

- General management includes meticulous attention to airway, breathing, and circulation. The patient should be placed on a continuous cardiac monitor, and an ECG should be obtained as soon as possible.
- QRS greater than 120 ms should be treated as described in the Sodium Channel Blockers section.
- Treatment is directed to maintain adequate end-organ perfusion with a goal of an MAP greater than 65 mm Hg.

Table 6
Treatment strategies for BB and CCB toxicity

Treatment	Indication	Dose	Comments
Calcium	• Decreased contractility	1 ampule calcium chloride or 3 ampules calcium gluconate	$CaCl_2$ requires central access
Glucagon	• Decreased contractility • Bradycardia	0.1-mg/kg bolus; continuous infusion at 0.1 mg/kg/h	Unlikely to be efficacious in CCB toxicity
Epinephrine	• Decreased contractility • Bradycardia • Decreased peripheral resistance	Initiate infusion at 0.25 μg/kg/min; double rate every 2 min until MAP of 65 mm Hg is obtained	Requires central access
Insulin (HIE)	• Decreased contractility	1-U/kg bolus; continuous infusion of 1 U/kg/h; may increase infusion rate by 1 U/kg/h	• Please consult local poison center for treatment guidelines. • Monitor glucose every 15 min until stable then hourly • May require dextrose infusion to maintain euglycemia • Insulin infusions must be concentrated to prevent volume overload
Extracorporeal cardiopulmonary support	• Intractable hypotension	ECMO Intra-aortic balloon pump	—
IFE	• Intractable hypotension	Intralipid bolus 1.5 mL/kg, followed by continuous infusion at 0.25 mL/kg/min	—
$NaHCO_3$ infusion	• Prolonged QRS (>120 ms)	1- to 2-mEq/kg (2–4 vials) $NaHCO_3$ bolus; followed by a continuous infusion of 150 mEq/l $NaHCO_3$ + 40 mEq KCL at 200 mL/h	Please see section titled Sodium Channel Blockers for details

Abbreviations: ECMO, extracorporeal membrane oxygenation; HIE, high-dose insulin with euglycemia.

- Hypotension due to BB should be treated with intravenous crystalloids, calcium, glucagon, direct-acting vasopressors, and high-dose insulin.
- Hypotension due to CCB should be treated with intravenous crystalloids, calcium, direct-acting vasopressors, and high-dose insulin.
- IFE therapy should be administered as salvage therapy for lipophilic drugs; optimal timing is unknown.
- Extracorporeal cardiopulmonary support should be strongly considered in any patient with cardiac collapse refractory to medical therapy.

CARDIOACTIVE STEROIDS
Introduction

Historically, cardioactive steroids were the cornerstone treatment of heart failure and to control ventricular response rates in atrial tachydysrhythmias. Owing to their narrow therapeutic index, the use of cardioactive steroids has declined, but both chronic and acute toxicity remain problematic today. Cardioactive steroid toxicity is most often encountered in the very young and the aged. Most pediatric acute overdoses are unintentional and result from dosing errors or mistaken ingestion of an adult's medication. Older adults are at particular risk for toxicity as a result of alteration in the absorption, protein binding, elimination of the cardioactive steroid itself, or interactions with other medications. The most commonly prescribed cardioactive steroid in North America is digoxin; other documented sources of cardioactive steroids include a variety of plants and the *Bufo* toad (**Table 7**).

Pathophysiology

Cardioactive steroids are positive inotropes. Cardioactive steroids inhibit active transport of sodium and potassium across the cell membrane during repolarization by binding to and inhibiting the sodium-potassium ATPase ($3Na^+-2K^+$ ATPase). This inhibition decreases sodium efflux, increases cytosolic sodium concentration, and decreases the transmembrane sodium gradient that drives the sodium-calcium antiporter. Thus, intracellular calcium increases, thereby enhancing calcium-induced calcium release from the myocyte's sarcoplasmic reticulum. The end result is an increase in the force of cardiac muscle contraction.[16]

Cardioactive steroids both increase and shorten the repolarization intervals of cardiac muscle. Concomitant rise in vagally mediated parasympathetic tone decreases conduction through the SA and AV nodes. These effects are reflected on the ECG by PR interval prolongation and a decreased ventricular response rate to atrial stimuli. Cardioactive steroids also effect ventricular repolarization via increased intracellular calcium, manifested by QT interval shortening and ST-T wave forces opposite to the direction of the QRS forces (resulting in the characteristic scooped ST segments often termed the digitalis effect).

Hypokalemia (particularly at [K] <2.5 mEq/L) impairs the activity of $3Na^+-2K^+$ ATPase and also enhances myocardial automaticity, thereby increasing the likelihood of dysrhythmia.[17,18]

Clinical manifestations
Overview Cardioactive steroid toxicity may present in a protean manner and depends on a variety of factors. Individual patient factors (such as age, the presence of

Table 7	
Natural sources of cardioactive steroid toxicity	
Digitalis purpurea	Foxglove
Convallaria majalis	Lilly of the valley
Apocynum cannabinum	Dogbane
Urginea maritima	Red squill
Nerium oleander	Oleander
Thevetia peruviana	Yellow oleander
Bufo alvarius	Colorado river toad
Chan Su	Aphrodisiac derived from the dried secretions of *Bufo* toads

comorbid conditions, and renal function), short- versus long-term ingestions, as well as the identity and magnitude of the specific drug ingested all play significant roles in determining clinical manifestations. Acute cardioactive steroid toxicity may result from unintentional, suicidal, homicidal, or recreational exposure to cardioactive steroids. The clinician must bear in mind that the presentation of the patient will vary based on the time of ingestion and dose. Chronic toxicity is often difficult to diagnose, secondary to its insidious onset and nonspecific symptoms.

Cardioactive steroid toxicity may result in nearly any dysrhythmia, with the exception of rapidly conducted supraventricular tachydysrhythmias (because of AV nodal blockade). Dysrhythmias from these substances result from a complex interplay on both the myocardium itself and the conduction system, the latter resulting from direct and autonomic actions of cardioactive steroids.

The most common sign of cardiac toxicity is an ectopic ventricular rhythm.[18] No single dysrhythmia is completely pathognomonic of cardioactive steroid toxicity, whereas bidirectional ventricular tachycardia is nearly so.[19] Cardioactive steroid toxicity should be suspected when there is evidence of increased automaticity combined with impaired SA/AV nodal conduction.

Acute toxicity As outlined earlier, many dysrhythmias are associated with cardioactive steroid toxicity. These rhythms are characterized by a depressed AV node and sensitized myocardium. These types of dysrhythmias are occasionally responsive to atropine.

Acutely, an asymptomatic period of minutes to hours typically follows a single toxic dose of cardioactive steroid. Symptoms usually begin with nausea, emesis, and/or abdominal discomfort. CNS effects of acute toxicity include confusion, somnolence, and weakness that are not associated with hemodynamic changes. The absence of GI symptoms several hours after exposure makes acute cardioactive steroid toxicity unlikely.

Chronic toxicity Bradydysrhythmias appearing later in acute toxicity and in chronic poisoning typically are the result of direct toxin action on cardiac myocytes rather than AV nodal blockade. Thus, these dysrhythmias are often nonresponsive to atropine. Ventricular tachydysrhythmias are more common in chronic than acute toxicity.

Chronic toxicity is nonspecific and may present with weakness, anorexia, abdominal pain, and nausea/emesis. Typically, chronic toxicity results from volume depletion, extrinsic or intrinsic renal insufficiency, electrolyte disturbances, or drug-drug interactions (the most common interactions are enumerated in **Box 2**). Neuropsychiatric symptoms are somewhat more common than in acute toxicity and may encompass confusion, drowsiness, delirium, hallucinations, photophobia, chromatopsia (abnormal color vision, typically described as purple or yellow haloes around lights), and decreased visual acuity.[20,21]

Diagnostics

Cardioactive steroids increase serum potassium concentration by inhibiting the $3Na^+$-$2K^+$ ATPase, resulting in inhibition of potassium uptake by skeletal muscle, the body's largest potassium reservoir; thus, elevated serum potassium concentration may occur in patients with acute cardioactive steroid toxicity.[17] In fact, hyperkalemia is the single most important prognostic criteria in acute ingestion; serum potassium concentration is a better predictor of mortality than initial ECG changes or serum drug concentration.[22,23]

Serum digoxin concentrations are measured as either total or free digoxin. Most laboratories are capable of assaying only total digoxin. Under normal circumstances,

---

Box 2
Digoxin drug-drug interactions and causes of false positive digoxin levels

Digoxin drug-drug Interactions

- angiotensin-converting-enzyme inhibitor (ACEI)
- Amiodarone
- Carvedilol
- Diltiazem
- Quinidine
- Spironolactone
- Verapamil

Medical conditions and drugs associated with false-positive results of digoxin levels

- Pregnancy
- Acromegaly
- Hypothermia
- Impaired renal clearance
- Elevated bilirubin levels
- Spironolactone

---

total digoxin measurement is adequate because serum concentrations correlate with cardiac concentrations.[24] However, after digoxin-specific Fab administration, there is a large elevation in the total digoxin concentration because the cardioactive steroid is drawn out of tissues, inactivated, and trapped in the intravascular space. If measurement of active digoxin is necessary after administering digoxin-specific Fab, a free digoxin concentration must be obtained.

It is critical to consider the timing of ingestion when interpreting digoxin concentrations. Digoxin is absorbed and distributed over several hours, making interpretation of concentrations obtained predistribution fraught with peril.[25] In general, a digoxin concentration should be assessed no sooner than 6 hours after acute ingestion, to allow for distribution. Possible exceptions to this general rule include attempting to demonstrate exposure to a cardioactive steroid in a suicide attempt or possible pediatric poisoning.

Supratherapeutic digoxin concentration cannot be used as the sole indicator of toxicity; a significant overlap in digoxin concentration often exists between patients with and without toxicity. In general, patients with significant digoxin toxicity have postdistribution serum concentrations greater than 2 ng/mL.

Interpretation of serum digoxin levels poses a challenge in the setting of nondigoxin cardioactive steroids. At most centers, digoxin concentrations are the only estimation available for acute measurement of cardioactive steroids. Most assays cross-react, albeit unpredictably, with nondigoxin cardioactive steroids (eg, oleander poisoning); therefore, a positive level may assist a clinician in qualifying exposure to a nondigoxin cardioactive steroid. However, the numerical result cannot be equated to digoxin equivalents.[26–28]

False-positive results may occur in unexposed patients. Endogenous digoxin-like immunoreactive substance which is structurally and functionally similar to exogenous cardioactive steroids,[29] as well as exogenous and endogenous substances that cross-react with the digoxin assay may cause false-positive results (see **Box 2**).

Management

Gastrointestinal decontamination

Initial efforts can be directed toward prevention of further xenobiotic absorption with administration of activated charcoal. Many cardioactive steroids, including digoxin, undergo enterohepatic recirculation. Therefore, late and repeated activated charcoal administration may provide some benefit in reducing systemic levels.[30–33] However, standard caveats to the use of activated charcoal (ie, this therapy is contraindicated in those with active emesis, ileus, bowel obstruction, and altered mental status) apply in these cases.

Fluid and electrolyte therapy

Volume depletion Volume depletion and renal insufficiency are common causes of chronic cardioactive steroid toxicity. Almost 70% of total body digoxin is renally eliminated.[17] In hemodynamically stable patients with mild to moderate chronic toxicity, as-needed volume repletion and correction of volume/electrolyte status is advisable before administration of digoxin-specific F_{ab}.

Calcium is beneficial in most hyperkalemic individuals; however, calcium administration in the setting of cardioactive steroid poisoning has traditionally been contraindicated. A small number of case reports and studies purport a synergistic effect of calcium and cardioactive steroids on the heart resulting in dysrhythmias and the dreaded stone heart (severe hypercontractility rapidly progressing to refractory cardiac standstill, a sort of cardiac tetany). Stone heart is proposed to occur because of inhibition of calcium efflux from myocytes after an increase in the concentration gradient. Although the existence of stone heart is somewhat dubious, calcium administration in the setting of cardioactive-steroid-associated hyperkalemia is best avoided.

Advanced management

Digoxin-specific Fab fragment administration is definitive therapy for those with life-threatening cardioactive steroid toxicity. These fragments cause a rapid decrease in free serum digoxin concentration, increased renal clearance of cardioactive steroids, a decrease in serum potassium concentration, and a clear mortality benefit when properly administered (**Box 3**). Progressive bradydysrhythmia such as second-/third-degree heart block unresponsive to atropine and severe ventricular dysrhythmias in the setting of known or suspected cardiac steroid exposure should be treated with Fab. Any patient with a potassium concentration greater than 5 mEq/L in the setting of acute ingestion should also be treated with Fab.

Dosing of Fab depends on total body digoxin load. There are 2 major ways to estimate the required dose of Fab. The first is to use the serum digoxin concentration (or ingested dose) and use a mathematical formula, and the second is to use an empirical dose based on the average requirements for acute/chronic toxicity in adults (**Table 8**). Digoxin-specific Fab was designed to bind to digoxin and digitoxin, the 2 most commonly prescribed cardioactive steroids. There are structural similarities between all cardioactive steroids, however, and Fab indeed binds to and inactivates a variety of

---

Box 3
Indications for digoxin-specific Fab

- Life-threatening dysrhythmia due to digoxin
- Hemodynamic instability due to digoxin
- Potassium concentration greater than 5 mEq/L in acute toxicity

Table 8
Dosing for digoxin-specific Fab

Empirical dosing for acute toxicity	10 vials
Empirical dosing for chronic toxicity	1 vial
Dose based on serum level	# Vials = concentration (ng/mL) × weight (kg)/100
Dose based on amount ingested	# Vials = amount ingested (mg) × 0.8/0.5 (mg/vial)

nondigoxin compounds. Larger doses may be required in cases that involve other cardioactive steroids. Dosing should follow the empirical dosing guidelines, with initial therapy being 10 to 20 vials.

Lidocaine and phenytoin are second-line drugs that are rarely used for the management of ventricular tachydysrhythmias. These agents may be used as first-line therapies in extreme circumstances, or as Fab is being procured/prepared. The use of these agents counteracts the enhanced ventricular automaticity present in cardioactive steroid toxicity without slowing AV nodal conduction. If used, phenytoin can be infused slowly (50 mg/min) or administered as 100-mg aliquots every 5 minutes until dysrhythmia control is achieved, 1 g has been given in adults (15–20 mg/kg in pediatric patients), or Fab is administered.

Transcutaneous and transvenous cardiac pacing have not demonstrated definitive efficacy in managing dysrhythmias associated with cardioactive steroid toxicity.[23,34] Hemodialysis (HD) and hemoperfusion (HP) are ineffective in eliminating cardioactive steroids secondary to their large volume of distribution and high protein binding.[35]

- General management includes meticulous attention to airway, breathing, and circulation. The patient should be placed on a continuous cardiac monitor, and an ECG should be obtained as soon as possible.
- Any dysrhythmia may be seen in digoxin toxicity with the exception of supraventricular tachycardias.
- Many pharmaceuticals interact with cardioactive steroids.
- Potassium level is the best predictor of mortality in acute overdose.
- Digoxin-specific Fab is indicated for K^+ greater than 5 mEq/L in acute toxicity, life-threatening dysrhythmia, or hemodynamic instability.
- Dosing of digoxin-specific Fab may be empirical, based on the dose ingested or the digoxin level.
- Transcutaneous and transvenous cardiac pacing is unlikely to be efficacious.
- HD and HP are ineffective in eliminating cardioactive steroids.

β-AGONISTS AND METHYLXANTHINES
Background

Four β-receptor subtypes exist, each with a different physiologic effect based on their tissue distribution. Of these, the β_1-receptor is found primarily on myocardium, whereas the β_2-receptor resides on smooth muscle in the bronchioles, uterus, and vasculature. β-Agonists have a wide range of use medically and are used as bronchodilators, tocolytics, and vasopressors. In general, β_2-receptor agonists are phenylethylamine derivatives with β-adrenergic activity. Structural similarities make them selective for specific ARs (**Box 4**).

As their name implies, methylxanthines are derivatives of xanthine with varying patterns of methylated nitrogen groups. The 3 methylxanthines of clinical importance are caffeine, theophylline, and theobromine; they are most commonly found in coffee,

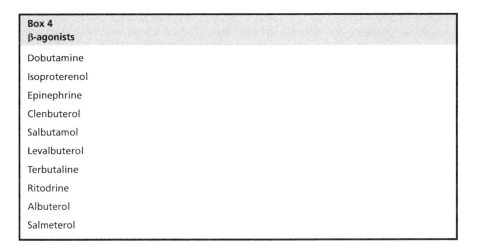

Box 4
β-agonists

Dobutamine

Isoproterenol

Epinephrine

Clenbuterol

Salbutamol

Levalbuterol

Terbutaline

Ritodrine

Albuterol

Salmeterol

tea, chocolate, soft drinks, and guarana. Methylxanthines not only cause the release of catecholamines but also inhibit phosphodiesterase and antagonize adenosine receptors.

Methylxanthines, such as caffeine, are commonly used to increase alertness, improve athletic performance, and promote weight loss.[36,37] Clinically, caffeine is used to treat headaches, as well as neonatal apnea and bradycardia.[38,39] Historically, theophylline or its salt aminophylline was a mainstay of treatment of asthma and chronic obstructive pulmonary disease; however, more-selective and better-tolerated selective β_2-agonists and inhaled corticosteroids have largely supplanted its use in adult respiratory disorders. Theophylline has likewise been used for neonatal apnea and bradycardia.[40] Theobromine toxicity is primarily reported in the veterinary literature.[41]

Pathophysiology

β-ARs are G protein complex (G_s)-linked receptors that activate adenylate cyclase, which leads to various downstream effects. Activation of β_1-receptors, found primarily in cardiac tissue, increases cardiac inotropy and chronotropy with resultant increased myocardial oxygen demand. β_2-Receptors are found throughout the body and have a variety of effects on various organs and tissue including dilation of both coronary and skeletal muscle arteries. The net result of nonspecific β agonism is increased cardiac output with maintained or slightly increased systolic blood pressure and a decrease in diastolic blood pressure. Widened pulse pressure with or without hypotension may occur with excessive stimulation. Physiologically, methylxanthines have similar CV and metabolic effects because of their mechanism of action, namely, by indirectly agonizing β-receptors and inhibiting phosphodiesterases.[42,43]

In addition to their β-agonist properties, methylxanthines are adenosine receptor antagonists. Adenosine receptors are ubiquitous throughout the body and can be conceptualized as the body's feedback inhibitor; they serve to prevent unchecked stimulation. For example, in the CNS, adenosine receptor stimulation suppresses seizures by inhibiting release of excitatory neurotransmitters and thereby terminates excessive neuroexcitation.[44] Similarly, in the heart, adenosine halts cardiac activity while dilating coronary arteries. The net effect of adenosine receptor agonism is decreased oxygen consumption and increased local nutrient delivery.[45] Thus, with inhibition of adenosine, the opposite is expected. Adenosine antagonism results in generalized excitation and decreased blood flow. In the CNS, adenosine antagonism therapeutically increases arousal and attention, and in overdose, it leads to unchecked neuroexcitation and seizure activity. In the heart, methylxanthines can cause a variety of tachydysrhythmias (ie, SVT).

Finally, with their shared mechanism of AR stimulation, both β-agonists and methylxanthines have similar metabolic and endocrinologic effects. Both of these cause hypokalemia, hypomagnesemia, hypophosphatemia, hyperglycemia, metabolic acidosis, elevated lactate levels, hyperthermia, and leukocytosis.[46–48]

Clinical Manifestations

Cardiovascular

Cardiac toxicity and hemodynamic perturbations are major components of β-agonist and methylxanthine toxicity (**Table 9**). Tachydysrhythmias are common with methylxanthines and β-agonist toxicity. Sinus tachycardia and Premature ventricular contraction are the most common dysrhythmias.[49] Dysrhythmias associated with β₂-agonists, although reported, are usually supraventricular in origin and infrequently lead to significant outcomes, whereas methylxanthines are more likely to cause malignant dysrhythmias.[50–54] Vasodilatation induced by β₂-receptor agonism also contributes to tachycardia and manifests in widened pulse pressures, bounding pulses, and overt hypotension.

Myocardial ischemia, infarction, and necrosis have been reported with methylxanthine and β₂-agonist use, misuse, and abuse.[55,56] Methylxanthines increase cardiac oxygen demand while simultaneously impairing coronary artery vasodilation, leading to demand ischemia.[57] Moreover, β₂-agonists (such as clenbuterol) may be directly myotoxic, inducing apoptosis and necrosis.[58] Indeed, elevated troponin

Table 9		
Comparison of toxicities of beta agonists and methylxanthines		
	β-Agonists	**Methylxanthines**
CV	Tachydysrhythmias	Tachydysrhythmias
	Widened pulse pressure	Widened pulse pressure
	Hypotension	Hypotension
	Myocardial necrosis (clenbuterol)	Myocardial ischemia/infarction
	Myocardial ischemia/infarction	
Neurologic	Anxiety	Seizures (can be difficult to control)
	Tremor	Altered mental status
		Anxiety
Gastrointestinal	Nausea and vomiting	Nausea and vomiting
		Emesis may be difficult to control
Electrolytes	Hypokalemia	Hypokalemia
	Hyperglycemia	Hyperglycemia
	Hypophosphatemia	Hypophosphatemia
	Hypomagnesemia	Hypomagnesemia
	Metabolic acidosis	Metabolic acidosis
Neuromuscular	Tremor	Tremor
	Myoclonus	Myoclonus
	Hypertonicity	Hypertonicity
	Fasciculations	Fasciculations
	Rhabdomyolysis	Rhabdomyolysis
	Compartment syndrome	Compartment syndrome

concentrations have been documented in cases of both therapeutic administration of β_2-adrenergic agents as well as overdose.[55,59,60]

Central nervous system
Methylxanthines can lead to notoriously difficult-to-control seizures.[61–63] Patients may present with a single seizure, with multiple seizures, or in status epilepticus leading to further metabolic derangements including profound metabolic acidosis, elevated lactate concentration, rhabdomyolysis, hypoxia, and hypercapnea.[64] Selective β_2-agonists on the other hand, do not cross the BBB and have no direct effect on the CNS.

Gastrointestinal
Methylxanthines can cause severe and refractory vomiting in overdose.[65,66] β_2-Agonists can likewise cause nausea and vomiting; however, the GI distress caused by these agents is typically less severe than that associated with methylxanthines.

Metabolic
Metabolic derangements seen with β-agonist and methylxanthine toxicity are a consequence of both primary and secondary effects. For example, methylxanthines directly cause hypokalemia via β_2-agonism; additionally, they also cause severe emesis leading to contraction alkalosis and kaliuresis. Severe hypokalemia may worsen acidemia and cause muscle weakness and respiratory insufficiency. Metabolic acidosis can be observed in both methylxanthines and β_2-agonist toxicity and can occur without hypoxia, shock, or seizures.[46,67–69] Increased muscular activity, seizures, and increased basal metabolic rate may result in hyperthermia, rhabdomyolysis, and renal failure.[70,71] Hyperglycemia and leukocytosis are also common but rarely of consequence.

Management
As with all poisonings, management should be tailored to the individual. Consultation with a regional poison center for assistance is advised considering the potentially life-threatening toxicity from these agents. Immediate and reliable intravenous access is critical, and all poisoned patients should be placed on a continuous cardiopulmonary monitor. Core temperature should be assessed and aggressive cooling should be initiated when appropriate. An ECG should be obtained as early as possible.

Primary treatment of methylxanthine-induced tachydysrhythmias and hypotension centers on benzodiazepine and fluid administration. In the setting of refractory hypotension, direct-acting vasopressors should be used. Although counterintuitive in the setting of hypotension, administration of a β-blocker may counteract the β_2-mediated vasodilation and significantly improve hemodynamic parameters.[72,73] Esmolol has the advantage of a short half-life and can be easily titrated. The potential for CV collapse is a potential concern when initiating BB therapy in unstable patients, but has not been reported. Intravenous CCBs have been used and found to be effective in animal models of theophylline toxicity.[74] However, these medications may promote further vasodilation and hypotension. The judicious use of intravenous crystalloids is appropriate to increase preload in the face of profound vasodilation.

Although considered a first-line agent for supraventricular tachycardias, adenosine and electrical cardioversion are likely to be ineffective in the treatment of methylxanthine-associated SVT. Methylxanthines are adenosine antagonists and remain in the circulation for hours, whereas intravenous adenosine has an extremely short duration of action. Electrical cardioversion is effective in resetting focally abnormal areas of depolarization but is not effective in correcting global aberrant electrical activity because of drug effect.

Treatment of neuroexcitation is of critical importance in the setting of methylxanthine toxicity. High-dose benzodiazepines and barbiturates may be necessary but may further exacerbate hypotension. Repetitive and escalating dosing should be used until seizures terminate. Propofol administration can be considered after the airway has been secured. If the patient is intubated and sedated with propofol, continuous electroencephalography should be considered. As with most other toxin-induced seizures, other antiepileptics have no role in methylxanthine poisoning.[75–77]

Electrolyte abnormalities such as mild hypokalemia may be well tolerated; however, any evidence of ECG changes or severe hypokalemia should be treated given the increased predisposition for cardiac dysrhythmias. Because potassium has been shifted intracellularly, administration of β-antagonists may be sufficient. Furthermore, aggressive replacement of potassium may lead to hyperkalemia as the drug effect abates.

Traditional dosing of antiemetic medications may be insufficient to control the emesis associated with methylxanthine toxicity, and higher dosing of these medications may be necessary (ondansetron and metoclopramide). Phenothiazines should be used with caution, because the QTc prolongation caused by hypokalemia and hypomagnesemia may be further exacerbated by potassium channel blockade. In addition, these drugs may act synergistically with methylxanthines to lower the seizure threshold.[78]

The potential for refractory emesis and seizure activity often precludes administration of activated charcoal despite evidence that multidose activated charcoal (MDAC), often called gut dialysis, significantly reduces the half-life of theophylline.[79–81] If the patient is intubated or is able to tolerate repeat dosing, MDAC administration can be considered, particularly if the patient is located at a center that cannot perform HD. The benefit of whole bowel irrigation (WBI) is controversial in the treatment of sustained-release preparations of theophylline.

Enhanced elimination with HP or HD is recommended in patients with severe methylxanthine toxicity.[82–84] Caffeine, theophylline, and theobromine are all amenable to extracorporeal removal. The recommended indications for HD are highlighted in **Box 5**.[85] HP may not be available in all institutions, and high-flux HD may be equally efficacious. Seizure, dysrhythmia, and hypotension identify the subset of patients that have the greatest need for extracorporeal removal and should not be considered contraindications to HD. Infants with severe toxicity who are unable to tolerate HD may respond to exchange transfusion and MDAC.[83,86,87]

- General management includes meticulous attention to airway, breathing, and circulation. The patient should be placed on a continuous cardiac monitor, and an ECG should be obtained as soon as possible.
- Hyperthermic patients should be aggressively cooled.

Box 5
Suggested indications for charcoal HP or HD in methylxanthine toxicity

Any symptomatic patient with a serum theophylline or caffeine concentration >90 ug/mL

Serum theophylline or caffeine concentration greater than 40 μg/mL and any 1 of the following:

Seizures

Hypotension unresponsive to fluids

Ventricular dysrhythmias

Emesis unresponsive to medications

- Hypotension should be treated with fluid resuscitation and direct-acting vasopressors with phenylephrine as the preferred agent.
- Esmolol may significantly improve hemodynamic parameters.
- Seizures should be aggressively treated with benzodiazepines, barbiturates, propofol, or ketamine.
- Vomiting may be refractory and may require high doses of antiemetics for control.
- MDAC should be strongly considered to decrease the duration of toxicity if conditions are appropriate.
- Extracorporeal removal with HD, HP, or exchange transfusion may be required in patients with severe toxicity.

CENTRAL α_2-AGONISTS
Introduction

α_2-Adrenergic agonists and imidazolines are a class of commonly prescribed medications (**Box 6**) that have a variety of medical and nonmedical uses (**Box 7**). Imidazolines are commonly used over-the-counter vasoconstrictors; these agents may cross the BBB and stimulate both CNS α_2-AR and imidazoline receptors (IRs). Simulation of these receptors results in decreased sympathetic outflow, decreased vasomotor tone, sedation, and decreased heart rate. α_2-Adrenergic agents have a narrow therapeutic index and are often included in the one-pill-can-kill list of pediatric poisons.[88] Toxic manifestations include CNS depression, bradycardia, hypotension, respiratory depression, miosis, hyporeflexia, and hypothermia.

Pathophysiology

α_2-ARs are located both presynaptically and postsynaptically in the CNS and in peripheral vasculature. At present, 3 subtypes of α_2-AR and 3 classes of IR exist. α_2-

---

Box 6
Commonly encountered α_2-agonists and imidazolines

Clonidine (Catapres, Kapvay, Nexiclon, Duraclon)

Tizanidine (Zanaflex, Sirdalud)

Brimonidine (Alphagan)

Apraclonidine (Iopidine)

Xylazine (veterinary use)

Guanfacine (Tenex, Intuniv)

Guanabenz (Wytensin)

Methyldopa (Aldomet, Aldoril, Dopamet, Dopegyt)

Tetrahydrozoline (OptiClear, Tyzine)

Dexmedetomidine (Precedex)

Oxymetazoline (Afrin, Dristan, Navisln, Logicin, Zicam, Vicks Sinex, SinuFrin, Visine, Operil, Sudafed OM, Dimetapp, Mucinex Full Force, Oxyspray)

Naphazoline (Clear Eyes, Allersol, Nafazair, VasoClear, Estivin II, redness relief eye drops, Allerest Eye Drops, Ocu-Zoline, Vasocon, Nazal, Albalon, Privine, Naphcon, Degest 2, AK-Con)

Lofexidine (BritLofex)

Xylometazoline (Triaminic, Otrivin)

Box 7
Medical and nonmedical applications of imidazolines and α_2-adrenergic agonists*

Psychiatry

Attention-deficit/hyperactivity disorder

Pervasive developmental disorder

Autism

Tourette syndrome

Tic disorder

Neuropathic pain disorder

Mania

Anxiety

Posttraumatic stress disorder

Rage reactions

Opioid withdrawal

Smoking cessation

Ophthalmology

Glaucoma

Eye irritation

Otolaryngology

Nasal congestion

Epistaxis

Neurology

Migraine headache

Restless leg syndrome

Neuropathic pain disorder

Motor spasticity

Sedation

Anesthesia

Sedation

Pain control

CV

Hypertension

Others

Dysmenorrhea

Drug-facilitated sexual assault

* may not be indications approved by the US Food and Drug Administration.

ARs are found throughout the brain including the locus coeruleus, medulla, and the prefrontal cortex. IRs are located in the brainstem. The I_1 receptor is responsible for vasomotor modulation in the periphery by the CNS. The α_2-ARs are thought to be more responsible for the sedating side effects. Stimulation and interaction of both

α_2-ARs and IRs in the rostral ventrolateral medulla are likely necessary for the brady-cardia and hypotension seen clinically.[89] Stimulation of presynaptic α_2-AR and IR in the CNS inhibits the release of various neurotransmitters, including norepinephrine, epinephrine, dopamine, serotonin, and γ-aminobutyric acid. Thus, central α_2- and IR agonism decreases sympathetic outflow; this effect is termed sympatholysis and leads to CNS depression, bradycardia, hypothermia, and vasodilation.

Clinical Manifestations

Clinically, α_2-agonists cause lethargy, miosis, bradycardia, respiratory depression, hy-pothermia, and hypotension. This presentation may be indistinguishable from that of opioid intoxication, and naloxone is often given in undifferentiated patients. Because both α_2-agonists and imidazolines are readily absorbed through the GI tract and are able to cross the BBB, clinical effects are often seen within 15 minutes of ingestion; toxicity usually resolves within 24 to 48 hours.[90–92]

Respiratory depression and sedation may be significant enough to require intuba-tion. Interestingly, and in contrast to toxicity from opioids, those poisoned by α_2-agonists frequently respond to stimulation alone. Premature extubation can occur as the constant noxious stimulation of the tracheal tube causes enough arousal and agitation that clinicians liberate the patient from mechanical ventilation. However, once the noxious stimulus is removed, the patient may require reintubation secondary to recurrence of hypoventilation.

Although hypotension is often the ultimate result of toxicity, initial hypertension is re-ported.[93–95] This elevation in blood pressure, thought to be due to peripheral α_1- and α_2-AR agonism, is usually transient, asymptomatic, and does not require treatment. The degree of hypertension is correlated with the significance of the exposure, and higher serum concentrations better correlate with development of hypertension.[96,97] Thus although most cases of elevated blood pressures seen are asymptomatic, massive overdoses with resultant severe-range blood pressures can lead to end-organ manifestations including myocardial infarction, subarachnoid hemorrhage, altered mental status, and seizures.[94,98,99] With respect to heart rate, sinus brady-cardia is the most common bradydysrhythmia.[100,101] Tachycardia should not be ex-pected and suggests a coingestion or an alternate diagnosis.

Special considerations

Brimonidine and apraclonidine are α_2-agonist topical ophthalmic medications used to decrease intraocular pressure. Despite favorable pharmacologic characteristics when compared with clonidine, therapeutic use in children for congenital glaucoma has resulted in many cases of toxicity. Accidental ingestion has likewise led to toxicity.[102–104]

Management

Given the often-similar presentation of α_2-agonists and opioid toxicity, naloxone is often empirically used with varying results.[105–108] Although administration of empirical naloxone to anyone presenting with somnolence, miosis, and life-threatening respira-tory depression should be encouraged, adequate response should not be assumed and the emergency physician should be prepared to secure the airway. Furthermore, although stimulation alone may satisfactorily restore the respiratory drive temporarily, intubation may still be necessary if the patient becomes apneic when stimulation is ceased.[97]

If the patient does respond to naloxone, repeat dosing and an infusion may be required given naloxone's relatively short half-life when compared with that of the offending agents.[107] Patient response is unpredictable as the cause of naloxone response is likely multifactorial. Mitigating factors include age, baseline sympathetic tone, baseline concentration of endogenous opioids, and individual differences in receptors.[97]

As discussed previously, initial hypertension is often asymptomatic with the exception of massive exposures and does not require treatment. If treatment is required, the use of long-acting antihypertensive agents is contraindicated because of the transitory nature of the hypertension. Given the accompanying bradycardia, agents with significant nodal blocking characteristics (eg, verapamil, esmolol) should be avoided in favor of direct vasodilators such as nitrates. During the hypertensive phase, no attempt should be made to treat sinus bradycardia with atropine.

In terms of hypotension, reasonable amounts of intravenous crystalloid should be administered, with consideration lent to volume status and comorbid conditions such as heart failure. If the patient is refractory to multiple boluses or the patient's volume status or cardiac physiology cannot tolerate fluid therapy, dopamine should be initiated. Dopamine does not require central venous administration and is less deleterious than direct-acting vasopressors in the case of extravasation. High doses and the use of multiple vasopressors are generally not required. If this should occur, the clinician should consider other causes or the possibility of coingestants causing hypotension.

WBI is reasonable in the case of symptomatic clonidine patch ingestion, and it has been successfully used in case reports and has little associated morbidity.[109] The usual contraindications of obstruction, ileus, hemorrhage, and perforation apply.

- General management includes meticulous attention to airway, breathing, and circulation. The patient should be placed on a continuous cardiac monitor, and an ECG should be obtained as soon as possible.
- Typical presentation is sedation, miosis, respiratory depression, hypotension, and bradycardia.
- Hypertension may be seen initially and should only be treated with short-acting agents if end-organ damage is suspected.
- Naloxone may reverse respiratory depression.
- Fluid resuscitation and atropine are first-line treatments for symptomatic bradycardia.
- Dopamine is the preferred vasopressor because of its safety profile.

ACKNOWLEDGMENTS

Our thanks to Anthony Pizon for coining the term cardiotoxicodynamics.

REFERENCES

1. Roden DM, Balser JR, George AL Jr, et al. Cardiac ion channels. Annu Rev Physiol 2002;64:431–75.
2. Lafuente-Lafuente C, Longas-Tejero MA, Bergmann JF, et al. Antiarrhythmics for maintaining sinus rhythm after cardioversion of atrial fibrillation. Cochrane Database Syst Rev 2012;(5):CD005049.
3. Kim SY, Benowitz NL. Poisoning due to class IA antiarrhythmic drugs. Quinidine, procainamide and disopyramide. Drug Saf 1990;5(6):393–420.
4. Oliphant LD, Goddard M. Tocainide-associated neutropenia and lupus-like syndrome. Chest 1988;94(2):427–8.

5. Cole JB, Stellpflug SJ, Engebretsen KM. Asystole immediately following intravenous fat emulsion for overdose. J Med Toxicol 2014;10(3):307–10.
6. Levine M, Skolnik AB, Ruha AM, et al. Complications following antidotal use of intravenous lipid emulsion therapy. J Med Toxicol 2014;10(1):10–4.
7. Nelson L, Goldfrank LR. Goldfrank's toxicologic emergencies. Chapters 60 & 61. 9th edition. New York: McGraw-Hill Medical; 2011. xxviii, 1940.
8. Kerns W 2nd. Management of beta-adrenergic blocker and calcium channel antagonist toxicity. Emerg Med Clin North Am 2007;25(2):309–31 [abstract: viii].
9. Jang DH, Spyres MB, Fox L, et al. Toxin-induced cardiovascular failure. Emerg Med Clin North Am 2014;32(1):79–102.
10. Brass BJ, Winchester-Penny S, Lipper BL. Massive verapamil overdose complicated by noncardiogenic pulmonary edema. Am J Emerg Med 1996;14(5): 459–61.
11. Sami Karti S, Ulusoy H, Yandi M, et al. Non-cardiogenic pulmonary oedema in the course of verapamil intoxication. Emerg Med J 2002;19(5):458–9.
12. Siddiqi TA, Hill J, Huckleberry Y, et al. Non-cardiogenic pulmonary edema and life-threatening shock due to calcium channel blocker overdose: a case report and clinical review. Respir Care 2014;59(2):e15–21.
13. Levine M, Curry SC, Padilla-Jones A, et al. Critical care management of verapamil and diltiazem overdose with a focus on vasopressors: a 25-year experience at a single center. Ann Emerg Med 2013;62(3):252–8.
14. Kline JA, Raymond RM, Leonova ED, et al. Insulin improves heart function and metabolism during non-ischemic cardiogenic shock in awake canines. Cardiovasc Res 1997;34(2):289–98.
15. Kline JA, Tomaszewski CA, Schroeder JD, et al. Insulin is a superior antidote for cardiovascular toxicity induced by verapamil in the anesthetized canine. J Pharmacol Exp Ther 1993;267(2):744–50.
16. McGarry SJ, Williams AJ. Digoxin activates sarcoplasmic reticulum Ca(2+)-release channels: a possible role in cardiac inotropy. Br J Pharmacol 1993; 108(4):1043–50.
17. Kelly RA, Smith TW. Recognition and management of digitalis toxicity. Am J Cardiol 1992;69(18):108G–18G [discussion: 118G–9G].
18. Rosen MR, Wit AL, Hoffman BF. Electrophysiology and pharmacology of cardiac arrhythmias. IV. Cardiac antiarrhythmic and toxic effects of digitalis. Am Heart J 1975;89(3):391–9.
19. Smith SW, Shah RR, Hunt JL, et al. Bidirectional ventricular tachycardia resulting from herbal aconite poisoning. Ann Emerg Med 2005;45(1):100–1.
20. Cooke DM. The use of central nervous system manifestations in the early detection of digitalis toxicity. Heart Lung 1993;22(6):477–81.
21. Gorelick DA, Kussin SZ, Kahn I. Paranoid delusions and auditory hallucinations associated with digoxin intoxication. J Nerv Ment Dis 1978;166(11):817–9.
22. Bismuth C, Gaultier M, Conso F, et al. Hyperkalemia in acute digitalis poisoning: prognostic significance and therapeutic implications. Clin Toxicol 1973;6(2): 153–62.
23. Bismuth C, Motte G, Conso F, et al. Acute digitoxin intoxication treated by intracardiac pacemaker: experience in sixty-eight patients. Clin Toxicol 1977;10(4): 443–56.
24. Doherty JE, Perkins WH, Flanigan WJ. The distribution and concentration of tritiated digoxin in human tissues. Ann Intern Med 1967;66(1):116–24.
25. Selzer A. Role of serum digoxin assay in patient management. J Am Coll Cardiol 1985;5(5 Suppl A):106A–10A.

26. Cheung K, Hinds JA, Duffy P. Detection of poisoning by plant-origin cardiac glycoside with the Abbott TDx analyzer. Clin Chem 1989;35(2):295–7.
27. Cheung K, Urech R, Taylor L, et al. Plant cardiac glycosides and digoxin Fab antibody. J Paediatr Child Health 1991;27(5):312–3.
28. Radford DJ, Cheung K, Urech R, et al. Immunological detection of cardiac glycosides in plants. Aust Vet J 1994;71(8):236–8.
29. Haddy FJ. Endogenous digitalis-like factor or factors. N Engl J Med 1987; 316(10):621–3.
30. de Silva HA, Fonseka MM, Pathmeswaran A, et al. Multiple-dose activated charcoal for treatment of yellow oleander poisoning: a single-blind, randomised, placebo-controlled trial. Lancet 2003;361(9373):1935–8.
31. Lalonde RL, Deshpande R, Hamilton PP, et al. Acceleration of digoxin clearance by activated charcoal. Clin Pharmacol Ther 1985;37(4):367–71.
32. Levy G. Gastrointestinal clearance of drugs with activated charcoal. N Engl J Med 1982;307(11):676–8.
33. Pond S, Jacobs M, Marks J, et al. Treatment of digitoxin overdose with oral activated charcoal. Lancet 1981;2(8256):1177–8.
34. Taboulet P, Baud FJ, Bismuth C, et al. Acute digitalis intoxication–is pacing still appropriate? J Toxicol Clin Toxicol 1993;31(2):261–73.
35. Warren SE, Fanestil DD. Digoxin overdose. Limitations of hemoperfusion-hemodialysis treatment. JAMA 1979;242(19):2100–1.
36. Ganio MS, Klau JF, Casa DJ, et al. Effect of caffeine on sport-specific endurance performance: a systematic review. J Strength Cond Res 2009;23(1): 315–24.
37. Jurgens TM, Whelan AM, Killian L, et al. Green tea for weight loss and weight maintenance in overweight or obese adults. Cochrane Database Syst Rev 2012;(12):CD008650.
38. Derry CJ, Derry S, Moore RA. Caffeine as an analgesic adjuvant for acute pain in adults. Cochrane Database Syst Rev 2012;(3):CD009281.
39. Henderson-Smart DJ, De Paoli AG. Methylxanthine treatment for apnoea in preterm infants. Cochrane Database Syst Rev 2010;(12):CD000140.
40. Henderson-Smart DJ, Steer PA. Caffeine versus theophylline for apnea in preterm infants. Cochrane Database Syst Rev 2010;(1):CD000273.
41. Strachan ER, Bennett A. Theobromine poisoning in dogs. Vet Rec 1994; 134(11):284.
42. Echeverri D, Montes FR, Cabrera M, et al. Caffeine's vascular mechanisms of action. Int J Vasc Med 2010;2010:834060.
43. Hess P, Wier WG. Excitation-contraction coupling in cardiac Purkinje fibers. Effects of caffeine on the intracellular [Ca2+] transient, membrane currents, and contraction. J Gen Physiol 1984;83(3):417–33.
44. Paul S, Elsinga PH, Ishiwata K, et al. Adenosine A(1) receptors in the central nervous system: their functions in health and disease, and possible elucidation by PET imaging. Curr Med Chem 2011;18(31):4820–35.
45. Mustafa SJ, Morrison RR, Teng B, et al. Adenosine receptors and the heart: role in regulation of coronary blood flow and cardiac electrophysiology. Handb Exp Pharmacol 2009;(193):161–88.
46. Bernard S. Severe lactic acidosis following theophylline overdose. Ann Emerg Med 1991;20(10):1135–7.
47. Schnack C, Podolsky A, Watzke H, et al. Effects of somatostatin and oral potassium administration on terbutaline-induced hypokalemia. Am Rev Respir Dis 1989;139(1):176–80.

48. Wong CS, Pavord ID, Williams J, et al. Bronchodilator, cardiovascular, and hypokalaemic effects of fenoterol, salbutamol, and terbutaline in asthma. Lancet 1990;336(8728):1396–9.
49. Avci S, Sarikaya R, Buyukcam F. Death of a young man after overuse of energy drink. Am J Emerg Med 2013;31(11):1624.e3–4.
50. Breeden CC, Safirstein BH. Albuterol and spacer-induced atrial fibrillation. Chest 1990;98(3):762–3.
51. Cook P, Scarfone RJ, Cook RT. Adenosine in the termination of albuterol-induced supraventricular tachycardia. Ann Emerg Med 1994;24(2):316–9.
52. Duane M, Chandran L, Morelli PJ. Recurrent supraventricular tachycardia as a complication of nebulized albuterol treatment. Clin Pediatr 2000;39(11):673–7.
53. Keller KA, Bhisitkul DM. Supraventricular tachycardia: a complication of nebulized albuterol. Pediatr Emerg Care 1995;11(2):98–9.
54. Trachsel D, Newth CJ, Hammer J. Adenosine for salbutamol-induced supraventricular tachycardia. Intensive Care Med 2007;33(9):1676.
55. Fisher AA, Davis MW, McGill DA. Acute myocardial infarction associated with albuterol. Ann Pharmacother 2004;38(12):2045–9.
56. Forman J, Aizer A, Young CR. Myocardial infarction resulting from caffeine overdose in an anorectic woman. Ann Emerg Med 1997;29(1):178–80.
57. Higgins JP, Babu KM. Caffeine reduces myocardial blood flow during exercise. Am J Med 2013;126(8):730.e1–8.
58. Burniston JG, Chester N, Clark WA, et al. Dose-dependent apoptotic and necrotic myocyte death induced by the beta2-adrenergic receptor agonist, clenbuterol. Muscle Nerve 2005;32(6):767–74.
59. Chiang VW, Burns JP, Rifai N, et al. Cardiac toxicity of intravenous terbutaline for the treatment of severe asthma in children: a prospective assessment. J Pediatr 2000;137(1):73–7.
60. Huckins DS, Lemons MF. Myocardial ischemia associated with clenbuterol abuse: report of two cases. J Emerg Med 2013;44(2):444–9.
61. Shum S, Seale C, Hathaway D, et al. Acute caffeine ingestion fatalities: management issues. Vet Hum Toxicol 1997;39(4):228–30.
62. Eldridge FL, Paydarfar D, Scott SC, et al. Role of endogenous adenosine in recurrent generalized seizures. Exp Neurol 1989;103(2):179–85.
63. Fredholm BB. Theophylline actions on adenosine receptors. Eur J Respir Dis Suppl 1980;109:29–36.
64. Dettloff RW, Touchette MA, Zarowitz BJ. Vasopressor-resistant hypotension following a massive ingestion of theophylline. Ann Pharmacother 1993;27(6):781–4.
65. Amitai Y, Lovejoy FH Jr. Characteristics of vomiting associated with acute sustained release theophylline poisoning: implications for management with oral activated charcoal. J Toxicol Clin Toxicol 1987;25(7):539–54.
66. Shannon M. Life-threatening events after theophylline overdose: a 10-year prospective analysis. Arch Intern Med 1999;159(9):989–94.
67. Hagley MT, Traeger SM, Schuckman H. Pronounced metabolic response to modest theophylline overdose. Ann Pharmacother 1994;28(2):195–6.
68. Koul PB, Minarik M, Totapally BR. Lactic acidosis in children with acute exacerbation of severe asthma. Eur J Emerg Med 2007;14(1):56–8.
69. Maury E, Ioos V, Lepecq B, et al. A paradoxical effect of bronchodilators. Chest 1997;111(6):1766–7.
70. Campana C, Griffin PL, Simon EL. Caffeine overdose resulting in severe rhabdomyolysis and acute renal failure. Am J Emerg Med 2014;32(1):111.e3–4.

71. Wrenn KD, Oschner I. Rhabdomyolysis induced by a caffeine overdose. Ann Emerg Med 1989;18(1):94–7.
72. Price KR, Fligner DJ. Treatment of caffeine toxicity with esmolol. Ann Emerg Med 1990;19(1):44–6.
73. Gaar GG, Banner W Jr, Laddu AR. The effects of esmolol on the hemodynamics of acute theophylline toxicity. Ann Emerg Med 1987;16(12):1334–9.
74. Whitehurst VE, Joseph X, Vick JA, et al. Reversal of acute theophylline toxicity by calcium channel blockers in dogs and rats. Toxicology 1996;110(1–3):113–21.
75. Jacobs MH, Senior RM. Theophylline toxicity due to impaired theophylline degradation. Am Rev Respir Dis 1974;110(3):342–5.
76. Jacobs MH, Senior RM, Kessler G. Clinical experience with theophylline. Relationships between dosage, serum concentration, and toxicity. JAMA 1976; 235(18):1983–6.
77. Marquis JF, Carruthers SG, Spence JD, et al. Phenytoin-theophylline interaction. N Engl J Med 1982;307(19):1189–90.
78. Shaw EB, Dermott RV, Lee R, et al. Phenothiazine tranquilizers as a cause of severe seizures. Pediatrics 1959;23(3):485–92.
79. Berlinger WG, Spector R, Goldberg MJ, et al. Enhancement of theophylline clearance by oral activated charcoal. Clin Pharmacol Ther 1983;33(3):351–4.
80. Ohning BL, Reed MD, Blumer JL. Continuous nasogastric administration of activated charcoal for the treatment of theophylline intoxication. Pediatr Pharmacol 1986;5(4):241–5.
81. True RJ, Berman JM, Mahutte CK. Treatment of theophylline toxicity with oral activated charcoal. Crit Care Med 1984;12(2):113–4.
82. Holstege CP, Hunter Y, Baer AB, et al. Massive caffeine overdose requiring vasopressin infusion and hemodialysis. J Toxicol Clin Toxicol 2003;41(7):1003–7.
83. Shannon M, Wernovsky G, Morris C. Exchange transfusion in the treatment of severe theophylline poisoning. Pediatrics 1992;89(1):145–7.
84. Shannon MW. Comparative efficacy of hemodialysis and hemoperfusion in severe theophylline intoxication. Acad Emerg Med 1997;4(7):674–8.
85. Nelson L, Goldfrank LR. Goldfrank's toxicologic emergencies. Chapter 65. 9th edition. New York: McGraw-Hill Medical; 2011. xxviii, 1940.
86. Osborn HH, Henry G, Wax P, et al. Theophylline toxicity in a premature neonate– elimination kinetics of exchange transfusion. J Toxicol Clin Toxicol 1993;31(4): 639–44.
87. Perrin C, Debruyne D, Lacotte J, et al. Treatment of caffeine intoxication by exchange transfusion in a newborn. Acta Paediatr Scand 1987;76(4):679–81.
88. Michael JB, Sztajnkrycer MD. Deadly pediatric poisons: nine common agents that kill at low doses. Emerg Med Clin North Am 2004;22(4):1019–50.
89. Ernsberger P, Giuliano R, Willette RN, et al. Role of imidazole receptors in the vasodepressor response to clonidine analogs in the rostral ventrolateral medulla. J Pharmacol Exp Ther 1990;253(1):408–18.
90. Klein-Schwartz W. Trends and toxic effects from pediatric clonidine exposures. Arch Pediatr Adolesc Med 2002;156(4):392–6.
91. Spiller HA, Bosse GM, Adamson LA. Retrospective review of tizanidine (Zanaflex) overdose. J Toxicol Clin Toxicol 2004;42(5):593–6.
92. Spiller HA, Klein-Schwartz W, Colvin JM, et al. Toxic clonidine ingestion in children. J Pediatr 2005;146(2):263–6.
93. Domino LE, Domino SE, Stockstill MS. Relationship between plasma concentrations of clonidine and mean arterial pressure during an accidental clonidine overdose. Br J Clin Pharmacol 1986;21(1):71–4.

94. Frye CB, Vance MA. Hypertensive crisis and myocardial infarction following massive clonidine overdose. Ann Pharmacother 2000;34(5):611–5.
95. Perruchoud C, Bovy M, Durrer A, et al. Severe hypertension following accidental clonidine overdose during the refilling of an implanted intrathecal drug delivery system. Neuromodulation 2012;15(1):31–4 [discussion: 34].
96. Kobinger. Central alpha-adrenergic systems as targets for hypotensive drugs. Rev Physiol Biochem Pharmacol 1978;81:39–100.
97. Rangan C, Everson G, Cantrell FL. Central alpha-2 adrenergic eye drops: case series of 3 pediatric systemic poisonings. Pediatr Emerg Care 2008;24(3): 167–9.
98. Johnson ML, Visser EJ, Goucke CR. Massive clonidine overdose during refill of an implanted drug delivery device for intrathecal analgesia: a review of inadvertent soft-tissue injection during implantable drug delivery device refills and its management. Pain Med 2011;12(7):1032–40.
99. Pomerleau AC, Gooden CE, Fantz CR, et al. Dermal Exposure to a Compounded Pain Cream Resulting in Severely Elevated Clonidine Concentration. J Med Toxicol 2014;10(1):61–4.
100. Luciani A, Brugioni L, Serra L, et al. Sino-atrial and atrio-ventricular node dysfunction in a case of tizanidine overdose. Vet Hum Toxicol 1995;37(6):556–7.
101. Osterhoudt KC, Henretig FM. Sinoatrial node arrest following tetrahydrozoline ingestion. J Emerg Med 2004;27(3):313–4.
102. Hoffmann U, Kuno S, Franke G, et al. Adrenoceptor agonist poisoning after accidental oral ingestion of brimonidine eye drops. Pediatr Crit Care Med 2004;5(3): 282–5.
103. Soto-Perez-de-Celis E, Skvirsky DO, Cisneros BG. Unintentional ingestion of brimonidine antiglaucoma drops: a case report and review of the literature. Pediatr Emerg Care 2007;23(9):657–8.
104. Sztajnbok J. Failure of naloxone to reverse brimonidine-induced coma in an infant. J Pediatr 2002;140(4):485–6 [author reply: 486].
105. Ahmad SA, Scolnik D, Snehal V, et al. Use of naloxone for clonidine intoxication in the pediatric age group: case report and review of the literature. Am J Ther 2015;22(1):e14–6.
106. Banner W Jr, Lund ME, Clawson L. Failure of naloxone to reverse clonidine toxic effect. Am J Dis Child 1983;137(12):1170–1.
107. Cook P. Clonidine-induced unconsciousness: reversal with naloxone. Anaesth Intensive Care 1987;15(4):470–1.
108. Niemann JT, Getzug T, Murphy W. Reversal of clonidine toxicity by naloxone. Ann Emerg Med 1986;15(10):1229–31.
109. Horowitz R, Mazor SS, Aks SE, et al. Accidental clonidine patch ingestion in a child. Am J Ther 2005;12(3):272–4.

Atrial Fibrillation

Eric Goralnick, MD, MS[a],*, Laura J. Bontempo, MD, MEd[b]

KEYWORDS

- Atrial fibrillation • Atrial flutter • Cardioembolic stroke

KEY POINTS

- Atrial fibrillation (AF) is the most common dysrhythmia diagnosed in US emergency departments.
- Rate control and rhythm control management strategies carry equal mortality and stroke risk.
- All patients with AF must have their cardioembolic risk assessed, even if sinus rhythm is restored.
- Novel oral anticoagulants (NOAs) may be considered instead of vitamin K antagonists (VKAs) for anticoagulation in patients with nonvalvular AF.

OVERVIEW

AF is a supraventricular tachyarrhythmia that results from the chaotic depolarization of atrial tissue. AF is the most common sustained cardiac dysrhythmia and the most common dysrhythmia diagnosed in US emergency departments (EDs).[1] AF affects between 1% and 2% of the general population, with a peak prevalence of 10% in those older than 80 years.[2,3] It is estimated that by 2050 nearly 16 million US patients will have AF.[4]

AF is an independent risk factor for stroke, congestive heart failure (HF), and overall mortality.[5] Rates of ischemic stroke in nonvalvular AF average 5% annually, 2 to 7 times the rate in the population of patients without AF.[6] In a 20-year follow-up study of patients with AF, women had a 5-fold increased risk of cardiovascular events and men has a 2-fold increase compared with patients without AF. Most of the adverse events were related to stroke and HF.[7] Overall mortality in patients with AF is almost double that of patients with normal sinus rhythm.[8]

Disclosure: none.
[a] Department of Emergency Medicine, Brigham and Women's Hospital, Harvard Medical School, 75 Francis Street, Boston, MA 02115, USA; [b] Department of Emergency Medicine, University of Maryland School of Medicine, 6th Floor, Suite 200, 110 South Paca Street, Baltimore, MD 21201, USA
* Corresponding author.
E-mail address: egoralnick@partners.org

Emerg Med Clin N Am 33 (2015) 597–612
http://dx.doi.org/10.1016/j.emc.2015.04.008
0733-8627/15/$ – see front matter © 2015 Elsevier Inc. All rights reserved.
emed.theclinics.com

In addition to its significant health impact, AF also places a formidable economic burden on the health care system, accounting for $6.65 billion annually in direct and indirect costs.[9]

There are many terms used to describe the various types of AF. The classification scheme endorsed by the American College of Cardiology Foundation (ACCF), American Heart Association (AHA), and the European Society of Cardiology (ESC) is based on the duration of the episode of AF, its recurrences, and the patient's clinical course[10] (**Table 1**). Emergency medicine (EM) physicians are often tasked with management of new-onset or paroxysmal AF.

Management strategies have traditionally encompassed rate control, rhythm control, and anticoagulation, but a lack of solid evidence has led to wide variation in ED physician practice.[11]

The recommendations included below are derived from a combination of existing guidelines, additional evidence, and consensus.

CAUSES

It is imperative for the EM physician to identify and treat the serious and reversible underlying causes of AF.

AF is most commonly associated with cardiovascular disease. Hypertension, coronary artery disease, cardiomyopathy, valvular disease, myocarditis, and pericarditis are the most common associations. AF may also occur after cardiac surgery.

Dangerous causes of AF that must be considered are myocardial infarction (MI), pulmonary embolism (PE), and hyperthyroidism. If these are the suspected causes of the dysrhythmia, then the AF is secondary and the primary cause should be addressed first.

AF may also result from another supraventricular tachycardia, Wolff-Parkinson-White (WPW) syndrome, in which rapid hemodynamic collapse may occur as a result of accessory pathway conduction. The management of AF with WPW focuses exclusively on the treatment of WPW. Many of the standard treatments of AF (such as β-blockers and nondihydropyridine calcium channel antagonists) are contraindicated with this cause.

Hyperthyroidism, hypokalemia, sympathomimetic use, electrocution, and pulmonary disorders, including pulmonary embolism and obstructive sleep apnea, are all noncardiac secondary causes of AF. Excessive alcohol intake, termed holiday heart syndrome, another noncardiac cause of AF, typically occurs after an alcohol binge in someone who is not accustomed to drinking large volumes of alcohol.

AF in patients younger than 60 years with no underlying cardiovascular disease is termed lone AF. This condition is particularly common in patients with paroxysmal AF, wherein no underlying cardiac disease is identified in up to 45% of cases.[12]

Table 1 AF classification	
Term	**Definition**
Recurrent	≥2 episodes
Paroxysmal	Duration≤7 d, spontaneous resolution
Persistent	Duration>7 d; not self-terminating
Permanent	Duration>7 d & cardioversion has failed or not been attempted
Lone	Age<60 y; no clinical or echocardiographic evidence of cardiopulmonary disease

Used for episodes of AF greater than 30 s without a reversible cause.

DIAGNOSIS

The uncoordinated activity of the atria results in irregular passage of impulses through the atrioventricular (AV) node to the ventricle. The patient may experience palpitations because of the irregular, and often rapid, ventricular contractions. On examination, the clinician will find an irregularly irregular, likely tachycardic, pulse.

The electrocardiogram (ECG) of a patient in AF does not have discernable, independent P waves. Instead, the P waves are replaced by fibrillatory waves that are rapid oscillations that vary in shape and amplitude. Owing to the irregular conduction of these atrial fibrillatory impulses to the ventricles, QRS complexes occur with varying R-R intervals. Overall, this results in a rapid, narrow complex, irregular rhythm without discernable P waves (**Fig. 1**). The ECG of a patient with AF may show a rapid, wide complex rhythm if the AF is occurring in combination with a bundle branch block.

If the atrial impulses conduct to the ventricle via an accessory pathway or if the impulse is interrupted by a ventricular conduction block (right or left bundle), the QRS complex is wide. A sustained, rapid, irregular, wide complex tachycardia suggests AF with a bundle branch block or AF with conduction through an accessory pathway.

MANAGEMENT

When managing a patient with AF, the clinician must choose a strategy of rate control or rhythm control. Rhythm control is a strategy to terminate the AF and return the patient to normal sinus rhythm. A rate control strategy focuses on maintaining AF at a controlled ventricular rate. In the ED, the selection of management strategy primarily depends on patient stability, severity of symptoms, duration of symptoms, and clinician preference. In a hemodynamically unstable patient, a rhythm control strategy may be necessary regardless of other factors, including the duration of the AF.

The Atrial Fibrillation Follow-up Investigation of Rhythm Management (AFFIRM) study[13] and the Rate Control versus Electrical Cardioversion for Persistent Atrial Fibrillation (RACE) study[14] compared the outcomes of patients treated with a rate versus rhythm control strategy. The AFFIRM study, which enrolled over 4000 patients, found no difference in mortality or stroke rates between treatment arms. The RACE trial, which enrolled over 500 patients, also found no significant difference in survival or quality of life advantage between the 2 treatment arms.[15] Higher rates of thromboembolic events were seen in the rhythm control group in both studies; however, these events occurred in patients in whom adequate anticoagulation was not achieved.[14,15] The risk of a thromboembolic stroke when using a rhythm control strategy is equal to that of rate control plus anticoagulation.[16] The ACCF, AHA, and Heart Rhythm Society (HRS) thus now recommend that antithrombotic therapy be considered for patients who are managed with either a rate or a rhythm control strategy.[17]

For patients with AF in whom the duration of the AF is unknown or known to be greater than 48 hours, a rate control strategy is preferred until adequate

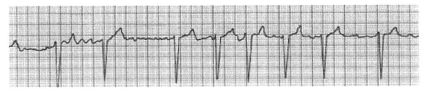

Fig. 1. Atrial fibrillation. (*From* Bontempo LJ, Goralnick E. Atrial fibrillation. Emerg Med Clin North Am 2011;29(4):748; with permission.)

anticoagulation is achieved or an intracardiac thrombus is ruled out through a trans-esophageal echocardiogram. In any patient with hemodynamic instability due to the AF, the dysrhythmia must be terminated and, therefore, a rhythm control strategy is necessary.

Selecting a rate control strategy in the ED and initiating appropriate anticoagulation still allows the selection of a rhythm control strategy, if desired, by the patient's follow-up physician in the outpatient setting. Early follow-up must be arranged because pharmacologic cardioversion is most effective within 7 days of the onset of an episode of AF.

Rate Control

The goal of a rate control strategy for AF is to control the ventricular rate of the dysrhythmia without actually terminating the AF.

In their 2006 guidelines, the ACCF, the AHA, and the ESC recommended a resting heart rate of 60 to 80 beats per minute and a moderate exercise heart rate of 90 to 115 beats per minute as an adequate end point for patients with rate-controlled AF.[16] In 2010, however, the need for strict heart rate control was challenged and a more lenient parameter of a resting heart rate less than 110 beats per minute was proposed.[18] A comparison of strict versus lenient approaches showed similar patient outcomes at 2 years and no significant difference in cardiovascular morbidity and mortality including the prevalence of AF symptoms, hospitalizations for HF, and stroke in patients with a left ventricular ejection fraction greater than 40%.[18,19] Even in the setting of HF, diastolic dysfunction, hypertrophic cardiomyopathy, hypotension, and pulmonary congestion, it is not proven that strict rate control offers any benefit over lenient control.[20] The 2011 guidelines now endorse that strict heart rate control shows no significant benefit over lenient control.[21] Lenient heart rate control parameters may be easier to achieve in the ED and maintain as an outpatient, thereby making rate control a simpler option for patients and health care providers. In follow-up, a patient's heart rate can be checked during visits to health care providers or via a 24-h ambulatory ECG monitor.

Rate control is primarily accomplished by using agents that prolong the refractory period of the AV node. The 2 main classes of medications used are β-blockers and nondihydropyridine calcium channel antagonists. Digoxin may be used as an adjunct agent, but because of its delayed therapeutic onset, its emergent utility is limited. Both β-blockers and calcium channel antagonists are effective in achieving rate control. In the AFFIRM trial, however, β-blockers were found to achieve strict heart rate control in 70% of patients, whereas calcium channel antagonists achieved rate control in 54% of patients.[15] In light of the new guidelines allowing lenient heart rate control, the benefit of a β-blocker versus a calcium channel antagonist as a rate-controlling agent must be reexamined. In the ED, rate control of AF with rapid ventricular response may be accomplished via the administration of either class of medications.

β-Blockers with class 1 recommendations are metoprolol, esmolol, and propranolol. The possible side effects of these drugs include hypotension, heart block, brady-cardia, bronchospasm, and HF.[16,17] β-Blockers, therefore, should be used cautiously in patients with AF and hypotension or HF from a depressed ejection fraction[16] (**Table 2**).

Calcium channel antagonists with class I recommendations are diltiazem and verapamil[16,17] (see **Table 2**). Both drugs have similar safety profiles including their effects on blood pressure.[22] Diltiazem is classically dosed at 0.25 mg/kg intravenously (IV) over 2 minutes, although doses less than 0.2 mg/kg have been shown to be effective with a decreased risk of hypotension.[23] In addition to hypotension, the possible

Table 2
Rate control agents for AF

Agent	IV Loading & Maintenance Dose	Oral Dose
β-Blockers		
Esmolol	500 μg/kg then 60–200 μg/kg/min	None
Metoprolol	5 mg every 5 min, up to 3 doses	25–100 mg bid
Propranolol	0.15 mg/kg	80–240 mg daily in divided doses
Calcium Channel Antagonists		
Diltiazem	0.25 mg/kg[a] then 5–15 mg/h	120–360 mg daily in divided doses
Verapamil	0.075–0.15 mg/kg	240–360 mg daily in divided doses
Other		
Digoxin	0.25 mg every 2 h; maximum = 1.5 mg	0.125–0.375 mg daily
Amiodarone	150 mg over 10 min then 0.5–1 mg/min	None

Abbreviation: IV, intravenous.
[a] Doses as low at 0.1 mg/kg may be effective.

side effects of calcium channel antagonists are heart block and HF because of their negative ionotropic effects. These antagonists, therefore, should not be used in the treatment of patients with decompensated HF. Calcium channel antagonists do not have the side effect of bronchospasm and may be preferred in patients with chronic obstructive pulmonary disease or asthma.

Digoxin works by enhancing vagal activity and increasing the AV node's refractory period, which, in turn, decreases the ventricular rate. The onset of action for IV digoxin is at least 60 minutes, and its peak effect can take up to 6 hours.[16] These pharmacokinetics make digoxin of limited utility in the acute management of AF with a rapid ventricular response. Digoxin is no longer recommended as a first-line agent in the management of paroxysmal AF. Digoxin is best used as an adjunct in patients treated with a β-blocker or calcium channel antagonist.[24,25] Digoxin also has a role in the long-term ventricular rate management of patients with persistent AF.[26]

Amiodarone is a second-line agent for the management of AF with rapid ventricular response and should be considered when first-line agents have failed.[16] Amiodarone works to lower the ventricular rate through its sympatholytic and calcium channel antagonist properties.[17]

Once rate control is obtained, the patient must be administered the oral equivalent of whichever agent achieved the rate control (see **Table 2**).

Rhythm Control

The goal of a rhythm control strategy is to terminate AF and restore and maintain sinus rhythm.

A critical piece of information for any emergency physician (EP) contemplating a rate control strategy is the duration of the patient's AF. The risk of a thromboembolic event increases when the duration of the AF exceeds 48 hours. If the duration of the AF is greater than 48 hours or is not known to be less than 48 hours, a rhythm control strategy should not be pursued from the ED. Instead, the ventricular response rate should be controlled (see section titled Rate Control) and anticoagulation initiated.

The 2 main modes of rhythm control are pharmacologic cardioversion and electrical cardioversion. The risk of a thromboembolic event is the same with both modes, and, therefore, the guidelines for anticoagulation are the same for both.[16]

Direct current electrical cardioversion (DCCV) can be attempted with a synchronized monophasic shock or a synchronized biphasic shock. Biphasic shocks have a higher success rate for restoration of sinus rhythm, and success is achieved using fewer joules. In a head-to-head study comparing the efficacy of synchronized monophasic to biphasic shocks in AF, biphasic shocks had a success rate of 94%, whereas monophasic shock had a success rate of 79%.[27] Biphasic shock waveforms are, therefore, the standard of care for DCCV of AF.[16]

The overall success rate of DCCV is 70% to 90%.[28,29] Predictors for successful cardioversion include shorter duration of AF, younger age, and lower thoracic impedance.[16,29] Patients with left atrial enlargement, underlying heart disease, and cardiomegaly are less likely to achieve DCCV successfully.[29] The rate of recurrence of AF after cardioversion is high with one study finding that only 23% of patients remained in sinus rhythm 1 year after successful cardioversion.[30] DCCV, however, is a low-risk procedure and does not incur the risk of adverse drug effects seen with pharmacologic agents. If hemodynamic stability permits, patients should be procedurally sedated before DCCV.

Pretreating a patient with the antidysrhythmic ibutilide (1 mg infused over 10 minutes then waiting 10 minutes before DCCV) facilitates successful cardioversion.

This pretreatment has also been shown to reduce the number of DCCV attempts and the amount of energy required for biphasic cardioversion.[31]

Pharmacologic attempts at cardioversion are less effective than DCCV using a biphasic waveform[16]; nonetheless, many agents are available for pharmacologic cardioversion. Of the options available, 4 agents have class I, level of evidence A recommendations from the ACCF, AHA, and HRS: flecainide, propafenone, ibutilide, and dofetilide[10] (**Table 3**).

Flecainide is a Vaughan-Williams class IC antiarrhythmic that acts through sodium channel inhibition. Flecainide can be given IV or orally and is more effective than amiodarone, propafenone, and placebo in converting AF to sinus rhythm.[32–35] After a single oral dose of 300 mg, the AF in 75% to 91% of patients converts within 8 hours.[36] Flecainide should not be used for patients with a history of acute coronary ischemia, structural heart disease, or cardiomyopathy.[37]

Table 3
Control in AF

Drug	AF Conversion Dose	Maintenance Dose	Comments
Flecanide	200 mg orally *or* 2 mg/kg IV over 10 min	50–100 mg bid	• May repeat oral dose if needed after 4 h • Avoid in patients with history of ACS, structural heart disease, or cardiomyopathy
Propafenone	600 mg orally *or* 2 mg/kg IV over 10 min	150–300 mg bid	Avoid in patients with history of ACS, structural heart disease, or cardiomyopathy
Ibutilide	1 mg IV over 10 min; may repeat once	—	Risk of torsades de pointes
Amiodarone	6 mg/kg IV over 60 min then 1.2 g over 24 h	600 mg daily for 1 wk then taper	• Slow onset • Risk of hypotension

Abbreviation: ACS, acute coronary syndrome.
From Bontempo LJ, Goralnick E. Atrial fibrillation. Emerg Med Clin North Am 2011;29(4):753; with permission.

Propafenone is also a class IC antiarrhythmic that can be given orally or IV. Oral propafenone has a cardioversion rate between 56% and 83% within 6 hours of administration. IV propafenone has a shorter onset of action and results in more cardioversions within the first 2 hours.[16] The safety profile of this drug is good with significant adverse side effects being uncommon.[38] The use of propafenone should be avoided in patients with structural heart disease, HF, and severe obstructive lung disease.[16]

Ibutilide is a class III antiarrhythmic that acts as a potassium channel blocker, prolonging the refractory period of the atrial and ventricular myocardium, the accessory pathway, and the AV node.[38] Ibutilide is given as a single IV dose, which may be repeated once if necessary. This drug has a conversion rate of 75% in recent-onset AF. For patients with atrial flutter, the conversion rate is greater than 80% within 30 minutes of administration.[39]

The most significant side effect of ibutilide is QT interval lengthening and subsequent ventricular dysrhythmias. There is a 4% risk of torsades de pointes and a 5% risk of monomorphic ventricular tachycardia. Patients at higher risk for torsades de pointes are those with small body size, a history of HF, nonwhite race, and female gender.[40] In addition, caution should be exercised for patients with ischemia, HF, and prior MI, because torsades de pointes can be refractory to treatment in these patients.

Most episodes of ibutilide-induced torsades de pointes occur within 1 hour after treatment and almost all will occur within 6 hours. Owing to these dysrhythmia risks, patients must be monitored for up to 6 hours after drug administration. Pretreating with 4 g of IV magnesium reduces the risk of both torsades de pointes and ventricular tachycardia. This pretreatment also improves the efficacy of ibutilide for cardioversion of AF.[41] Hypokalemia should also be corrected before ibutilide treatment.

Amiodarone is an antidysrhythmic with predominately Vaughan-Williams class III effects. This drug can be given orally or IV. Although amiodarone was not proven superior to flecainide or propafenone in the management of recent-onset AF, it has an acceptable safety profile for patients with left ventricle dysfunction or structural heart disease. Amiodarone should, therefore, be considered for use in patients who have contraindications to class IC agents, such as left ventricle systolic dysfunction and structural heart disease.[42]

Dofetilide is a class III antiarrhythmic; it is primarily used for patients with persistent AF and, therefore, is of limited use to the EP. In addition, owing to its complex dosing and potential to induce malignant dysrhythmias, patients require 72 hours of in-hospital monitoring after administration.[43] Dofetilide has been studied in multiple trials and is a moderately effective agent for pharmacocardioversion of patients with persistent AF.[44,45]

Dronedarone is a newer antidysrhythmic used to increase the time between recurrences of AF. Although it was shown to reduce the risk of hospitalization due to cardiovascular events in patients with AF, it does not play a role in the ED management of new-onset or paroxysmal AF.[46]

In addition to the above-mentioned agents, procainamide may also be considered. Procainamide has an ACCF/AHA/ESC class IIb recommendation with level of evidence B.[10] Use of procainamide for pharmacologic cardioversion, according to the Ottawa Aggressive Protocol (OAP), resulted in conversion to sinus rhythm in 59.9% of patients in AF and 28.1% of patients in atrial flutter.[47]

The OAP deserves special attention because it sequentially combined the use of pharmacocardioversion and DCCV for patients with recent-onset AF or atrial flutter. In this protocol, patients who presented to the Ottawa Hospital ED with recent-onset AF or atrial flutter were treated with a rhythm control strategy. Recent-onset

AF or flutter was defined as symptoms clearly present for fewer than 48 hours unless the patient was already therapeutically anticoagulated with warfarin for 3 weeks. Stable patients received 1 g of procainamide infused over 1 hour. If procainamide failed to convert the AF to sinus rhythm, or if pharmacologic cardioversion was not attempted (because of physician choice), DCCV was performed. DCCV was successful in 91% of patients in AF and 100% of patients in atrial flutter. The adverse event rate was low for all OAP patients, with the most common event being transient hypotension.[47]

The OAP successfully demonstrated the feasibility of a rhythm control strategy in the ED. Overall, 96.8% of the enrolled patients were discharged home and 93.3% left in sinus rhythm. The overall average ED length of stay for enrolled patients was 4.9 hours. Follow-up was conducted for 7 days after the index ED visit, and within this time AF relapsed in 8.6% of patients.[47] Patients who are rhythm controlled in the ED must, therefore, have close follow-up arranged, and consideration should be given to oral antiarrhythmic drugs for rhythm maintenance. In addition, anticoagulation needs to be initiated, as appropriate, even if the AF converts to sinus rhythm.

Anticoagulation

AF is the most common cause of cardioembolic stroke and confers an increased risk of morbidity and mortality when compared with non-AF-related stroke.[48] For patients with AF aged 80 to 89 years, the stroke risk is up to 8% per year.[7] Effective antithrombotic therapy is both a critical and controversial component of AF management.

The $CHADS_2$ scoring system was derived to predict cardioembolic stroke risk based on risk factors in patients with nonvalvular AF and to guide antithrombotic therapy[49] (**Table 4**). More recently, the CHA_2DS_2-VASc score was introduced to incorporate the additional stroke risk factors of female gender and vascular disease and to be more inclusive of age-related risk[50] (see **Table 4**). The main goal of the CHA_2DS_2-VASc score is to better identify patients with a risk of thromboembolic events low enough that antithrombotic therapy is not warranted.[51] The $CHADS_2$ and the CHA_2DS_2-VASc scores perform approximately equally in identifying patients who will develop stroke and thromboembolic events.[52,53]

The adjusted annual incidence of stroke in patients with AF without antithrombotic therapy increases with each additional point on the CHA_2DS_2-VASc scale (**Table 5**). A score of 2 or more confers a 2.2% annual stroke risk and, therefore, oral anticoagulation (OAC) is recommended. A CHA_2DS_2-VASc of 1 carries an adjusted stroke risk of

Table 4 $CHADS_2$ & CHA_2DS_2-VASc score		
Risk Factor	**$CHADS_2$ Score**	**CHA_2DS_2-VASc Score**
Congestive HF/LVEF ≤40%	1	1
Hypertension	1	1
Age ≥75 y	1	2
Diabetes mellitus	1	1
Stroke/TIA/thromboembolism	2	2
Vascular disease (MI, PAD, complex aortic plaque)	—	1
Age 65–74 y	—	1
Female gender	—	1
Maximum score	6	9

Abbreviations: LVEF, left ventricular ejection fraction; MI, myocardial infarction; PAD, peripheral artery disease; TIA, transient ischemic attack.

Table 5
CHA$_2$DS$_2$-VASc adjusted stroke rate & ESC Treatment Guidelines

CHA$_2$DS$_2$-VASc Score	Stroke Rate (% per year)	ESC Guidelines
0	0	No antithrombotic therapy
1	1.3	OAC (preferred) or ASA No antithrombotic therapy if score is because of female gender only
2	2.2	OAC
3	3.2	OAC
4	4.0	OAC
5	6.7	OAC
6	9.8	OAC
7	9.6	OAC
8	6.7	OAC
9	15.2	OAC

Abbreviations: ASA, aspirin; OAC, oral anticoagulation.

1.3% per year; the management of patients with this score is still debatable. The 2010 ESC guidelines stated that OAC or aspirin therapy was acceptable, but the newer 2012 guidelines recommend against aspirin as monotherapy.[51,54] The 2012 guidelines recommend no antithrombotic therapy for patients with a CHA$_2$DS$_2$-VASc score of 0, or 1 if the only risk factor is female gender.

There is an increased risk of thromboembolism and stroke in patients with AF for greater than 48 hours.[55] The incidence of thromboembolism or stroke in patients with AF of duration less than 48 hours is less than 1%.[56] Hemodynamically stable patients with AF duration less than 48 hours can undergo cardioversion and do not require anticoagulation before the procedure. Patients with AF duration greater than 48 hours should receive anticoagulation for 3 weeks before and 4 weeks after pharmacologic or electrical cardioversion. Patients who undergo transesophageal echocardiography (TEE) with no evidence of left atrial thrombus should continue anticoagulation for 4 weeks after a cardioversion procedure. Those with thrombus should use anticoagulation for 3 weeks and repeat a TEE to ensure thrombus resolution before cardioversion.[57] These guidelines apply to patients undergoing both pharmacologic and electrical cardioversion.

Even if a patient has sinus rhythm restored, the patient's thromboembolic risk must be addressed. The return of sinus rhythm does not guarantee the maintenance of sinus rhythm, and therefore a patient remains at increased risk for thromboembolic events.

Until recently, the only option for oral antithrombotic therapy in moderate- and high-risk patients was VKA (eg, warfarin). VKAs reduce the risk of ischemic stroke by 64%[58,59] but require regular monitoring and have labile drug and food interactions, pharmacogenetic variability, significant risk of major bleeding, and a narrow therapeutic window. The utility of VKAs has been challenged in the light of the advent of the NOAs.

NOAs fall into 2 classes: direct thrombin inhibitors and direct factor Xa inhibitors. At present, dabigatran etexilate (direct thrombin inhibitor), rivaroxaban (factor Xa inhibitor), and apixaban (factor Xa inhibitor) are the NOAs approved for use in the United States (**Table 6**).

Table 6 Novel oral anticoagulants	
Name	Classification
Dabigatran	Direct thrombin inhibitor
Rivaroxaban	Factor Xa inhibitor
Apixaban	Factor Xa inhibitor

Vitamin K antagonists

Warfarin is still the mainstay of anticoagulation treatment for patients with AF. The goal international normalized ratio (INR) of 2 to 3 for nonvalvular AF is achieved only two-thirds of the time in randomized controlled trials and even less in clinical practice.[60] Owing to the narrow therapeutic window, the INR should be determined weekly during the initiation of therapy.[17] The 2011 ACCF/AHA/HRS guidelines recommend VKA for patients with a $CHADS_2$ score of 2 more (class I, level of evidence A) or a CHA_2DS_2-VASc score greater than 1 (class IIa, level of evidence B).[17]

Direct thrombin inhibitors

Both the intrinsic coagulation pathway (involving factors XII, XI, IX, and VIII) and the extrinsic coagulation pathway (involving factor VII) end in the same common pathway, the activation of factor X to factor Xa. Factor Xa, along with factor Va, activates prothrombin (factor II) to thrombin (factor IIa). Thrombin not only activates fibrinogen into fibrin (factor Ia) but also activates factors V, VII, VIII, IX, and XIII. Direct thrombin inhibitors directly block thrombin formation and thereby inhibit coagulation.

Dabigatran is the only oral direct thrombin inhibitor with data from phase 3 trials for stroke prevention in patients with AF. The Randomized Evaluation of Long-Term Anti-coagulation Therapy (RE-LY) trial included 18,113 patients with AF. Stroke or systemic embolism occurred less frequently in patients taking 110 mg of dabigatran twice daily compared with those taking warfarin (1.1% vs 1.7%). The incidence of hemorrhagic stroke and intracranial hemorrhage were reduced in the patients on dabigatran; however, they had an increased incidence of gastrointestinal bleeding and MI.[51,61] Dabigatran is nonreversible, and this must also be considered when evaluating its risk/benefit ratio for a patient.

Factor Xa inhibitors

In the Rivaroxaban versus Warfarin in Nonvalvular Atrial Fibrillation (ROCKET-AF) study, more than 14,000 patients were evaluated to compare the efficacy of rivaroxaban to warfarin in preventing stroke and systemic embolism.[62] Rivaroxaban was found to be noninferior to warfarin. Rivaroxaban reduced the rates of hemorrhagic stroke, intracranial hemorrhage, and fatal bleeding but had an increased number of gastrointestinal bleed and bleeds requiring transfusion when compared with warfarin therapy.[51,62]

Apixaban was compared with warfarin in the Apixaban versus Warfarin in Patients with Atrial Fibrillation (ARISTOTLE) trial. Apixaban showed a reduction in stroke or systemic embolism when compared with warfarin, 1.27% versus 1.6%. Apixaban demonstrated reduced major bleeding and intracranial hemorrhage. Gastrointestinal bleeding rates were similar.[63]

Factor Xa inhibitors do not have reversal agents either, so this must also be considered when evaluating their risk/benefit ratio for individual patients.

Antiplatelet therapy

For patients who refuse to or are unable to tolerate OAC, aspirin plus clopidogrel should be considered. The Effect of Clopidogrel Added to Aspirin in Patients with Atrial Fibrillation (ACTIVE-A) study compared clopidogrel and aspirin to aspirin only treatment.[64] This study found that the combination of clopidogrel plus aspirin reduced the risk of major vascular events but increased the risk of major hemorrhage. In 2011, the AHA, ACCF, and ESC recommended considering the use of clopidogrel plus aspirin in patients with AF in whom OAC is unsuitable because of "patient preference or the physician's assessment of the patient's ability to safely sustain anticoagulation."[17] The ESC 2012 guidelines advise aspirin plus clopidogrel for patients who otherwise refuse any form of OAC.[51]

Disposition

Patients with newly detected AF and hemodynamic stability can be managed in the ED. If anticoagulation is addressed, and rate control achieved or sinus rhythm restored, further workup can be undertaken in the outpatient setting.[17]

ATRIAL FLUTTER

Atrial flutter is a separate electrophysiological entity from AF. Atrial flutter is characterized by rapid, regular atrial contractions that result in sawtooth P waves on the ECG (**Fig. 2**). These sawtooth atrial waves are termed flutter waves or F waves and typically occur at a rate between 240 and 320 contractions per minute. The resultant ventricular rate is typically 120 to 160 beats per minute. Most of the management guidelines pertaining to rate control, rhythm control, and anticoagulation discussed in this article also apply to atrial flutter.[17,65,66]

Atrial flutter is notoriously difficult to rate control, therefore a rhythm control strategy may be necessary. Ibutilide is the agent of choice for pharmacologic rhythm control with atrial flutter; however, DCCV may be necessary for sustained return to sinus rhythm. In a retrospective cohort study of 122 patients at 2 urban EDs, patients in atrial flutter who received DCCV successfully achieved normal sinus rhythm 91% of the time, whereas those who received antiarrhythmic pharmacotherapy achieved sinus rhythm only 27% of the time. Of those patients electrically cardioverted, nearly 20% required more than 150 J for successful restoration of sinus rhythm. Although 3 patients died within the 1-year follow-up period, no patient had a stroke.[67]

As in AF, even if a patient reverts to sinus rhythm, anticoagulation should be initiated as appropriate for the patient's level of thromboembolic risk.

Disposition

After rate or rhythm control is accomplished, underlying inciting events are addressed, anticoagulation is initiated, and close follow-up is established, patients with new-onset AF may be considered for discharge from the ED. Discharged patients should be symptom free or symptom controlled, hemodynamically stable, and without evidence of myocardial ischemia or other serious cause of their AF.

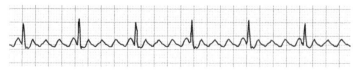

Fig. 2. Atrial flutter.

Follow-up is essential to identify potential underlying structural heart disease, monitor heart rate and rhythm, and ensure adequate anticoagulation, including INR monitoring. The duration of antidysrhythmic and anticoagulation therapy as well as the necessity of cardiac imaging also needs to be addressed in follow-up.

SUMMARY

AF is the most common dysrhythmia diagnosed in US EDs. When AF is first encountered, the EP must look for dangerous and treatable primary causes such as MI, PE, myocarditis, and hyperthyroidism.

The 2 main treatment strategies for AF that have been present for less than 48 hours are rate control and rhythm control. Either strategy confers the same mortality and stroke risk to the patient. If AF is present for more than 48 hours, a rate control strategy should be selected.

The CHA_2DS_2-VASc score can be used to determine the optimal anticoagulation for patients with AF. All patients with AF should have their cardioembolic risk addressed, even if sinus rhythm has been restored, because the maintenance of sinus rhythm is not guaranteed. NOAs may reduce or replace VKAs in the near future.

REFERENCES

1. McDonald AJ, Pelletier AJ, Ellinor PT, et al. Increasing US emergency department visit rates and subsequent hospital admissions for atrial fibrillation from 1993 to 2004. Ann Emerg Med 2008;51:58–65.
2. Go AS, Hylek EM, Phillips KA, et al. Prevalence of diagnosed atrial fibrillation in adults: national implications for rhythm management and stroke prevention: the AnTicoagulation and Risk Factors in Atrial Fibrillation (ATRIA) Study. JAMA 2001;285:2370–5.
3. Feinberg WM, Blackshear JL, Laupacis A, et al. Prevalence, age distribution, and gender of patients with atrial fibrillation. Analysis and implications. Arch Intern Med 1995;155:469–73.
4. Miyasaka Y, Barnes ME, Gersh BJ, et al. Secular trends in incidence of atrial fibrillation in Olmsted County, Minnesota, 1980 to 2000, and implications on the projections for future prevalence. Circulation 2006;114:119–25.
5. Lloyd-Jones D, Adams RJ, Brown TM, et al. Heart disease and stroke statistics— 2010 Update: a report from the American Heart Association. Circulation 2010; 121:e91.
6. Wolf PA, Abbott RD, Kannel WB, et al. Atrial fibrillation as an independent risk factor for stroke: the Framingham Study. Stroke 1991;22:983–8.
7. Stewart S, Hart CL, Hole DJ, et al. A population-based study of the long-term risks associated with atrial fibrillation: 20-year follow-up of the Renfrew/Paisley study. Am J Med 2002;113(5):359–64.
8. Krahn AD, Manfreda J, Tate RB, et al. The natural history of atrial fibrillation: incidence, risk factors, and prognosis in the Manitoba Follow-Up Study. Am J Med 1995;98:476–84.
9. Coyne KS, Paramore C, Grandy S, et al. Assessing the direct costs of treating nonvalvular atrial fibrillation in the United States. Value Health 2006;9:348–56.
10. Fuster V, Rydén LE, Cannom DS, et al. 2011 ACCF/AHA/HRS focused updates incorporated into the ACC/AHA/ESC 2006 guidelines for the management of patients with atrial fibrillation. A report of the American College of Cardiology Foundation/American Heart Association Task Force on Practice Guidelines. Circulation 2011;123:e269–367.

11. Stiell IG, Clement CM, Brison RJ, et al. Variation in management of recent-onset atrial fibrillation and flutter among academic hospital emergency departments. Ann Emerg Med 2011;57:13–21.
12. Page RL. Clinical practice. Newly diagnosed atrial fibrillation. N Engl J Med 2004; 351:2408–16.
13. Curtis AB, Gersh BJ, Corley SD, et al. Clinical factors that influence response to treatment strategies in atrial fibrillation: the Atrial Fibrillation Follow-up Investigation of Rhythm Management (AFFIRM) study. Am Heart J 2005;149:645–9.
14. Van Gelder IC, Hagens VE, Bosker HA, et al. A comparison of rate control and rhythm control in patients with recurrent persistent atrial fibrillation. N Engl J Med 2002;347:1834–40.
15. Wyse DG, Waldo AL, DiMarco JP, et al. A comparison of rate control and rhythm control in patients with atrial fibrillation. N Engl J Med 2002;347:1825–33.
16. Fuster V, Ryden LE, Cannom DS, et al. ACC/AHA/ESC 2006 guidelines for the management of patients with atrial fibrillation: a report of the American College of Cardiology/American Heart Association Task Force on Practice Guidelines and the European Society of Cardiology Committee for Practice Guidelines (Writing Committee to Revise the 2001 Guidelines for the Management of Patients With Atrial Fibrillation): developed in collaboration with the European Heart Rhythm Association and the Heart Rhythm Society. Circulation 2006;114: e257–354.
17. Fuster V, Rydén LE, Cannom DS, et al. 2011 ACCF/AHA/HRS focused updates incorporated into the ACC/AHA/ESC 2006 Guidelines for the management of patients with atrial fibrillation: a report of the American College of Cardiology Foundation/American Heart Association Task Force on Practice Guidelines developed in partnership with the European Society of Cardiology and in collaboration with the European Heart Rhythm Association and the Heart Rhythm Society. J Am Coll Cardiol 2011;57(11):e101–98.
18. Van Gelder IC, Groenveld HF, Crijns HJ, et al. Lenient versus strict rate control in patients with atrial fibrillation. N Engl J Med 2010;362:1363–73.
19. Wann LS, Curtis AB, January CT, et al. 2011 ACCF/AHA/HRS focused update on the management of patients with atrial fibrillation (updating the 2006 guideline): a report of the American College of Cardiology Foundation/American Heart Association Task Force on Practice Guidelines. Circulation 2011;123:104–23.
20. Rienstra M, Van Gelder IC. Ventricular rate control of atrial fibrillation in heart failure. Heart Fail Clin 2013 Oct;9(4):397–406.
21. Wann LS, Curtis AB, January CT, et al. 2011 ACCF/AHA/HRS focused update on the management of patients with atrial fibrillation (Updating the 2006 Guideline): a report of the American College of Cardiology Foundation/American Heart Association Task Force on Practice Guidelines. Heart Rhythm 2011;8(1):157–76.
22. Phillips BG, Gandhi AJ, Sanoski CA, et al. Comparison of intravenous diltiazem and verapamil for the acute treatment of atrial fibrillation and atrial flutter. Pharmacotherapy 1997;17:1238–45.
23. Lee J, Kim K, Lee CC, et al. Low-dose diltiazem in atrial fibrillation with rapid ventricular response. Am J Emerg Med 2011;29(8):849–54.
24. Farshi R, Kistner D, Sarma JS, et al. Ventricular rate control in chronic atrial fibrillation during daily activity and programmed exercise: a crossover open-label study of five drug regimens. J Am Coll Cardiol 1999;33:304–10.
25. Tamariz LJ, Bass EB. Pharmacological rate control of atrial fibrillation. Cardiol Clin 2004;22:35–45.

26. Patel NJ, Hoosien M, Deshmukh A, et al. Digoxin significantly improves all-cause mortality in atrial fibrillation patients with severely reduced left ventricular systolic function. Int J Cardiol 2013;169(5):e84–6.

27. Mittal S, Ayati S, Stein KM, et al. Transthoracic cardioversion of atrial fibrillation: comparison of rectilinear biphasic versus damped sine wave monophasic shocks. Circulation 2000;101:1282–7.

28. Gowda SA, Shah A, Steinberg JS, et al. Cardioversion of atrial fibrillation. Prog Cardiovasc Dis 2005;48:88–107.

29. Van Gelder IC, Crijns HJ, Van Gilst WH, et al. Prediction of uneventful cardioversion and maintenance of sinus rhythm from direct-current electrical cardioversion of chronic atrial fibrillation and flutter. Am J Cardiol 1991;68:41–6.

30. Siaplaouras S, Jung J, Buob A, et al. Incidence and management of early recurrent atrial fibrillation (ERAF) after transthoracic electrical cardioversion. Europace 2004;6:15–20.

31. Mazzocca G, Corbucci G, Venturini E, et al. Is pretreatment with ibutilide useful for atrial fibrillation cardioversion when combined with biphasic shock? J Cardiovasc Med (Hagerstown) 2006;7:124–8.

32. Donovan KD, Power BM, Hockings BE, et al. Intravenous flecainide versus amiodarone for recent-onset atrial fibrillation. Am J Cardiol 1995;75:693–7.

33. Donovan KD, Dobb GJ, Coombs LJ, et al. Efficacy of flecainide for the reversion of acute onset atrial fibrillation. Am J Cardiol 1992;70:50A–4A [discussion: 54A–5A].

34. Martinez-Marcos FJ, Garcia-Garmendia JL, Ortega-Carpio A, et al. Comparison of intravenous flecainide, propafenone, and amiodarone for conversion of acute atrial fibrillation to sinus rhythm. Am J Cardiol 2000;86:950–3.

35. Capucci A, Lenzi T, Boriani G, et al. Effectiveness of loading oral flecainide for converting recent-onset atrial fibrillation to sinus rhythm in patients without organic heart disease or with only systemic hypertension. Am J Cardiol 1992;70:69–72.

36. Khan IA. Oral loading single dose flecainide for pharmacological cardioversion of recent-onset atrial fibrillation. Int J Cardiol 2003;87:121–8.

37. National Collaborating Centre for Chronic Conditions (UK). Atrial fibrillation. National clinical guideline for management in primary and secondary care. London: Royal College of Physicians; 2006.

38. Glatter KA, Dorostkar PC, Yang Y, et al. Electrophysiological effects of ibutilide in patients with accessory pathways. Circulation 2001;104:1933–9.

39. Ando G, Di Rosa S, Rizzo F, et al. Ibutilide for cardioversion of atrial flutter: efficacy of a single dose in recent-onset arrhythmias. Minerva Cardioangiol 2004;52:37–42.

40. Gowda RM, Khan IA, Wilbur SL, et al. Torsade de pointes: the clinical considerations. Int J Cardiol 2004;96:1–6.

41. Steinwender C, Honig S, Kypta A, et al. Pre-injection of magnesium sulfate enhances the efficacy of ibutilide for the conversion of typical but not of atypical persistent atrial flutter. Int J Cardiol 2010;141:260–5.

42. Khan IA, Mehta NJ, Gowda RM, et al. Amiodarone for pharmacological cardioversion of recent-onset atrial fibrillation. Int J Cardiol 2003;89:239–48.

43. Singh S, Zoble RG, Yellen L, et al. Efficacy and safety of oral dofetilide in converting to and maintaining sinus rhythm in patients with chronic atrial fibrillation or atrial flutter: the Symptomatic Atrial Fibrillation Investigative Research on Dofetilide (SAFIRE-D) study. Circulation 2000;102:2385–90.

44. Falk RH, Pollak A, Singh SN, et al. Intravenous dofetilide, a class III antiarrhythmic agent, for the termination of sustained atrial fibrillation or flutter. Intravenous Dofetilide Investigators. J Am Coll Cardiol 1997;29:385–90.

45. Norgaard BL, Wachtell K, Christensen PD, et al. Efficacy and safety of intravenously administered dofetilide in acute termination of atrial fibrillation and flutter: a multicenter, randomized, double-blind, placebo-controlled trial. Danish Dofetilide in Atrial Fibrillation and Flutter Study Group. Am Heart J 1999;137:1062–9.

46. Hohnloser SH, Crijns HJ, van Eickels M, et al, ATHENA Investigators. Effect of dronedarone on cardiovascular events in atrial fibrillation. N Engl J Med 2009; 360:668–78.

47. Stiell IG, Clement CM, Perry JJ, et al. Association of the Ottawa Aggressive Protocol with rapid discharge of emergency department patients with recent-onset atrial fibrillation or flutter. CJEM 2010;12:181–91.

48. Marini C, De Santis F, Sacco S, et al. Contribution of atrial fibrillation to incidence and outcome of ischemic stroke: results from a population-based study. Stroke 2005;36:1115–9.

49. Gage BF, Waterman AD, Shannon W, et al. Validation of clinical classification schemes for predicting stroke: results from the National Registry of Atrial Fibrillation. JAMA 2001;285:2864–70.

50. Lip GH, Nieuwlaat R, Pisters R, et al. Refining clinical risk stratification for predicting stroke and thromboembolism in atrial fibrillation using a novel risk factor-based approach: the euro heart survey on atrial fibrillation. Chest 2010;137(2):263–72.

51. Camm AJ, Lip GY, De Caterina R, et al. 2012 focused update of the ESC guidelines for the management of atrial fibrillation: an update of the 2010 ESC guidelines for the management of atrial fibrillation–developed with the special contribution of the European Heart Rhythm Association. Europace 2012;14: 1385–413.

52. Friberg L, Rosenqvist M, Lip GY. Evaluation of risk stratification schemes for ischaemic stroke and bleeding in 182 678 patients with atrial fibrillation: the Swedish Atrial Fibrillation Cohort study. Eur Heart J 2012;33:1500–10.

53. Boriani G, Botto GL, Padeletti L, et al. Improving stroke risk stratification using the CHADS2 and CHA2DS2-VASc risk scores inpatients with paroxysmal atrial fibrillation by continuous arrhythmia burden monitoring. Stroke 2011;42:1768–70.

54. European Heart Rhythm Association, European Association for Cardio-Thoracic Surgery, Camm AJ, et al. Guidelines for the management of atrial fibrillation: the Task Force for the Management of Atrial Fibrillation of the European Society of Cardiology (ESC). Eur Heart J 2010;31(19):2369–429.

55. Raghavan AV, Decker WW, Meloy TD, et al. Management of atrial fibrillation in the emergency department. Emerg Med Clin North Am 2005;23:1127–39.

56. Weigner MJ, Caulfield TA, Danias PG, et al. Risk for clinical thromboembolism associated with conversion to sinus rhythm in patients with atrial fibrillation lasting less than 48 hours. Ann Intern Med 1997;126:615–20.

57. Klein AL, Murray RD, Grimm RA, et al. Role of transesophageal echocardiography-guided cardioversion of patients with atrial fibrillation. J Am Coll Cardiol 2001;37:691–704.

58. Hart RG, Pearce LA, Aguilar MI, et al. Meta-analysis: antithrombotic therapy to prevent stroke in patients who have nonvalvular atrial fibrillation. Ann Intern Med 2007;146:857–67.

59. Ansell J, Hirsh J, Hylek E, et al. Pharmacology and management of the vitamin K antagonists: American College of Chest Physicians Evidence-Based Clinical Practice Guidelines (8th Edition). Chest 2008;133:160S–98S.

60. Matchar DB, Samsa GP, Cohen SJ, et al. Improving the quality of anticoagulation of patients with atrial fibrillation in managed care organizations: results of the managing anticoagulation services trial. Am J Med 2002;113:42–51.

61. Wallentin L, Yusuf S, Ezekowitz MD, et al. Efficacy and safety of dabigatran compared with warfarin at different levels of international normalised ratio control for stroke prevention in atrial fibrillation: an analysis of the RE-LY trial. Lancet 2010;376:975–83.

62. Patel MR, Mahaffey KW, Garg J, et al, ROCKET AF Investigators. Rivaroxaban versus warfarin in nonvalvular atrial fibrillation. N Engl J Med 2011;365(10): 883–91.

63. Granger CB, Alexander JH, McMurray JJ, et al, ARISTOTLE Committees and Investigators. Apixaban versus Warfarin in Patients with Atrial Fibrillation. N Engl J Med 2011;365(11):981–92.

64. Connolly SJ, Pogue J, Hart RG, et al. Effect of clopidogrel added to aspirin in patients with atrial fibrillation. N Engl J Med 2009;360:2066–78.

65. Stiell IG, Clement CM, Symington C, et al. Emergency department use of intravenous procainamide for patients with acute atrial fibrillation or flutter. Acad Emerg Med 2007;14:1158–64.

66. Domanovits H, Schillinger M, Thoennissen J, et al. Termination of recent-onset atrial fibrillation/flutter in the emergency department: a sequential approach with intravenous ibutilide and external electrical cardioversion. Resuscitation 2000;45:181–7.

67. Scheuermeyer FX, Grafstein E, Heilbron B, et al. Emergency department management and 1-year outcomes of patients with atrial flutter. Ann Emerg Med 2011;57:564–71.e2.

Human Immunodeficiency Virus Infection–Related Heart Disease

 CrossMark

Thuy Van Pham, MD*, Mercedes Torres, MD

KEYWORDS

- HIV • AIDS • Anti-retroviral therapy (ART)
- Highly active anti-retroviral therapy (HAART) • Atrial fibrillation
- Prolonged QT syndrome • Acute coronary syndrome (ACS)
- Coronary artery disease (CAD) • Cardiomyopathy • Myocarditis
- Pericardial effusion • Valvular disease

KEY POINTS

- Medications of patients with known human immunodeficiency virus (HIV) infection/AIDS who present to the emergency department (ED) with an arrhythmia should be carefully reviewed.
- A lower threshold should be maintained to evaluate for acute coronary syndrome (ACS) and coronary artery disease (CAD) in patients with known HIV/AIDS who present with chest pain.
- Given its nonspecific symptoms, myocarditis should be included in the differential diagnosis for toxic-appearing HIV-infected patients who present with fever, upper respiratory illness (URI), and flulike symptoms.
- HIV-infected patients who present with acute-onset congestive heart failure (CHF) have a higher mortality rate than non-HIV-infected patients.
- Pericardial effusions in HIV-infected patients should be managed as in non-HIV-infected patients.
- HIV-infected patients have a high rate of valvular diseases, but most of these patients are asymptomatic.

INTRODUCTION

Since the introduction of antiretroviral therapy (ART) for HIV infection and AIDS in the mid-1990s, the natural history of HIV and AIDS has shifted from an acute infection to a

---

Disclosure: None.

Department of Emergency Medicine, University of Maryland School of Medicine, 110 South Paca Street, Sixth Floor, Suite 200, Baltimore, MD 21201, USA

* Corresponding author.

E-mail address: tpham@umem.org

Emerg Med Clin N Am 33 (2015) 613–622

http://dx.doi.org/10.1016/j.emc.2015.04.009

chronic disease. In the pre-ART era or areas of the world where ART is not readily available, opportunistic infections causing pericarditis and myocarditis contributed to the high morbidity of cardiovascular diseases (CVDs) in HIV-infected patients. In the post-ART era, arrhythmias, ACS, and CAD are the major CVDs affecting morbidity and mortality in these patients. CAD and associated ACS are the third most common cause of death in HIV-infected patients in the United States.[1] In addition to traditional risk factors such as smoking and family history, HIV has both direct and indirect effects on the heart; it causes an acute inflammatory response, leads to chronic cellular changes, and is an independent risk factor for CVD.[1–4] In addition, the antiretroviral medications used in the management and treatment of HIV/AIDS have significant cardiovascular side effects, including metabolic dysregulation that leads to dyslipidemia and atherosclerosis.[1–4] The pathophysiologic effects of HIV/AIDS on the heart are summarized in **Box 1**. Altogether, these factors have changed the course of CVD in HIV-infected patients.

As the growing population living with HIV ages, they accrue risk factors for other chronic diseases. The current prevalence of HIV/AIDS in the United States is greater than 1.1 million, with approximately 50,000 incident cases annually.[5] Between 2009 and 2010, patients with HIV/AIDS accounted for more than 1 million ED visits.[6] Emergency practitioners are on the front line in the management of patients with HIV/AIDS. As such, it is imperative to recognize the changing natural history of CVD in HIV-infected patients and its particular manifestations in this population.

DEFINITIONS

- HIV: 1 of 2 retroviruses (HIV-1, HIV-2) that affect and destroy helper T-cells of the human immune system
- AIDS: final stage of HIV disease leading to severe immunosuppression
- ART: medication that targets the HIV
- Highly active antiretroviral therapy (HAART): an antiretroviral regimen that contained a minimum of 3 antiretroviral drugs in combination. Common combinations: 2 nucleoside reverse transcriptase inhibitors (NRTIs) and a nonnucleoside reverse transcriptase inhibitor (NNRTI); 3 NRTIs; 2 NRTIs and a protease inhibitor (PI); 2 PIs and an NNRTI; 2 PIs and an NRTI; an NRTI, an NNRTI, and a PI.
- Centers for Disease Control and World Health Organization Stages of HIV/AIDS: **Table 1**

CORONARY ARTERY DISEASE AND ACUTE CORONARY SYNDROME

HIV-infected patients are at increased risk of CAD and ACS. The mean age for the first episode of ACS is 48 years in the HIV-infected population, approximately 10 years

---

Box 1
Pathophysiologic effects of HIV/AIDS on the cardiovascular system

Proatherogenic effects of the virus

Procoagulant effects of the virus

Metabolic dysregulation from ART

Data from Mavroudis CA, Majumder B, Loizides, S, et al. Coronary artery disease and HIV; getting to the HAART of the matter. Int J Cardiol 2013;167:1147–53. Available at: http://www.internationaljournalofcardiology.com/article/S0167-5273(12)01149-7/abstract.

Table 1 Stages of HIV/AIDS			
	A	**B**	**C**
	Asymptomatic, Acute HIV, Persistent Generalized Lymphadenopathy	**Symptomatic Conditions, Not A or C**	**AIDS-Indicator Conditions**
CD4 ≥500 cells/μL	A1	B1	C1
CD4 200–499 cells/μL	A2	B2	C2
CD4 <299 cells/μL	A3	B3	C3

From HIV classification: CDC and WHO staging systems. Available at: http://aidsetc.org/guide/hiv-classification-cdc-and-who-staging-systems. Accessed April 26, 2015.

earlier than the non-HIV-infected population.[1] Many factors contribute to this increased risk. HIV-infected patients have higher rates of traditional risk factors, such as age, history of CAD, smoking, dyslipidemia, diabetes, hypertension, and increased body mass index.[1,2] Adjusting for age, smoking, and cocaine abuse are the strongest risk factors for CAD and ACS among HIV-infected patients.[3,4] Smoking is the strongest predictor of CAD in HIV-infected patients, and the rate of smoking among this population is 2 to 3 times higher than in the general population.[4] Cocaine abuse is common in North America and Europe, and it has been associated with accelerated CAD secondary to vasospasm and atherosclerosis.[1,2] The virus also contributes to a chronic inflammatory process that accelerates atherosclerosis.[1,2]

Certain antiretroviral medications, especially PIs and NRTIs, have been linked to metabolic dysregulation (increased insulin resistance, dyslipidemia, and lipodystrophy) through a direct impact on lipid and glucose metabolism.[2,3,7] PIs lead to decreasing levels of high-density lipoproteins and to increasing levels of triglycerides.[2] The Data Collection in the Adverse Effects of Anti-HIV Drugs (D:A:D) study found an increased risk of CAD and ACS in patients taking PIs that was attributed to these dysmetabolic effects.[8] In patients who were at low risk for the development of CAD and ACS, PIs did not play a significant role in worsening disease progression.[8] Lifestyle modifications seemed to help decrease risk factors of certain medications in moderate- to high-risk patients.[8]

In the Strategies for Management of Antiretroviral Therapy (SMART) study, treatment interruption was associated with a 57% increased risk of ACS requiring intervention (percutaneous coronary intervention or bypass grafting) or resulting in death.[9] Although PIs are associated with dysmetabolic effects, their long-term benefits tend to outweigh their short-term risk factors.[2,3,7] Nonetheless, providers should be aware of this increased risk. Statins and fibrates are the first-line drugs in the management of dyslipidemia among HIV-infected patients. Caution is advised, as there are still drug-drug interactions that may occur between statins and PIs because of their shared metabolism via the cytochrome P450 system, which may lead to statin toxicity.[7] Pravastatin has the least risk of drug-drug interactions with PIs, with the exception of ritonavir and darunvir.[7] Although new ART is not typically started in the ED, providers should be aware of possible drug-drug interactions with common coprescriptions such as statins.

HIV has both direct and indirect effects on the heart itself. The virus has proatherogenic and procoagulopathic activities on smooth muscle cells that lead to accelerated atherosclerosis.[2,3,7] The virus induces both an acute and chronic inflammatory reaction at the cellular level.[2,3,7] HIV-infected patients also have increased levels of anticardiolipic and lupus anticoagulation factors.[2,3,7] Histopathologic studies reveal that the coronary arteries of deceased patients with AIDS had larger atherosclerotic plaques composed of higher proportions of extracellular lipid as compared with non-HIV-infected patients.[10] However, the duration of HIV infection, CD4 count, viral load, or the duration of antiretroviral therapy did not predict the extent of atherosclerotic disease.[10]

When patients with known HIV/AIDS present to the ED with chest pain, providers should have a lower threshold to evaluate for possible ACS. Multiple studies have shown that revascularization with percutaneous coronary intervention (PCI) or coronary artery bypass graft surgery is safe and effective, with no differences in short-term or long-term mortality compared with non-HIV/AIDS patients.[2,3,7] There is no difference in the rates of acute stent thrombosis between HIV-infected patients and non-HIV-infected patients who undergo PCI, but there is a higher rate of overall in-stent restenosis in HIV-infected patients, likely due to the aforementioned proinflammatory and procoagulopathic mechanisms.[3]

ARRHYTHMIAS

Patients with HIV/AIDS are at increased risk for electrocardiographic (ECG) abnormalities, such as sinus tachycardia, QTc prolongation, atrial fibrillation, and nonspecific ST-segment and T-wave changes.[11] The clinically concerning arrhythmias are PR prolongation, QTc prolongation, and atrial fibrillation, all of which can lead to atrial and ventricular tachydysrhythmias.[11] QTc prolongation is one of the most common arrhythmias reported in HIV-infected patients. It is associated with other chronic diseases such as diabetes, hypertension, and cirrhosis.[12] Among all HIV-infected patients, the prevalence of a prolonged QTc interval is as high as 28%; in patients with AIDS, the prevalence increases to 45%.[11] HIV exerts both direct and indirect effects on the cardiovascular system, including autonomic neuropathy, altering cardiac innervation.[11,12] Although the pathophysiology remains unclear, HIV-infected patients have a sympathovagal imbalance leading to increased sympathetic tone.[13] One theory suggests a direct effect of the virus on the central nervous system, notably the hippocampus, basal ganglia, and other regions of the hypothalamus.[13] Among HIV-infected patients with autonomic neuropathy, the prevalence of QTc prolongation increases to 65%.[12] Autonomic neuropathy occurs in early stages of HIV infection, but there is no correlation to CD4 counts or viral loads. However, there is an association between the duration of infection and an increased frequency of arrhythmias[12,13] (**Box 2**).

Box 2
Common medications used by patients with HIV/AIDS that cause QT prolongation

Pentamidine

Trimethoprim-sulfamethoxazole

Ciprofloxacin

Clarithromycin

Erythromycin

Ketoconazole

Methadone

Haloperidol

Certain antiretroviral drugs have also been linked to QTc prolongation, most notably PIs.[11,12,14] This class of medication blocks a type of potassium channel called a HERB receptor, prolonging the QTc interval and predisposing patients to associated life-threatening tachydysrhythmias such as torsade de pointes.[11,12,14] Certain PIs, such as indinavir, directly inhibit the GLUT-4 transporter that is expressed in neurons localized to the hypothalamic nuclei.[13] This transporter is involved in glucose-insulin regulation, and disruption leads to autonomic and metabolic dysregulation.[12,13] In 2009, the US Food and Drug Administration issued a warning based on isolated case reports that PIs carry an associated risk of QTc prolongation.[14] In response, multiple follow-up studies were conducted to investigate this association, including the SMART study. Investigators found no association between PI use and a prolonged QTc interval.[12,14,15] The only significant association with QTc prolongation was duration of HIV infection greater than 3 years.[12] PI use did have a dose-dependent prolongation of the PR interval but this normalized after discontinuation of the medication.[14]

Another common arrhythmia in HIV-infected patients is atrial fibrillation. In addition to traditional risk factors for atrial fibrillation, such as older age, white race, CAD, CHF, alcoholism, chronic kidney disease, and hypothyroidism, HIV is an independent factor.[15] The pathophysiology of this remains unclear, and the cause is most likely multifactorial.[11,12,15,16] As with the rest of the population, atrial fibrillation among HIV-infected patients is associated with increased morbidity and mortality due to strokes, heart failure, and death.[11,12,15,16] More severe AIDS, as measured by low CD4 levels and high viral load, increases the risk of developing atrial fibrillation.[15] A high viral load is associated with a 70% higher risk of atrial fibrillation.[15] This risk may be due to the changing physiology of the aging HIV-infected patient population and the chronic inflammatory changes that take place in cells secondary to viral presence and disease progression.[15] The workup and management of atrial fibrillation is unchanged as compared with the general population.

Providers should carefully review medications of patients with known HIV/AIDS who present to the ED with an arrhythmia. Although PIs have not been shown to have significant short-term effects on QTc prolongation, there is a dose-dependent effect on the PR interval. Providers should also consider the arrhythmogenic properties of medications they prescribe (eg, typical and atypical antipsychotics, certain antibiotics). It is always advisable to perform ECG for baseline interval assessment before initiating any new arrhythmogenic medications.

MYOCARDITIS AND CARDIOMYOPATHY

In clinical-pathological studies done in the pre-ART period, the estimated prevalence of dilated cardiomyopathy (DCM) among patients with AIDS was 30% to 40%, and the estimated annual incidence was 15.9 per 1000 patients.[17,18] DCM was thought to be associated with an inflammatory response to the virus leading directly to right and left ventricular dysfunction.[19] With the introduction of HAART, the prevalence of cardiomyopathy has decreased by 30% in developed countries.[19] This decrease has been attributed to a commensurate decline in opportunistic infections and myocarditis.[19]

However, the prevalence in countries without access to HAART remains high. The numbers have actually increased by 32% because of scant resources and additional nutritional deficiencies attributable to malnutrition and diarrhea (eg, selenium and vitamin B_{12}).[19] CHF in HIV-infected patients still carries a high morbidity and mortality. The prognosis is worse when the CHF is acute in onset: more than 50% of patients die from heart failure within 6 to 12 months of diagnosis.[17] Otherwise, the diagnosis, workup, and management of new-onset CHF in HIV-infected patients is the same as in non-HIV-infected patients.

The most common causes of cardiomyopathy in patients with AIDS are myocarditis and drug cardiotoxicity.[19] Myocarditis is defined as inflammation of the heart muscle characterized by a lymphocytic infiltrate with necrosis and/or degeneration of adjacent myocytes not typical of ischemic changes with CAD.[18] It has been documented in autopsy reports in up to 50% of patients who died with AIDS before the advent of HAART.[18] Although the histologic findings did not differ between HIV-infected patients and non-HIV-infected patients with DCM, other autopsy studies have demonstrated mild to moderate lymphocytic infiltrate in HIV-infected patients, whether or not they exhibit cardiac symptoms.[18] The most common opportunistic infections in patients with AIDS that cause myocarditis leading to cardiomyopathy are listed in **Box 3**.[18] Other pathogens are endemic to certain regions in the world. Because myocarditis can present with nonspecific symptoms, practitioners in the ED should keep this diagnosis in their differential in toxic-appearing HIV-infected patients who present with fever, URI, and flulike symptoms. These symptoms can precede CHF symptoms (eg, dyspnea on exertion, orthopnea) by days.[18] Patients may have elevated levels of cardiac enzymes such as troponin and myoglobin. Cardiac catheterization with myocardial biopsy is the gold standard for diagnosis of myocarditis.[18]

The medications taken by HIV-infected patients that are most associated with cardiotoxicity include zidovudine, doxorubicin, and foscarnet.[19] Zidovudine is commonly used in HARRT regimens. In a mouse model, it is associated with the destruction of cardiac mitochondrial structure that leads to diffuse dysfunction.[18,19] This same effect has yet to be observed in clinical or observational studies. Doxorubicin has a cumulative dose-related effect causing cardiotoxicity.[19] It is used in the treatment of Kaposi sarcoma and non-Hodgkin lymphoma.[19] Foscarnet, used to treat cytomegalovirus esophagitis, has a dose-dependent effect as well. Patients receiving these specific drugs will likely have opportunistic infections found only in end-stage AIDS; thus these patients carry twice the risk of developing cardiotoxicity.[19]

PERICARDIAL EFFUSION

In addition to an increased susceptibility to concomitant infections, HIV causes a serous effusive process involving the pleural and peritoneal surfaces that is due to a capillary leak syndrome from enhanced cytokine expression.[20] In the pre-HAART era, the incidence of pericardial effusion was 11% in HIV-infected patients.[17,20–22] It was one of the most common cardiac manifestations in this patient population and was an independent predictor of increased mortality (as high as 62% in 6 months).[17,20–22] Effusions were more common in patients with advanced AIDS, and most effusions were small and asymptomatic with unclear causes.[20,23] Since

---

Box 3
Opportunistic infections causing myocarditis

Toxoplasma gondii

Cryptococcus neoformans

Coccidioides immitis

Histoplasma capsulatum

Candida species

Aspergillus

the mid-1990s, the incidence of pericardial effusion has dramatically decreased.[21] In one observational study, only 2 of 802 HIV-infected patients developed a pericardial effusion during a 2-year period in an outpatient setting.[21] However, in resource-deficient areas of the world where ART is not readily available, HIV remains epidemic and pericardial effusion continues to be a major cause of increased mortality.[24] Most cases are due to tuberculosis (TB).[24] The number of cases of tuberculous pericarditis is increasing worldwide, especially in Africa, Asia, and Latin America.[24] The immune response elicited from the acid-fast bacilli in a delayed hypersensitivity reaction accounts for the morbidity and mortality associated with TB pericarditis.[24]

As in non-HIV-infected patients, dyspnea and edema are the most common presenting symptoms in patients with large pericardial effusions.[22] Larger effusions are associated with CHF, malignancies such as Kaposi sarcoma or non-Hodgkin lymphoma, TB, or other pulmonary infections.[17,22] The management of pericardial effusions in HIV-infected patients is similar to that in non-HIV-infected patients. Chest radiographs may show normal findings or an enlarged cardiac silhouette.[25–30] The ECG may show normal findings or nonspecific ST-T wave changes, but sinus tachycardia is the most common presentation.[25] Echocardiogram is the diagnostic modality of choice to identify a pericardial effusion.[25] Pericarditis and cardiac tamponade are rare presentations; emergent pericardiocentesis is not typically indicated even in symptomatic patients with moderate to large effusion unless the patient is hemodynamically unstable with evidence of cardiac tamponade.[22] In developing countries, if suspicion for TB pericarditis or pericardial effusion is high, pericardiocentesis may be considered as part of the initial workup to make the diagnosis.[24] Treatment of tuberculous pericarditis consists of the standard 4-drug anti-TB regimen for 6 months.[25] Surgical resection of the pericardium remains an appropriate option for constrictive pericarditis once medical treatments have failed.[24]

VALVULAR DISEASE

Valvular disease is a common finding in HIV-infected patients. Up to 78% of HIV-infected patients have pathologic function of one or more of the cardiac valves.[25] Tricuspid regurgitation is the most commonly seen abnormality, and the incidence increases with the duration of HIV infection.[25] However, unlike patients with other cardiac manifestations, most of these patients are asymptomatic or have mild presentations.[25] Clinically relevant valvular disorders are seen in only in 5% of HIV-infected patients.[25] There is no association between CD4 count or viral load and the incidence of valvular disease, although the rate of valvular disease is associated as HIV/AIDS progresses, especially in patients who have had an AIDS-defining disease.[25]

Infective endocarditis is a risk factor for valvular disease, and the rate of endocarditis has decreased since the introduction of ART. The incidence of endocarditis in HIV-infected patients is similar to that of other high-risk groups, notably patients who abuse intravenous drugs.[25] The prevalence of endocarditis is 6% to 34% in HIV-infected patients.[25] In patients without a history of intravenous drug abuse, marantic endocarditis occurs in 3% to 5% of patients with AIDS.[25] The initial workup and management of endocarditis in HIV-infected patients in the ED remains the same as for non-HIV-infected patients, including obtaining blood cultures and administering parenteral antibiotics.

SUMMARY

Since the introduction of ART, the natural course of HIV/AIDS has changed from an acute infection to a chronic disease. In the pre-ART era, HIV-infected patients had increased morbidity and mortality from opportunistic infections; in the post-ART era, these patients are at increased risk of chronic diseases such as ACS, CAD, cardiac arrhythmias, and cardiomyopathy. Emergency providers should recognize that HIV infection is a risk factor in itself for CVD entities.

REFERENCES

1. Boccara F. Acute coronary syndrome in HIV-infected patients. Does it differ from that in the general population? Arch Cardiovasc Dis 2010;103:567–9. Available at: http://ac.els-cdn.com/S1875213610001889/1-s2.0-S1875213610001889-main.pdf?_tid=c39df8e2-a07e-11e3-883c-00000aab0f26&acdnat=1393595386_6401eeb81e35c04dbd4e19c2661bdb21.
2. Triant VA. HIV infection and coronary heart disease: an intersection of epidemics. J Infect Dis 2012;205:355–61. Available at: http://www.ncbi.nlm.nih.gov/pmc/articles/PMC3349293/.
3. Boccara F, Lang S, Meuleman C, et al. HIV and coronary heart disease. J Am Coll Cardiol 2013;61(5):511–23. Available at: http://www.sciencedirect.com/science/article/pii/S0735109712047754.
4. Stein JH. Cardiovascular risk and dyslipidemia management in HIV-infected patients. Top Antivir Med 2012;20(4):129–33. Available at: http://www.iasusa.org/sites/default/files/tam/20-4-129.pdf.
5. HIV classification: CDC and WHO staging systems. Available at: http://aidsetc.org/guide/hiv-classification-cdc-and-who-staging-systems. Accessed April 26, 2015.
6. Mohared AM, Rothman RE, Hsieh YH. Emergency department (ED) utilization by HIV-infected ED patients in the United States in 2009 and 2010. HIV Med 2013; 14(10):605–13. Available at: http://www.medscape.com/viewarticle/812997.
7. Mavroudis CA, Majumder B, Loizides S, et al. Coronary artery disease and HIV; getting to the HAART of the matter. Int J Cardiol 2013;167:1147–53. Available at: http://www.internationaljournalofcardiology.com/article/S0167-5273(12)01149-7/abstract.
8. DAD Study Group, Friis-Moller N, Reiss P, et al. Class of antiretroviral drugs and the risk of myocardial infarction. N Engl J Med 2007;356(17):1723–35.
9. Strategies for Management of Antiretroviral Therapy (SMART) Study Group, El-Sadr WM, Lundgren J, et al. CD4+ count-guided interruption of antiretroviral treatment. N Engl J Med 2006;355(22):2283–96.
10. Micheletti RG, Fishbein GA, Fishbein MC, et al. Coronary atherosclerotic lesions in human immunodeficiency virus–infected patients: a histopathologic study. Cardiovasc Pathol 2009;18:28–36. Available at: http://www.sciencedirect.com/science/article/pii/S1054880708000021.
11. Sani MU, Okeahialam BN. QTc interval prolongation in patients with HIV and AIDS. J Natl Med Assoc 2005;97(12):1657–61. Available at: http://www.ncbi.nlm.nih.gov/pmc/articles/PMC2640718/pdf/jnma00868-0059.pdf.
12. Charbit B, Rosier A, Bollens D, et al. Relationship between HIV protease inhibitors and QTc interval duration in HIV-infected patients: a cross-sectional study. Br J Clin Pharmacol 2008;67(1):76–82. Available at: http://onlinelibrary.wiley.com/store/10.1111/j.1365-2125.2008.03332.x/asset/j.1365-2125.2008.03332.x.pdf?v=1&t=hs7ij74d&s=b08b7d94722a35d75f857f62d87aa1305f5a1bdb.
13. Chow DC, Wood R, Choi J, et al. Cardiovagal autonomic function in HIV-infected patients with unsuppressed HIV viremia. HIV Clin Trials 2011;12(3):141–50.
14. Soliman EZ, Lundgren JD, Roediger MP, et al. Boosted protease inhibitors and the electrocardiographic measures of QT and PR durations. AIDS 2011;25(3):

367–77. Available at: http://www.ncbi.nlm.nih.gov/pmc/articles/PMC3111078/?report=reader.

15. Hsu JC, Yongmei L, Marcus GM, et al. Atrial fibrillation and atrial flutter in human immunodeficiency virus-infected persons: incidence, risk factors, and association with markers of HIV disease severity. J Am Coll Cardiol 2013; 61(22):2288–95. Available at: http://www.sciencedirect.com/science/article/pii/S0735109713013065.

16. Fisher SD, Kanda BS, Miller TL, et al. Cardiovascular disease and therapeutic drug-related cardiovascular consequences in HIV-infected patients. Am J Cardiovasc Drugs 2011;11(6):383–94. Available at: http://link.springer.com/article/10.2165/11594590-000000000-00000.

17. Barbarini G, Barbaro G. Incidence of the involvement of the cardiovascular system in HIV infection. AIDS 2003;17(1):46–50. Available at: http://www.ncbi.nlm.nih.gov/pubmed/12870530.

18. Barbaro G. HIV-associated cardiomyopathy: etiopathogenesis and clinical aspects. Herz 2005;30(6):486–92. Available at: http://link.springer.com/article/10.1007/s00059-005-2728-z.

19. Barbaro G, Barbarini G. Human immunodeficiency virus and cardiovascular risk. Indian J Med Res 2011;134(6):898–903. Available at: http://www.ncbi.nlm.nih.gov/pmc/articles/PMC3284097/.

20. Khunnawat C, Mukerji S, Havlichek D, et al. Cardiovascular manifestations in human immunodeficiency virus-infected patients. Am J Cardiol 2008;102(5):635–42. Available at: http://www.ajconline.org/article/S0002-9149(08)00793-5/abstract.

21. Lind A, Reinsh N, Neuhaus K, et al, the HIV-HEART Study on behalf of the Competence Network of Heart Failure and the Competence Network of HIV/AIDS. Pericardial effusion of HIV-infected patients - results of a prospective multicenter cohort study in the era of antiretroviral therapy. Eur J Med Res 2011;16:480–3. Available at: http://www.ncbi.nlm.nih.gov/pmc/articles/PMC3351804/.

22. Mishra R. Cardiac emergencies in patients with HIV. Emerg Med Clin North Am 2010;28(2):273–82. Available at: http://www.sciencedirect.com/science/article/pii/S0733862710000064.

23. Silva-Cardoso J, Moura B, Martins L, et al. Pericardial involvement in human immunodeficiency virus infection. Chest 1999;115:418–22. Available at: http://journal.publications.chestnet.org/article.aspx?articleid=1076832.

24. Mayosi BM, Burgess LJ, Doubell AF. Tuberculous pericarditis. Circulation 2005; 112:3608–16. Available at: http://circ.ahajournals.org/content/112/23/3608.long.

25. Cheitlin M. Cardiac and vascular disease in HIV infected patients. In: UpToDate Walham (MA): UpToDate; 2014. Assessed October, 2013.

26. Reinsch N, Esser S, Gelbrich G, et al, on behalf of the German Competence Network Heart Failure and the German Competence Network for HIV/AIDS. Valvular manifestations of human immunodeficiency virus infection – results from the prospective, multicenter HIV-HEART study. J Cardiovasc Med 2013;14:733–9. Available at: http://www.ncbi.nlm.nih.gov/pubmed/?term=Valvular+manifestations+of+human+immunodeficiency+virus+infection+-+results+from+the+prospective,+multicenter+HIV-HEART+Study.

27. Mangili A, Polak JF, Skinner SC, et al. HIV infection and progression of carotid and coronary atherosclerosis: the CARE study. J Acquir Immune Defic Syndr 2011; 58:148–53. Available at: http://www.ncbi.nlm.nih.gov/pubmed/?term=HIV+Infection+and+Progression+of+Carotid+and+Coronary+Atherosclerosis:+The+CARE+Study.

28. Moayedi S, Torres M. Cardiac disease in special populations: HIV, pregnancy and cancer. In: Mattu A, Brady WJ, Bresler MJ, et al, editors. Cardiovascular emergencies. Dallas (TX): American College of Emergency Physicians; 2014.
29. Fuchs SC, Alencastro PR, Ikeda ML, et al. Risk of coronary heart disease among HIV-infected patients - a multicenter study in Brazil. ScientificWorldJournal 2013; 2013:1–8. Available at: http://www.hindawi.com/journals/tswj/2013/163418/.
30. Islam FM, Wu J, Jansson J, et al. Relative risk of cardiovascular disease among people living with HIV: a systematic review and meta-analysis. HIV Med 2012;3: 453–68. Available at: http://onlinelibrary.wiley.com/doi/10.1111/j.1468-1293.2012. 00996.x/abstract.

Management of Crashing Patients with Pulmonary Hypertension

John C. Greenwood, MD[a],*, Ryan M. Spangler, MD[b]

KEYWORDS

- Pulmonary hypertension • Right ventricular failure • Cardiogenic shock

KEY POINTS

- Management goals for patients with pulmonary hypertension (PH) are to optimize preload and volume status, maintain right ventricular function, prevent right coronary artery malperfusion, reduce right ventricular afterload, and reverse the underlying cause whenever possible.
- Right ventricular failure is a hallmark finding in patients with decompensated PH.
- The bedside echocardiogram is the most useful tool when evaluating patients with PH and suspected right heart failure.
- Atrial fibrillation, atrial flutter, and atrioventricular nodal reentrant tachycardia are the most common dysrhythmias in patients with PH. Rhythm control is preferred over rate control in patients with severe PH.
- Unmonitored continuous fluid administration should be avoided in patients with PH because it often worsens pressure overload of the right heart.

INTRODUCTION

Critically ill patients with pulmonary hypertension (PH) often seem well, but they can decompensate dramatically in a short time. PH has several causes, classes, and complications; but the natural progression eventually leads to right ventricular (RV) failure, which can be extraordinarily difficult to manage. The purpose of this review is to discuss the causes, signs, and symptoms of PH as well as its management strategies and emergent complications. Treatment options are often limited, so it is imperative

Funding sources: nothing to disclose.
Conflict of interest: nothing to disclose.
[a] Department of Emergency Medicine, Ground floor, Ravdin Hospital of the University of Pennsylvania, 3400 Spruce Street, Philadelphia, PA 19104, USA; [b] Department of Emergency Medicine, University of Maryland School of Medicine, 110 South Paca Street, 6th Floor, Baltimore, MD 21201, USA
* Corresponding author.
E-mail address: johncgreenwood@gmail.com

Emerg Med Clin N Am 33 (2015) 623–643
http://dx.doi.org/10.1016/j.emc.2015.04.012
0733-8627/15/$ – see front matter © 2015 Elsevier Inc. All rights reserved.

that the emergency department (ED) physician can recognize and manage these patients in a timely fashion.

CLASSIFICATION

PH is defined by an elevated mean pulmonary artery pressure (PAP) ($\geq$25 mm Hg) during right heart catheterization (normal, 14–20 mm Hg).[1,2] The first classification of PH was published by the World Health Organization (WHO) in 1973. The classification has been revised several times since then. The current structure, with 5 groups (**Table 1**), is based on cause, physiology, pathology, and treatment (**Fig. 1**).

Group 1 PH is defined by a pulmonary wedge pressure of 15 mm Hg or less, indicating isolated pulmonary arterial hypertension (PAH) and normal left ventricular (LV) function.[2] This group has a much lower prevalence than the others.[3] In 1970, the histologic differences between this group and the others were delineated.[4] The difference is thought to be the result of a variety of homeostatic imbalances related to vasoactive chemicals, growth factors, and prothrombotic and antithrombotic

Table 1 Current classification of PH	
Group 1	PAH 1.1 Idiopathic PAH 1.2 Heritable PAH 1.3 Drug and toxin induced 1.4 Associated with connective tissue disorders, HIV infection, portal hypertension, congenital heart disease, schistosomiasis
Group 1′	Pulmonary venoocclusive disease and/or pulmonary capillary hemangiomatosis
Group 2	PH caused by left heart disease 2.1 Left ventricular systolic dysfunction 2.2 Left ventricular diastolic dysfunction 2.3 Valvular disease 2.4 Congenital/acquired left heart inflow/outflow tract obstruction and congenital cardiomyopathies
Group 3	PH caused by lung diseases and/or hypoxia 3.1 Chronic obstructive pulmonary disease 3.2 Interstitial lung disease 3.3 Other pulmonary diseases with mixed restrictive and obstructive pattern 3.4 Sleep-disordered breathing 3.5 Alveolar hypoventilation disorders 3.6 Chronic exposure to high altitude 3.7 Developmental lung diseases
Group 4	Chronic thromboembolic PH
Group 5	PH with unclear multifactorial mechanisms 5.1 Hematologic disorders: chronic hemolytic anemia, myeloproliferative disorders, splenectomy 5.2 Systemic disorders: sarcoidosis, pulmonary histiocytosis, lymphangioleiomyomatosis 5.3 Metabolic disorders: glycogen storage disease, Gaucher disease, thyroid disorders 5.4 Others: tumoral obstruction, fibrosing mediastinitis, chronic renal failure, segmental PH

Abbreviations: HIV, human immunodeficiency virus; PAH, pulmonary arterial hypertension.

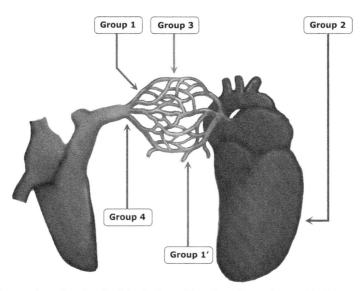

Fig. 1. Anatomic and pathophysiological considerations for patients with PH.

chemicals in the pulmonary vasculature.[5] Group 1 is broken into subgroups based on cause.

Several drugs have been implicated as causing PAH and can be important in assessing patients' overall risk of disease (**Table 2**).[6] In the 1960s, an epidemic of PAH was linked to appetite-suppressing drugs. Toxic rapeseed oil and selective serotonin reuptake inhibitors have been implicated as risk factors for the development of PAH.[7–9] Chin and colleagues[10] found that nearly 30% of the patients with PAH in their study had a history of stimulant use (methamphetamine, amphetamine, cocaine); however, direct causation has not been proven.

Heritable PAH is associated with several acquired and congenital conditions as well as connective tissue disorders, infection with the human immunodeficiency virus (HIV), portal hypertension, and congenital heart defects.[11] Patients with a history of scleroderma or with congenital heart disease are at a particularly high risk of mortality when diagnosed with PAH.[12,13] Schistosomiasis is the most prevalent cause of PAH worldwide, with mortality approaching 15% at 3 years.[14,15]

Pulmonary venoocclusive disease (PVOD) and pulmonary capillary hemangiomatosis (PCH) share the unique category of group 1'. This distinction was made because,

Table 2
Drugs that can cause PH

Definite Association	Likely Association	Possible Association
Aminorex	Amphetamines	Cocaine
Fenfluramine	L-tryptophan	Phenylpropanolamine
Dexfenfluramine	Methamphetamines	St. John's wort
Toxic rapeseed oil	Dasatinib	Chemotherapeutic agents
Benfluorex	—	Interferon α and β
Selective serotonin reuptake inhibitor	—	Amphetaminelike drugs

although PVOD and PCH often cause pathologic changes similar to those seen in group 1 PAH and have similar risk factors, they can cause physical examination findings distinct from those associated with idiopathic PAH.[16] Clinical outcomes in these patients also tend to be worse than for those with group 1 PAH.[17]

Most patients with PH will be classified as group 2 PH, which is often a result of significant left heart disease or left-sided valvular abnormalities.[18] Untreated LV systolic or diastolic dysfunction as well as mitral regurgitation, mitral stenosis, and aortic stenosis can all cause chronically elevated pulmonary vascular pressures, leading to the development of PH. The inciting factor is the backward transmission of pressures resulting from valvular or LV dysfunction, causing what is initially a transient increase in pulmonary vascular pressure. However, over time, this increased pressure results in vascular remodeling and a new fixed PH.[19]

Group 3 encompasses several primary pulmonary disorders (eg, emphysema/chronic obstructive pulmonary disease and interstitial lung disease) plus causes of chronic hypoxemia (eg, living at high altitude and cystic fibrosis). Hypoxemia itself constricts the pulmonary vasculature through a variety of neurohormonal and cellular mechanisms, which, over time, leads to vascular hypertrophy and sustained PH.[20] Most group 3 patients have mild pulmonary pressure elevation but rarely go on to develop severe PH (mean PAP >40 mm Hg).[21,22]

Group 4 PH, referred to as chronic thromboembolic PH (CTEPH), occurs in approximately 4% of patients after acute pulmonary embolism (PE).[23] It is thought that PH develops in patients with chronic PE as a result of persistent macrovascular obstruction that causes small vessel arteriopathy, leading to persistent small vessel pulmonary vasoconstriction and thrombosis in situ.[24,25]

Group 5 comprises multiple forms of PH with unknown cause. These forms include hematologic, systemic, metabolic, and mechanical disorders. The 2 diseases in this category that are most commonly implicated are sarcoidosis and thyroid disease.[26,27]

RIGHT VENTRICULAR DYSFUNCTION

In healthy patients, the RV is a thin-walled, crescent-shaped structure that shares the intraventricular septum with the LV. Together, the free wall and the septum contribute equally to RV function. The free wall of the RV is highly elastic and responds readily to changes in volume, whereas the LV is less compliant and more suited to overcome changes in pressure. Normally, the RV is required to generate only 25% of the stroke work because of the low resistance of the pulmonary vasculature.[28] The principle of ventricular interdependence is important, as superficial myocardial fibers encircle both ventricles and the RV and LV work collectively in series to maintain cardiac output. Because the ventricles share an intraventricular septum, and both are contained within the same pericardial cavity (except in patients who have undergone cardiac surgery), any disruption in the size or shape of these cavities can have deleterious effects on cardiac output.[29,30]

Unlike the LV, the thin, compliant RV is unable to overcome large changes in afterload. In the presence of chronic PH, the RV is subjected to pressure overload because of excessive pulmonary vascular resistance (PVR). Chronic elevations in PVR cause the RV to undergo both adaptive (preserved systolic and diastolic function) and maladaptive remodeling (causing RV dysfunction).

Sustained elevations in PVR cause a pressure-induced growth of RV cardiomyocytes and proliferation of a collagen-based extracellular matrix.[31–33] RV enlargement encroaches on LV filling, decreasing cardiac output. Reduced RV function is often characterized by uncoupling of the RV and pulmonary vasculature, leading to disruption of the normal relationship between the RV and the pulmonary arterial tree.[34] Changes in the anatomic structure of the RV eventually result in systolic and diastolic dysfunction of both ventricles as well as increase the risk of dysrhythmias related to abnormal conduction.[35,36]

Perfusion of the right coronary artery (RCA) is severely impaired in patients with advanced PH.[37] The blood supply of the RV's free wall varies according to the anatomic dominance of the coronary system. In approximately 80% of the general population, the RCA provides perfusion to the RV.[38,39] The left anterior descending coronary artery supplies the anterior two-thirds of the septum, and the posterior descending artery supplies the inferoposterior third.[28]

Under normal circumstances, the RCA is perfused during both systole and diastole.[40] As RV remodeling progresses in patients with chronic PH, elevation in RV wall tension and transmural pressure impairs RCA systolic perfusion to the point that blood flow occurs almost exclusively during diastole.[37,41–43] Malperfusion of the RCA leads to RV ischemia and an increased risk of arrhythmias and can rapidly precipitate RV failure.

EMERGENCY DEPARTMENT PRESENTATION

PH in patients presenting to the ED can be very difficult to recognize and diagnose. In general, the symptoms are highly nonspecific and slow to progress. Therefore, patients often go undiagnosed and are managed improperly for a long time, even if they are symptomatic. Despite increasing clinical education and awareness, 20% of cases of symptomatic PAH are undiagnosed for more than 2 years.[3,44]

Of even greater concern is that most patients with PAH do not receive a diagnosis until they are severely debilitated (WHO functional classes III and IV) and have a much higher risk of death.[3,45,46] It is critical to assess for PH risk factors (**Table 3**) is an important tool.

Many of the presenting complaints associated with PH are nonspecific. The most common is dyspnea, either on exertion or at rest, occurring in 60% to 99% of cases.[3,44,47] Other presenting symptoms include peripheral edema, chest pain, syncope, lightheadedness, palpitations, and fatigue.[48,49] Syncope or presyncope suggests more severe disease. It is seen in up to one-third of patients with PH and has a variety of mechanisms, including fixed cardiac output, arrhythmias, and cardiac ischemia.

In addition to the patients' history, several clues suggesting PH can be picked up on the physical examination. A midsystolic murmur, early systolic click, left parasternal lift, and prominent jugular pulsation are all associated with increased PAP.[47,50] An accentuated P2 heart sound is found in almost 90% of patients.[51] Central cyanosis from Eisenmenger syndrome, clubbing caused by chronic lung disease,

Table 3 Risk factors for PH		
Definite	**Likely**	**Possible**
Drugs and toxins[a]	Portal hypertension	Pregnancy
Female sex	Connective tissue disorder	Systemic hypertension
HIV infection	Congenital systemic-pulmonary cardiac shunts	Thyroid disorder

[a] See **Table 2**.

Adapted from Galiè N, Torbicki A, Barst R, et al. Guidelines on diagnosis and treatment of pulmonary arterial hypertension. Eur Heart J 2004;25:2243–78.

hepatomegaly, spider angiomas, or signs of scleroderma and other connective tissue disorders might also be seen. Hypotension, decreased pulse pressure, and cool extremities could indicate impending cardiovascular collapse.

DIAGNOSTIC STUDIES

When evaluating ED patients with suspected PH, several laboratory and diagnostic studies can be useful (**Table 4**). Electrocardiography, chest radiography, and computed tomography (CT) are commonly performed and should be considered.

Laboratory Testing

Laboratory assessment of symptomatic patients with PH is often critical and should be directed toward excluding cardiac ischemia and new end-organ dysfunction and assessing global perfusion. Specific tests to be considered include measurement of troponin I to look for signs of myocardial strain and ischemia as well as a lactic acid to evaluate for systemic hypoperfusion. Laboratory testing for electrolyte imbalances, anemia, liver function, and coagulopathy can provide prognostic information as well as give clues to an underlying correctable disturbance.[46,52]

Measurement of B-type natriuretic peptide (BNP) can be helpful in the acute setting if the current level can be compared with previous values. This comparison can indicate RV dysfunction in acutely decompensated patients.[53,54] An increase in the BNP or troponin value or worsening renal function is associated with a higher mortality rate.[46,55]

Electrocardiogram

The electrocardiogram (ECG) is a cheap, rapid, and valuable diagnostic tool for patients with known or suspected PH. Common ECG findings in patients with PH are listed in **Box 1**. They are often the result of significant right heart dysfunction.

Right axis deviation is found in 70% of patients with PH, along with signs of RV hypertrophy, such as an incomplete right bundle branch block or a tall R wave in V1.[56] A tall P wave in the inferior leads can indicate right atrial enlargement.[57] Signs of RV strain include ST depressions and T-wave inversions in the inferior and right precordial lead.[57] The mortality rate may be increased among patients with PH and evidence of right ventricular hypertrophy (defined by the WHO criteria) and dysfunction.[57]

The most common arrhythmias in patients with PH are supraventricular tachycardias, including AV nodal reentrant tachycardia, atrial fibrillation, and atrial flutter.[48] It is imperative to recognize any dysrhythmia and treat it quickly. Atrial fibrillation is

Table 4 Testing for suspected PH	
Emergency Testing	**Beyond the ED**
ECG	VQ scan
Chest film	MRI
Echocardiography	Pulmonary function tests
CT scan	6-min walk test
Troponin	Right heart catheterization
BNP	Genetic testing

Abbreviations: BNP, B-type natriuretic peptide; CT, computed tomography; ECG, electrocardiogram.

Box 1
Common ECG findings associated with PH

Normal sinus rhythm

Right-axis deviation

Right bundle branch block

rSR′ in V1

qR V1

Large inferior P waves

ST depression or T-wave inversion inferiorly and in the V1

RV hypertrophy

---

particularly malignant in patients with PH and is associated with a mortality rate exceeding 80%.[48] Tachydysrhythmias are particularly problematic, as the loss of an atrial kick can impair ventricular filling, leading to a reduction of cardiac output and rapid cardiovascular collapse (**Fig. 2**).

Chest Radiography

A chest radiograph should be obtained in any symptomatic patient with suspected PH. Common findings on the anterior-posterior view include enlarged hilar pulmonary arterial shadow, pulmonary venous congestion, increased peripheral vascular markings (pruning), prominent right heart border, and right atrial enlargement. A common radiologic phenomenon is vascular pruning, characterized as enlarged proximal pulmonary arterial shadows that have an early, dramatic taper toward the periphery (**Fig. 3**).[47] In the lateral view, obliteration of the retrosternal space could indicate RV enlargement caused by dilation or hypertrophy. However, the absence of these findings does not exclude PH as a possible diagnosis, as they are not universally present.[47,58]

Computed Tomography

CT of the chest can be helpful when evaluating patients with suspected PH because it can show structural abnormalities of the heart and lung as well as vascular abnormalities if performed with intravenous contrast or angiography. RV enlargement, hypertrophy, and dysfunction can be well visualized on a CT scan. Other findings suggestive of PH include a main pulmonary artery diameter greater than 30 mm.[60] In fact, there is a 96% positive predictive value for PH if the maximum transverse diameter of the main pulmonary artery is greater than the diameter of the proximal ascending thoracic aorta (**Fig. 4**).[60]

For any patient with new cardiopulmonary symptoms and known PH, early chest CT should be considered strongly to evaluate for a new PE. Patients with chronic PH are at higher risk for acute PE caused by preexisting RV dysfunction and reduced pulmonary vascular flow. Even small acute PE can cause hemodynamic deterioration in these patients. Current CT scans are valuable, as they can often differentiate old from new thrombotic material.

Echocardiography

Echocardiography is one of the most useful diagnostic tools for the emergency physician when evaluating patients with suspected PH. A rapid, bedside transthoracic

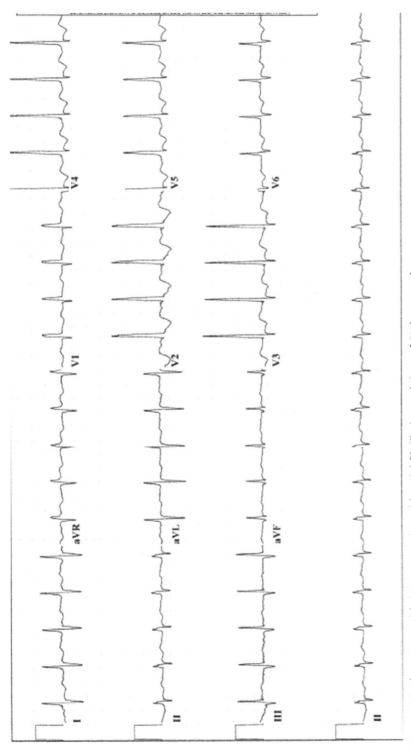

Fig. 2. ECG of a patient with PAH, presenting with atrial fibrillation and signs of RV hypertrophy.

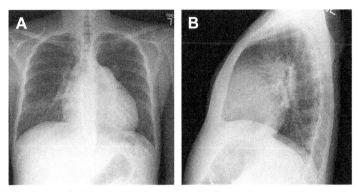

Fig. 3. (*A*) Evidence of right atrial enlargement and vascular pruning on posteroanterior chest radiograph of patient with PAH. (*B*) Obliteration of the retrosternal space on lateral chest radiography indicating RV hypertrophy or enlargement.

echocardiogram (TTE) often provides critical diagnostic information about the functional status of the right and left sides of the heart. Evaluation of the RV is the single most important component of the echocardiographic examination.

In the presence of elevated pulmonary pressures, patients often develop right atrial and RV dilation. In contrast to PH secondary to acute PE, in which the RV is dilated and thin, the RV in most patients with PH is thickened (**Fig. 5**) (seen in almost all standard TTE views).

Other signs of RV dysfunction include an RV:LV ratio greater than 1 in the apical 4-chamber view or an RV end-diastolic diameter greater than 20 mm with or without inspiratory collapse of the inferior vena cava.[61] Signs of RV pressure overload can be found by focusing on the shape of the intraventricular septum in the parasternal short-axis view. The classic D sign can be seen as the septum shifts paradoxically toward the LV during early diastole. Complete bowing of the septum into the LV is a poor prognostic sign and can indicate severe RV overload or end-stage disease, impairing LV filling (**Fig. 6**).[49,59]

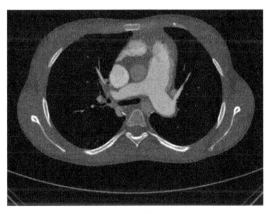

Fig. 4. Chest CT scan showing signs of PH, including vascular pruning and a main pulmonary artery diameter greater than the proximal ascending aorta.

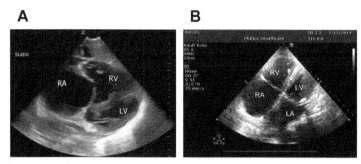

Fig. 5. (A) Evidence of chronic PH caused by dilated and hypertrophied RV with a dilated RA. (B) Evidence of acute PH with dilated and thin RV and atrium. LA, left atrium; RA, right atrium.

INITIAL MANAGEMENT

In general, the primary management goals should focus on identifying the underlying cause and improving RV function. Patients with symptomatic PH can progress rapidly to obstructive shock, cardiogenic shock, or cardiac arrest. RV systolic dysfunction, secondary LV dysfunction, severe tricuspid regurgitation, and arrhythmias can contribute to low cardiac output and hypotension. Specific attention should be directed toward optimizing intravascular volume (preload), RV systolic function, RCA perfusion, and RV afterload. It is important to note that guidelines for the management of patients with PH have not been published, so most current recommendations are based on expert opinion.

Preload and Volume Status

Intravascular volume assessment in patients with PH can be extraordinarily difficult. Traditional methods of assessing fluid responsiveness, such as central venous pressure, pulse pressure variation, and stroke volume variation, are unreliable in patients with RV dysfunction.[62,63] Elevation in plasma atrial natriuretic peptide and BNP seems to increase proportionately to the extent of RV dysfunction in patients with PH.[54,64] The traditional gold standard for the diagnosis and management of PH and RV

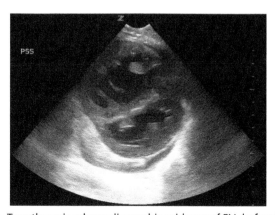

Fig. 6. The D sign. Transthoracic echocardiographic evidence of RV dysfunction and pressure overload.

dysfunction is pulmonary artery catheterization (PAC). Although PAC can aid in diagnosis, its routine use has not been shown to improve patient outcomes.[65,66]

The goal of fluid resuscitation in patients with PH is to ensure adequate, but not excessive, RV preload. Most patients with PH have elevated right heart pressures at baseline but can augment their cardiac output with intravenous fluid administration.[67] As a result, most experts agree that aggressive volume loading should be avoided in patients with evidence of increased RV filling pressures. Administering intravenous fluids to patients with a measured right atrial pressure or central venous pressure of greater than 10 to 15 mm Hg can worsen right heart performance by further distending the RV, increasing the septal shift toward the LV, and consequently worsen cardiac output by further distorting ventricular interdependence.[68]

For hemodynamically stable patients with volume overload, diuretic therapy can be considered, with a goal of maintaining a negative fluid balance, as many patients have an overstretched RV operating on the flat portion of the Frank-Starling curve. Diuretics have been a conventional therapy for patients with PH related to pulmonary vascular disease or LV failure.[69] Common agents, such as furosemide or bumetanide, may be used in patients with an adequate glomerular filtration rate and should be adjusted according to the patients' hemodynamic response.

For hypotensive patients with PH, or those who seem to be hypovolemic, a 500-mL bolus of an isotonic crystalloid solution should be administered. Repeated boluses may be administered but should be monitored to confirm a favorable hemodynamic response. RV failure and hypotension are more often the result of increased RV afterload and hypervolemia rather than volume depletion.[70] Continuous, unmonitored fluid administration is not recommended. Many unstable patients with PH who are hypervolemic require early initiation of vasopressor and inotropic medications rather than repeated fluid boluses.

Optimize Right Ventricular Systolic Function

In addition to preload optimization, RV systolic function should be maximized. Inotropic therapy is often required for patients with advanced PH and should be considered if there is evidence of inadequate oxygen delivery or volume overload that cannot be managed with diuretics alone.

The two most commonly used inotropic medications are dobutamine and milrinone. Dobutamine is a selective β_1-agonist that increases myocardial contractility, reduces PVR and systemic vascular resistance (SVR), and improves PA/RV coupling. It is the preferred inotropic medication for patients with PH.[69,71,72] Dobutamine is superior to vasopressors (eg, norepinephrine) alone in patients with process-induced right heart failure.[72] In normotensive patients with PH with RV dysfunction, a dobutamine infusion should be initiated at 2 mcg/kg/min and titrated to a maximum of 10 mcg/kg/min. Infusion rates greater than 10 mcg/kg/min should be avoided, as they have been shown to increase RV afterload and produce reflexive tachycardia and are associated with an increased mortality rate.[72,73] It is important to anticipate complications, such as systemic hypotension, secondary to dobutamine's $\beta2$-mediated systemic vasodilatory properties. If hypotension does occur, vasopressor therapy should be initiated rapidly.

Milrinone is a selective phosphodiesterase-3 inhibitor that increases contractility by increasing cyclic AMP levels and the concentration of intracellular calcium. In patients with pulmonary vascular dysfunction in the setting of multifactorial PH, LV failure, postventricular assist, or cardiac transplantation, milrinone has been shown to reduce pulmonary pressures and improve RV function.[74–76] A milrinone infusion can be started at 0.375 mcg/kg/min and titrated to a maximum of 0.75 mcg/kg/min. The use of milrinone is also limited by systemic hypotension at higher doses and might require the coadministration of vasopressor therapy.

Maintain Right Coronary Artery Perfusion

Preservation of RCA perfusion to prevent RV ischemia requires a mean arterial blood pressure that is greater than the PAP. If PVR exceeds SVR, RCA perfusion will occur only during diastole, which leads to increased RV ischemia.[37] In hypotensive patients with PH, vasopressor therapy should be instituted promptly to increase the SVR:PVR ratio and preserve coronary blood flow.

Little has been published regarding the use of specific vasopressors in the setting of PH. Norepinephrine is considered by many to be the vasopressor of choice, as it improves RV function through increases in SVR and cardiac output. In a comparison with dopamine, norepinephrine was found to have a lower 28-day mortality rate in patients with cardiogenic shock and a reduced rate of tachydysrhythmias.[77] The initial dosage of norepinephrine is 0.05 mcg/kg/min. Although there is no true maximum dose of norepinephrine, higher doses have been reported to cause pulmonary vasoconstriction, a detrimental effect for patients with impaired RV function.

Vasopressin is an intriguing vasopressor option, given its minimal effect on PVR. At lower doses, vasopressin may in fact cause pulmonary vasodilation through the production of endothelium-mediated nitric oxide (NO), but its role in managing decompensated patients with PH requires further investigation.[69] Phenylephrine is a potent α1-adrenergic agonist and a strong arteriolar vasoconstrictor that can worsen RV pressure overload in patients with chronic PH.[78,79] In general, phenylephrine should be avoided in patients with PH because it increases mean PAP and PVR, thereby worsening RV systolic function.

Reduce Right Ventricular Afterload

Increased RV afterload caused by excessive PAP is often the central cause of decompensation in patients with PH. RV afterload can be reduced by ensuring adequate oxygenation, avoiding prolonged hypercapnia, minimizing acidosis, and administering pulmonary vasodilators. Prolonged hypoxemia and hypercapnia are common precipitants of increased PVR.[80–82] Supportive therapy should begin with supplemental oxygen to maintain the arterial oxygen saturation greater than 90%.[70,83] Adequate oxygenation has been shown to selectively dilate pulmonary vasculature and improve cardiac output, regardless of the primary cause of PH.[84] Continuous positive airway pressure or noninvasive, bilevel positive airway pressure ventilation may be considered and can be particularly helpful when managing patients with group 2 or group 3 PH but should be used with caution if there is a concern for inadequate preload.

Every attempt should be made to avoid endotracheal intubation and mechanical ventilation. Initiation of positive-pressure ventilation in unstable patients with PH can have negative hemodynamic effects by increasing PVR and reducing venous return. If mechanical ventilation is required, etomidate is the preferred induction agent because of its minimal effect on SVR, PVR, and cardiac contractility. The use of lung-protective ventilator settings is recommended to avoid ventilator-associated lung injury and increases in PVR. Permissive hypercapnia should be avoided, as it can increase PVR by approximately 50% and mean PAP by approximately 30%.[85] Plateau pressures should be monitored frequently, the goal plateau pressure being less than 30 cm H_2O. Excessive plateau pressures can cause direct compression of the pulmonary vasculature, further increasing PVR.

Nitric oxide

Inhaled NO (iNO) is a potent pulmonary vasodilator that can be administered by face mask as a temporizing measure to prevent intubation or during mechanical ventilation. Local effects of iNO include a reduction in PAP and PVR, improved oxygenation, and reversal of hypoxic vasoconstriction without affecting SVR or cardiac output.[71,86] iNO therapy seems to have a short-term benefit in patients with acute right heart failure secondary to PH but does not seem to provide an overall mortality benefit other than for patients with acute postoperative PH.[87,88] Abrupt discontinuation of iNO therapy can result in rebound PH and, therefore, should be avoided. Prolonged iNO therapy has also been associated with methemoglobinemia, so it is recommended that serum concentrations should be determined before initiation of therapy and monitored every 6 hours during treatment.[59]

Continuous infusions of pulmonary vasodilators are rarely administered to treatment-naïve or hemodynamically unstable patients with PH in the ED. Given their frequent use in patients with stable PAH, it is important for the emergency physician to be familiar with them. The pulmonary vasodilators that are commonly used in PH are prostanoids, phosphodiesterase inhibitors, and endothelin receptor antagonists. For any patient with PH presenting to the ED, it is critical to determine if any of these medications have been discontinued abruptly. If so, the medication must be reinitiated as soon as possible to prevent rebound PH and cardiovascular collapse.[89,90] In all cases, these medications can be restarted through a peripheral intravenous catheter and do not require immediate central venous access.

Prostanoids

Most patients with previously diagnosed, advanced PAH are receiving continuous prostanoid therapy. Epoprostenol, treprostinil, and iloprost cause pulmonary vasodilation and have both antiplatelet and antiproliferative effects. Their effects are often limited by hypotension as well as nausea, flushing, headache, and diarrhea.[91] Prostacyclin treatment should be avoided in patients with significant LV dysfunction, as initiation can lead to the development of worsening pulmonary edema and further reduce LV function.[92]

Epoprostenol was the first therapy approved for use in advanced PAH and classically is the initial treatment of choice. It is administered continuously through a peripherally inserted central catheter. This drug has an extremely short half-life of just 2 to 5 minutes.[93,94] Treprostinil can be administered through a continuous intravenous infusion or subcutaneously. In contrast to epoprostenol, the half-life of treprostinil is approximately 4 to 5 hours, making it a more attractive alternative for outpatient management. The initial dosages and half-lives of prostanoids are listed in **Table 5**. If infusion pump malfunction or catheter occlusion occurs, both epoprostenol and treprostinil can be administered through a peripheral intravenous catheter. In patients

| Table 5 | | | | |
| Prostenoid infusions for use in PAH | | | | |
Drug	Starting Dosage	Target Dosage	Half-life	Steady State
Epoprostenol (IV)	2.0 μg/kg/min	20–40 μg/kg/min	2–5 min[a]	15 min
Treprostinil (SC)	1.25 μg/kg/min	40 μg/kg/min	4.0–4.5 h	10 h
Treprostinil (IV)	1.25 μg/kg/min	40 μg/kg/min	4.0–4.5 h	10 h

Abbreviations: IV, intravenous; SC, subcutaneous.
[a] At a temperature of 37°C and a pH of 7.4.

with PAH on chronic prostacyclin therapy, treatment can be reinitiated at the home infusion rate if they are hemodynamically stable. If they are unstable, or presenting with vasodilatory or mixed shock, lower infusion rates can be considered; but it is important to weigh the risks of worsening systemic hypotension with the benefits of treatment.

Phosphodiesterase inhibitors

Phosphodiesterase-5 (PDE-5) inhibitors (eg, sildenafil) increase cyclic GMP signaling and can potentiate the effects of NO. PDE-5 inhibitors can reduce PVR acutely, increase cardiac output, and reduce pulmonary capillary wedge pressure. Although these agents can improve clinical end points in stable patients with chronic PAH, their use has not been evaluated in setting of acute RV failure, so they should not be used in the acute setting.[70,89]

ADDITIONAL CONSIDERATIONS
Dysrhythmias

Atrial dysrhythmias represent one of the most common precipitants of acute decompensation in patients with PH. Supraventricular tachydysrhythmias, specifically atrial fibrillation and atrial flutter, are the most prevalent, with an annual incidence of 2.8% in patients with PAH or inoperable CTEPH.[48] More than 80% of patients with PH presenting with atrial fibrillation or atrial flutter experience hemodynamic compromise or acute RV failure. The incidence of tachydysrhythmias in patients with PH is an independent predictor of death.[48,95] In general, most patients with atrial fibrillation or atrial flutter should be managed aggressively with electrical or chemical cardioversion to restore sinus rhythm.[48] Rate control with β-adrenergic receptor antagonists or calcium channel blockers is not recommended, as these medications can impair cardiac contractility, leading to cardiogenic shock.

Anemia

Underlying hemoglobinopathies and significant anemia can worsen RV ischemia in the setting of PH. In decompensated patients with PH, the transfusion risks along with consideration of the patients' volume status must be weighed against the potential benefit, as specific transfusion thresholds are not well established. General practice would suggest to maintain a hemoglobin level greater than7 g/dL; however, the ideal level in patients with RV failure secondary to PH has never been studied.[96] Theoretically, reduced oxygen-carrying capacity secondary to worsening anemia or specific hemoglobinopathies could exacerbate RV ischemia. Some investigators have suggested that hemoglobin levels should be maintained at greater than 10 g/dL.[70,97]

Anticoagulation

Anticoagulation therapy is a mainstay of outpatient treatment of patients with idiopathic PAH and CTEPH. A goal international normalized ratio of 2.0 to 3.0 in patients with CTEPH has been suggested and of 1.5 to 2.5 in those receiving long-term continuous prostacyclin therapy.[2,98] Oral anticoagulation therapy has been associated with improved outcomes; however, specific therapeutic targets have not been well established.[83] Data for anticoagulation of patients with PH in the acute setting are also lacking. If an acute venothromboembolic event is suspected to be the precipitant cause of clinical decompensation, unfractionated heparin should be initiated, starting at 18 units/kg/h, with a goal activated partial thromboplastin time of 1.5 to 2.5 times the control.

Mechanical Circulatory Support

The use of extracorporeal life support (ECLS) or extracorporeal membrane oxygenation (ECMO) has been reported as salvage therapy for patients with PH in refractory shock.[95,99,100] The purpose of ECLS is to provide a bridge to definitive treatment, such as transplantation or initiation of pulmonary vasodilator therapy.[101] For severely hypoxic patients with early signs of RV failure, percutaneous venovenous ECMO can be initiated rapidly and improve hemodynamics significantly by reversing hypoxic pulmonary vasoconstriction and the deleterious effects of severe acidemia. In the setting of imminent cardiovascular collapse, percutaneous venoarterial ECMO can be performed to provide both cardiovascular and pulmonary support. After ECMO is initiated, many patients experience a rapid reversal of hemodynamics, decreased vasopressor requirements, reduced inotropic dependence, improved gas exchange, and increased end-organ perfusion.[102] The use of ECLS in patients with PH is extremely resource intensive and should be considered on a case-by-case basis.

SUMMARY

Patients with PH are some of the most critically ill patients in the ED. The diagnosis is often delayed until patients are highly dysfunctional before receiving appropriate treatment. Careful attention must be directed toward addressing volume status, optimizing RV function, maintaining RCA perfusion, and reducing RV afterload. Continuous infusion of a prostanoid, such as epoprostenol, is used only in patients with significant end-stage disease and should only be initiated after a thorough work-up and evaluation as in-patients. If the administration is stopped abruptly, it must be restarted immediately to avoid rapid deterioration and cardiovascular collapse. ECMO support can be considered, on a case-by-case basis, for patients in extreme shock related to severe PH and RV failure.

ACKNOWLEDGMENTS

The authors would like to thank and acknowledge Linda J. Kesselring, MS, ELS for copyediting the article and incorporating revisions into the final article.

REFERENCES

1. Badesch DB, Champion HC, Sanchez MA, et al. Diagnosis and assessment of pulmonary arterial hypertension. J Am Coll Cardiol 2009;54(1 Suppl):S43–54.
2. Galiè N, Hoeper M, Humbert M, et al. Guidelines for the diagnosis and treatment of pulmonary hypertension. The Task Force for the Diagnosis and Treatment of Pulmonary Hypertension of the European Society of Cardiology (ESC) and the European Respiratory Society (ERS), endorsed by the International Society of Heart and Lung Transplantation (ISHLT). Eur Heart J 2009;30:2493–537.
3. Humbert M, Sitbon O, Chaouat A, et al. Pulmonary arterial hypertension in France: results from a national registry. Am J Respir Crit Care Med 2006;173: 1023–30.
4. Wagenvoort CA, Wagenvoort N. Primary pulmonary hypertension: a pathologic study of the lung vessels in 156 clinically diagnosed cases. Circulation 1970;42: 1163–84.
5. Farber HW, Loscalzo J. Pulmonary arterial hypertension. N Engl J Med 2004; 351:1655–65.
6. Walker A, Langleben D, Korelitz J, et al. Temporal trends and drug exposures in pulmonary hypertension: an American experience. Am Heart J 2006;152:521–6.

7. Garcia-Dorado D, Miller DD, Garcia EJ, et al. An epidemic of pulmonary hypertension after toxic rapeseed oil ingestion in Spain. J Am Coll Cardiol 1983;1: 1216–22.

8. Chambers CD, Hernandez-Diaz S, Van Marter LJ, et al. Selective serotonin-reuptake inhibitors and risk of persistent pulmonary hypertension of the newborn. N Engl J Med 2006;354:579–87.

9. Kieler H, Artama M, Engeland A, et al. Selective serotonin reuptake inhibitors during pregnancy and risk of persistent pulmonary hypertension in the newborn: population based cohort study from the five Nordic countries. BMJ 2012;344:d8012.

10. Chin KM, Channick RN, Rubin LJ. Is methamphetamine use associated with idiopathic pulmonary arterial hypertension. Chest 2006;130:1657–63.

11. Simmonneau G, Robbins I, Beghetti M, et al. Updated clinical classification of pulmonary hypertension. J Am Coll Cardiol 2009;54:S43–54.

12. Tyndall AJ, Bannert B, Vonk M, et al. Causes and risk factors for death in systemic sclerosis: a study from the EULAR Scleroderma Trials and Research (EUSTAR) database. Ann Rheum Dis 2010;69:1809–15.

13. Lowe BS, Therrien J, Ionescu-Ittu R, et al. Diagnosis of pulmonary hypertension in the congenital heart disease adult population: impact on outcomes. J Am Coll Cardiol 2011;58:538–46.

14. Lapa M, Dias B, Jardim C, et al. Cardiopulmonary manifestations of hepatosplenic schistosomiasis. Circulation 2009;119:1518–23.

15. dos Santos Fernandes CJ, Jardim CV, Hovnanian A, et al. Survival in schistosomiasis-associated pulmonary arterial hypertension. J Am Coll Cardiol 2010;56:715–20.

16. Holcomb BW Jr, Loyd JE, Ely EW, et al. Pulmonary veno-occlusive disease: a case series and new observations. Chest 2000;118:1671–9.

17. Montani D, Achouh L, Dorfmuller P, et al. Pulmonary veno-occlusive disease: clinical, functional, radiologic, and hemodynamic characteristics and outcome of 24 cases confirmed by histology. Medicine (Baltimore) 2008;87:220–33.

18. Oudiz RJ. Pulmonary hypertension associated with left-sided heart disease. Clin Chest Med 2007;28(1):233–41.

19. Park MH, Mehra MR. Pulmonary hypertension: the great leveler. J Am Coll Cardiol 2012;59:232–4.

20. Fishman AP. Hypoxia on the pulmonary circulation: how and where it acts. Circ Res 1976;38:221–31.

21. Weitzenblum E, Hirth C, Ducolone A, et al. Prognostic value of pulmonary artery pressure in chronic obstructive pulmonary disease. Thorax 1981;36:752–8.

22. Chaouat A, Bugnet A, Kadaoui N, et al. Severe pulmonary hypertension and chronic obstructive pulmonary disease. Am J Respir Crit Care Med 2005;172: 189–94.

23. Pengo V, Lensing AWA, Prins MH, et al. Incidence of chronic thromboembolic pulmonary hypertension after pulmonary embolism. N Engl J Med 2004;350: 2257–64.

24. Egermayer P, Peacock AJ. Is pulmonary embolism a common cause of chronic pulmonary hypertension? Limitations of the embolic hypothesis. Eur Respir J 2000;15:440–8.

25. Moser KM, Bloor CM. Pulmonary vascular lesions occurring in patients with chronic major vessel thromboembolic pulmonary hypertension. Chest 1993; 103:685–92.

26. Curnock AL, Dweik RA, Higgins BH, et al. High prevalence of hypothyroidism in patients with primary pulmonary hypertension. Am J Med Sci 1999;318:289–92.

27. Shorr AF, Helman DL, Davies DB, et al. Pulmonary hypertension in advanced sarcoidosis: epidemiology and clinical characteristics. Eur Respir J 2005;25: 783–8.
28. Voelkel NF, Quaife RA, Leinwand LA, et al. Right ventricular function and failure: report of a National Heart, Lung, and Blood Institute working group on cellular and molecular mechanisms of right heart failure. Circulation 2006;114:1883–91.
29. Stojnic BB, Brecker SJ, Xiao HB, et al. Left ventricular filling characteristics in pulmonary hypertension: a new mode of ventricular interaction. Br Heart J 1992;68:16–20.
30. Pinsky MR. Recent advances in the clinical application of heart-lung interactions. Curr Opin Crit Care 2002;8:26–31.
31. Baicu CF, Stroud JD, Livesay VA, et al. Changes in extracellular collagen matrix alter myocardial systolic performance. Am J Physiol Heart Circ Physiol 2003; 284:H122–32.
32. Janicki JS, Brower GL, Gardner JD, et al. Cardiac mast cell regulation of matrix metalloproteinase-related ventricular remodeling in chronic pressure or volume overload. Cardiovasc Res 2006;69:657–65.
33. Bogaard HJ, Abe K, Vonk Noordegraaf A, et al. The right ventricle under pressure: cellular and molecular mechanisms of right-heart failure in pulmonary hypertension. Chest 2009;135:794–804.
34. Brimioulle S, Wauthy P, Ewalenko P, et al. Single-beat estimation of right ventricular end-systolic pressure-volume relationship. Am J Physiol Heart Circ Physiol 2003;284:H1625–30.
35. Khan R, Sheppard R. Fibrosis in heart disease: understanding the role of transforming growth factor-beta in cardiomyopathy, valvular disease and arrhythmia. Immunology 2006;118:10–24.
36. Louie EK, Lin SS, Reynertson SI, et al. Pressure and volume loading of the right ventricle have opposite effects on left ventricular ejection fraction. Circulation 1995;92:819–24.
37. van Wolferen SA, Marcus JT, Westerhof N, et al. Right coronary artery flow impairment in patients with pulmonary hypertension. Eur Heart J 2008;29:120–7.
38. Farrer-Brown G. Vascular pattern of myocardium of right ventricle of human heart. Br Heart J 1968;30:679–86.
39. Dell'Italia LJ. The right ventricle: anatomy, physiology, and clinical importance. Curr Probl Cardiol 1991;16:653–720.
40. Haupt HM, Hutchins GM, Moore GW. Right ventricular infarction: role of the moderator band artery in determining infarct size. Circulation 1983;67:1268–72.
41. Nootens M, Wolfkiel CJ, Chomka EV, et al. Understanding right and left ventricular systolic function and interactions at rest and with exercise in primary pulmonary hypertension. Am J Cardiol 1995;75:374–7.
42. Gibbons Kroeker CA, Adeeb S, Shrive NG, et al. Compression induced by RV pressure overload decreases regional coronary blood flow in anesthetized dogs. Am J Physiol Heart Circ Physiol 2006;290(6):H2432–8.
43. Gómez A, Bialostozky D, Zajarias A, et al. Right ventricular ischemia in patients with primary pulmonary hypertension. J Am Coll Cardiol 2001;38:1137–42.
44. Ling Y, Johnson MK, Kiely DG, et al. Changing demographics, epidemiology, and survival of incident pulmonary arterial hypertension: results from the Pulmonary Hypertension Registry of the United Kingdom and Ireland. Am J Respir Crit Care Med 2012;186:790–6.
45. Badesch DB, Raskob GE, Elliott CG, et al. Pulmonary arterial hypertension: baseline characteristics from the REVEAL Registry. Chest 2010;137:376–87.

46. Benza RL, Miller DP, Gomberg-Maitland M, et al. Predicting survival in pulmonary arterial hypertension: insights from the Registry to Evaluate Early and Long-term Pulmonary Arterial Hypertension Disease Management (REVEAL). Circulation 2010;122:164–72.

47. Rich S, Dantzker DR, Ayres SM, et al. Primary pulmonary hypertension: a national prospective study. Ann Intern Med 1987;107:216–23.

48. Tongers J, Schwerdtfeger B, Klein G, et al. Incidence and clinical relevance of supraventricular tachyarrhythmias in pulmonary hypertension. Am Heart J 2007; 153:127–32.

49. Raymond RJ, Hinderliter AL, Willis PW, et al. Echocardiographic predictors of adverse outcomes in primary pulmonary hypertension. J Am Coll Cardiol 2002;39:1214–9.

50. Gaine SP, Rubin LJ. Primary pulmonary hypertension. Lancet 1998;352:719–25.

51. Zhang J, Wang G, Wang Q. Clinical primary pulmonary hypertension: a retrospective study of 50 cases. Zhonghua Nei Ke Za Zhi 1996;35:322–5 [in Chinese].

52. Kruger S, Graf J, Merx NW, et al. Brain natriuretic peptide predicts right heart failure in patients with acute pulmonary embolism. Am Heart J 2004;147:60–5.

53. Nagaya N, Nishikimi T, Okano Y, et al. Plasma brain natriuretic peptide levels increase in proportion to the extent of right ventricular dysfunction in pulmonary hypertension. J Am Coll Cardiol 1998;31:202–8.

54. Nagaya N, Nishikimi T, Uematsu M, et al. Plasma brain natriuretic peptide as a prognostic indicator in patients with primary pulmonary hypertension. Circulation 2000;102:865–70.

55. Jing ZC, Xu XQ, Han ZY, et al. Registry and survival in Chinese patients with idiopathic and familial pulmonary arterial hypertension. Chest 2007;132:373–9.

56. Bossone E, Paciocco G, Iarussi D, et al. The prognostic role of the ECG in primary pulmonary hypertension. Chest 2002;121:513–8.

57. McGoon M, Gutterman D, Steen V, et al. Screening, early detection, and diagnosis of pulmonary arterial hypertension: ACCP Evidence-Based Clinical Practice Guideline. Chest 2004;126:14S–34S.

58. Heresi G, Tang WH, Aytekin M, et al. Sensitive cardiac troponin I predicts poor outcomes in pulmonary arterial hypertension. Eur Respir J 2012;39:939–44.

59. Matthews JC, Mclaughlin V. Acute right ventricular failure in the setting of acute pulmonary embolism or chronic pulmonary hypertension: a detailed review of the pathophysiology, diagnosis, and management. Curr Cardiol Rev 2008;4: 49–59.

60. Tan RT, Kuzo R, Goodman LR, et al. Utility of CT scan evaluation for predicting pulmonary hypertension in patients with parenchymal lung disease. Medical College of Wisconsin Lung Transplant Group. Chest 1998;113:1250–6.

61. Jardin F, Dubourg O, Bourdarias J. Echocardiographic pattern of acute cor pulmonale. Chest 1997;111:209–17.

62. Daudel F, Tüller D, Krähenbühl S, et al. Pulse pressure variation and volume responsiveness during acutely increased pulmonary artery pressure: an experimental study. Crit Care 2010;14:R122.

63. Wyler von ballmoos M, Takala J, Roeck M, et al. Pulse-pressure variation and hemodynamic response in patients with elevated pulmonary artery pressure: a clinical study. Crit Care 2010;14:R111.

64. Charloux A, Chaouat A, Piquard F, et al. Renal hyporesponsiveness to brain natriuretic peptide: both generation and renal activity of cGMP are decreased in patients with pulmonary hypertension. Peptides 2006;27:2993–9.

65. Hadian M, Pinsky MR. Evidence-based review of the use of the pulmonary artery catheter: impact data and complications. Crit Care 2006;10(Suppl 3):S8.
66. Harvey S, Harrison DA, Singer M, et al. Assessment of the clinical effectiveness of pulmonary artery catheters in management of patients in intensive care (PAC-Man): a randomised controlled trial. Lancet 2005;366(9484):472–7.
67. Price LC, Wort SJ, Finney SJ, et al. Pulmonary vascular and right ventricular dysfunction in adult critical care: current and emerging options for management: a systematic literature review. Crit Care 2010;14:R169.
68. Vonk-Noordegraaf A, Haddad F, Chin KM, et al. Right heart adaptation to pulmonary arterial hypertension: physiology and pathobiology. J Am Coll Cardiol 2013; 62(25 suppl):D22–33.
69. Zamanian RT, Haddad F, Doyle RL, et al. Management strategies for patients with pulmonary hypertension in the intensive care unit. Crit Care Med 2007; 35:2037–50.
70. Hoeper MM, Granton J. Intensive care unit management of patients with severe pulmonary hypertension and right heart failure. Am J Respir Crit Care Med 2011; 184:1114–24.
71. Vizza CD, Rocca GD, Roma AD, et al. Acute hemodynamic effects of inhaled nitric oxide, dobutamine and a combination of the two in patients with mild to moderate secondary pulmonary hypertension. Crit Care 2001;5:355–61.
72. Kerbaul F, Rondelet B, Motte S, et al. Effects of norepinephrine and dobutamine on pressure load-induced right ventricular failure. Crit Care Med 2004;32:1035–40.
73. Sztrymf B, Souza R, Bertoletti L, et al. Prognostic factors of acute heart failure in patients with pulmonary arterial hypertension. Eur Respir J 2010;35:1286–93.
74. Eichhorn EJ, Konstam MA, Weiland DS, et al. Differential effects of milrinone and dobutamine on right ventricular preload, afterload and systolic performance in congestive heart failure secondary to ischemic or idiopathic dilated cardiomyopathy. Am J Cardiol 1987;60:1329–33.
75. Kihara S, Kawai A, Fukuda T, et al. Effects of milrinone for right ventricular failure after left ventricular assist device implantation. Heart Vessels 2002;16:69–71.
76. Oztekin I, Yazici S, Oztekin DS, et al. Effects of low-dose milrinone on weaning from cardiopulmonary bypass and after in patients with mitral stenosis and pulmonary hypertension. Yakugaku Zasshi 2007;127:375–83.
77. De Backer D, Biston P, Devriendt J, et al. Comparison of dopamine and norepinephrine in the treatment of shock. N Engl J Med 2010;362:779–89.
78. Kwak YL, Lee CS, Park YH, et al. The effect of phenylephrine and norepinephrine in patients with chronic pulmonary hypertension. Anaesthesia 2002;57: 9–14
79. Rich S, Gubin S, Hart K. The effects of phenylephrine on right ventricular performance in patients with pulmonary hypertension. Chest 1990;98:1102–6.
80. Moudgil R, Michelakis ED, Archer SL. Hypoxic pulmonary vasoconstriction. J Appl Physiol 2005;98:390–403.
81. Balanos GM, Talbot NP, Dorrington KL, et al. Human pulmonary vascular response to 4 h of hypercapnia and hypocapnia measured using Doppler echocardiography. J Appl Physiol 2003;94:1543–51.
82. Mekontso Dessap A, Charron C, Devaquet J, et al. Impact of acute hypercapnia and augmented positive end-expiratory pressure on right ventricle function in severe acute respiratory distress syndrome. Intensive Care Med 2009;35: 1850–8.
83. Laughlin VV, Archer SL, Badesch DB, et al. ACCF/AHA 2009 expert consensus document on pulmonary hypertension: a report of the American College of

Cardiology Foundation Task Force on Expert Consensus Documents and the American Heart Association: developed in collaboration with the American College of Chest Physicians, American Thoracic Society, Inc., and the Pulmonary Hypertension Association. Circulation 2009;119:2250–94.

84. Roberts DH, Lepore JJ, Maroo A, et al. Oxygen therapy improves cardiac index and pulmonary vascular resistance in patients with pulmonary hypertension. Chest 2001;120:1547–55.

85. Viitanen A, Salmenpera M, Heinonen J. Right ventricular response to hypercarbia after cardiac surgery. Anesthesiology 1990;73:393–400.

86. Cockrill BA, Kacmarek RM, Fifer MA, et al. Comparison of the effects of nitric oxide, nitroprusside, and nifedipine on hemodynamics and right ventricular contractility in patients with chronic pulmonary hypertension. Chest 2001;119: 128–36.

87. Bhorade S, Christenson J, O'Connor M, et al. Response to inhaled nitric oxide in patients with acute right heart syndrome. Am J Respir Crit Care Med 1999;159: 571–9.

88. George I, Xydas S, Topkara VK, et al. Clinical indication for use and outcomes after inhaled nitric oxide therapy. Ann Thorac Surg 2006;82:2161–9.

89. Barst RJ, Rubin LJ, Long WA, et al. A comparison of continuous intravenous epoprostenol (prostacyclin) with conventional therapy for primary pulmonary hypertension. N Engl J Med 1996;334:296–301.

90. Rubenfire M, McLaughlin VV, Roblee A, et al. Transition from epoprostenol to treprostinil in pulmonary arterial hypertension: a controlled trial. Chest 2007; 132:757–63.

91. Papierniak ES, Lowenthal DT, Mubarak K. Pulmonary arterial hypertension: classification and therapy with a focus on prostaglandin analogs. Am J Ther 2012; 19:300–14.

92. Califf RM, Adams KF, Mckenna WJ, et al. A randomized controlled trial of epoprostenol therapy for severe congestive heart failure: the Flolan International Randomized Survival Trial (FIRST). Am Heart J 1997;134:44–54.

93. Anderson JR, Nawarskas JJ. Pharmacotherapeutic management of pulmonary arterial hypertension. Cardiol Rev 2010;18:148–62.

94. Safdar Z. Treatment of pulmonary arterial hypertension: the role of prostacyclin and prostaglandin analogs. Respir Med 2011;105:818–27.

95. Olsson KM, Nickel NP, Tongers J, et al. Atrial flutter and fibrillation in patients with pulmonary hypertension. Int J Cardiol 2013;167:2300–5.

96. Hebert PC, Blajchman MA, Marshall J, et al. A multicenter, randomized, controlled clinical trial of transfusion requirements in critical care. Transfusion Requirements in Critical Care Investigators, Canadian Critical Care Trials Group. N Engl J Med 1999;340:409–17.

97. Ruiter G, Lankhorst S, Boonstra A, et al. Iron deficiency is common in idiopathic pulmonary arterial hypertension. Eur Respir J 2011;37:1386–91.

98. Kearon C, Akl EA, Comerota AJ, et al. Antithrombotic therapy for VTE disease: antithrombotic therapy and prevention of thrombosis, 9th ed: American College of Chest Physicians evidence-based clinical practice guidelines. Chest 2012; 141(2 Suppl):e419S–94S.

99. Conrad SA, Rycus PT, Dalton H. Extracorporeal life support registry report 2004. ASAIO J 2005;51:4–10.

100. de Perrot M, Granton JT, McRae K, et al. Impact of extracorporeal life support on outcome in patients with idiopathic pulmonary arterial hypertension awaiting lung transplantation. J Heart Lung Transpl 2011;30:997–1002.

101. Srivastava MC, Ramani GV, Garcia JP, et al. Veno-venous extracorporeal membrane oxygenation bridging to pharmacotherapy in pulmonary arterial hypertensive crisis. J Heart Lung Transpl 2010;29:811–3.
102. Sayer GT, Baker JN, Parks KA. Heart rescue: the role of mechanical circulatory support in the management of severe refractory cardiogenic shock. Curr Opin Crit Care 2012;18:409–16.

Cardiogenic Shock

Joshua B. Moskovitz, MD, MPH, MBA*, Zachary D. Levy, MD,
Todd L. Slesinger, MD

KEYWORDS

- Cardiogenic shock • Heart failure • Congestive heart failure • Acute heart failure
- Cardiac failure

KEY POINTS

- Cardiogenic shock is defined as a state of hypoperfusion and end-organ dysfunction resulting from profoundly decreased cardiac output.
- Acute MI and left ventricular failure is the most common cause overall; less commonly, shock may be precipitated by acute valvular dysfunction and aortic dissection, both of which are surgical emergencies.
- Patients in cardiogenic shock require urgent evaluation for reperfusion therapies, including coronary artery bypass graft and PCI.
- Norepinephrine is the preferred agent for patients in cardiogenic shock who require pressor support; dobutamine and milrinone are second-line adjuncts that may worsen hypotension when used in isolation.
- In the emergency setting, IABP and percutaneous LVAD placement may be used as temporizing measures to improve patient hemodynamics while awaiting definitive treatment.

INTRODUCTION

Overall mortality in acute coronary syndrome (ACS) has dropped significantly in the past several decades, from 10.4% in 1990 to 6.3% in 2006.[1] The improvement in survival among patients with ACS can be attributed, in part, to advances in pharmacologic and mechanical interventions.[2–4] Many of these therapies target cardiogenic shock, a relatively common complication of ACS with an associated mortality rate between 50% and 80%.[2] Despite the need for well-defined, evidence-based treatment algorithms in this critically ill patient population, there is a paucity of data. This article describes the pathophysiology of cardiogenic shock, organizes treatment considerations, and catalogues advances in current practice.

No financial disclosures or conflicts of interest.
Department of Emergency Medicine, Hofstra North Shore-LIJ School of Medicine, 300 Community Drive, Hempstead, NY 11030, USA
* Corresponding author. Department of Emergency Medicine, North Shore University Hospital, 300 Community Drive, Hempstead, NY 11030.
E-mail address: joshmoskovitz@gmail.com

Emerg Med Clin N Am 33 (2015) 645–652
http://dx.doi.org/10.1016/j.emc.2015.04.013   emed.theclinics.com

PATHOPHYSIOLOGY

Cardiogenic shock is best described as a state of heart failure that results in inadequate cardiac output, hypoperfusion, and end-organ dysfunction. Defining features of cardiogenic shock appear in **Table 1**. The diagnosis was historically made via pulmonary artery catheterization, but noninvasive echocardiography is increasingly used.[5,6] In addition to hypotension, clinical signs may include cool extremities, decreased urine output, mottled skin, and altered mental status.

Ultimately, cardiogenic shock involves left and/or right ventricular dysfunction. The causes of ventricular failure are numerous, including acute myocardial infarction (MI), myocarditis/pericarditis, cardiomyopathies, acute or chronic valvular dysfunction, aortic dissection, myocardial contusion, and myocardial depression from septic shock.[7] Mechanical etiologies of cardiogenic shock (including valvular rupture and aortic dissection) are true surgical emergencies, requiring prompt diagnosis and surgical referral. These conditions often carry a poor prognosis.[8] The most common overall cause of cardiogenic shock, however, is left ventricular dysfunction in the setting of ACS involving the left-sided coronary arteries.[7] This article focuses predominantly on MIs as a cause of cardiogenic shock, and the various treatment options that emergency physicians should consider.

The primary insult is typically an infarct causing either reversible ischemia or irreversible injury to the left ventricle. As a result, coronary perfusion decreases, thereby decreasing cardiac output. The drop in cardiac output results in hypoperfusion, triggering catecholamine release to improve contractility and blood pressure. This, in turn, increases myocardial oxygen demand.[5] The result is a cycle of decreasing myocardial blood supply with increasing myocardial oxygen demand, a chain reaction that can manifest as rapid clinical deterioration.

Right ventricular MI accompanies inferior wall ischemia in up to 50% of cases, and generally does not exist in the absence of left ventricular MI. Hemodynamic stability in right ventricular MI is variable; some patients remain asymptomatic, whereas others experience severe hypotension and cardiogenic shock. Right ventricular MIs are more often complicated by arrhythmias, including complete atrioventricular or sinoatrial blocks.[9] It is important to consider right ventricular extension when evaluating a patient with inferior wall ischemia, and right precordial leads may be necessary when obtaining an electrocardiogram to evaluate for extension of an inferior wall MI. ST-segment elevation in lead V4R greater than 1 mm is reportedly 100% sensitive and 87% specific for right ventricular infarction.[9]

Several risk factors have been associated with increased mortality in cardiogenic shock in the setting of MI, include advanced age (>75) and increased serum lactate (>6.5 mmol/L).[10] Indeed, elevated serum lactate has previously been identified as an independent predictor of the development of cardiogenic shock.[11] Failed reperfusion and history of prior MI have also been identified as high-risk features.[12]

Table 1 Definition of cardiogenic shock	
Persistent hypotension	Systolic BP <90 or MAP >30 below baseline
Severe reduction in cardiac index	<1.8 L/min/m^2 without support
Adequate or elevated filling pressure	LV end diastolic pressure >18 mm Hg RV end diastolic pressure >10–15 mm Hg

Abbreviations: BP, blood pressure; LV, left ventricular; MAP, mean arterial pressure; RV, right ventricular.

TREATMENT STRATEGIES

Revascularization addresses the underlying pathology by restoring coronary blood flow to perfuse myocardial tissue that is still viable. Time is of the essence: animal models have demonstrated that nearly 50% of salvageable myocardium is lost within the first hour of coronary artery occlusion, and two-thirds within 3 hours.[2]

The recently published National Institute for Health and Care Excellence guideline recommends that patients with ST-segment elevation myocardial infarction in the presence of cardiogenic shock presenting within 12 hours of symptom onset should receive coronary angiography with primary percutaneous coronary intervention (PCI).[13] For patients presenting greater than 12 hours after the onset of the ST-segment elevation myocardial infarction, the likelihood of benefit may be limited and the consensus group recommends that decisions be made on a case-by-case basis.[13] The SHOCK trial compared coronary artery bypass grafting with PCI for patients in cardiogenic shock in the setting of acute MI, and found comparable favorable survival rates.[14]

These patients require urgent evaluation by a cardiologist and/or cardiothoracic surgeon to assess whether reperfusion is a viable option. In the meantime, an array of temporizing medical and mechanical interventions should be considered.

MEDICAL MANAGEMENT

The drugs most commonly used in the management of cardiogenic shock are inotropic agents, exerting their effect by increasing myocardial contractile performance. Examples of inotropic agents are listed in **Table 2** and include digoxin, dopamine, dobutamine, norepinephrine, milrinone, and levosimendan.

Digitalis

The inotropic powers of foxglove extract have been known for more than 200 years. Digoxin, the most commonly available cardiac glycoside, exerts its effect through inhibition of the sodium-potassium ATPase, increasing intracellular calcium concentrations and promoting more forceful myocardial contraction. It is notable for having little to no effect on systemic blood pressure and renal function, and has many protective neurohormonal effects.[15] It has not, however, been shown to reduce all-cause mortality in heart failure, despite symptom relief and improvement in hemodynamics.[16]

Adrenergics

Dopamine, dobutamine, and norepinephrine are all adrenergic agents used in the treatment of cardiogenic shock. Dopamine acts via β-adrenergic receptors to increase inotropy and heart rate, and at higher doses induces peripheral vasoconstriction via α-activation. Dobutamine is a synthetic agent that was developed to activate β-adrenergic receptors without causing peripheral vasoconstriction or triggering the

Table 2	
Examples of inotropic agents	
Medication Class	**Common Examples**
Cardiac glycosides	Digoxin, oubain
Adrenergics	Norepinephrine, dopamine, dobutamine
Phosphodiesterase inhibitors	Milrinone, amrinone
Calcium sensitizers	Levosimendan, pimobendan

release of endogenous catecholamines. Dobutamine can effectively increase cardiac output and reduce left ventricular end-diastolic pressure, but hypotension may result because of unopposed peripheral β_2 stimulation, and tolerance is observed with prolonged infusions.[17]

Norepinephrine is an endogenous adrenergic agent that acts at α- and β-receptors, and causes an increase in inotropy, chronotropy, and peripheral vasoconstriction. When compared with dopamine in cardiogenic shock, norepinephrine was found to be as effective as dopamine in improving hemodynamic parameters, but carried less risk of adverse arrhythmias and improved 28-day mortality.[18] Based on the available evidence, norepinephrine is the preferred first-line adrenergic agent in cardiogenic shock.

Phosphodiesterase Inhibitors

Milrinone is a noncatecholamine inotropic agent that inhibits the breakdown of cyclic AMP and promotes an increase in intracellular calcium in cardiac myocytes. Similar to dobutamine, milrinone improves contractility and cardiac output at the risk of increased systemic hypotension. It has not been shown to improve outcomes when routinely used in acute exacerbations of congestive heart failure.[19]

Calcium Sensitizers

As the name implies, calcium sensitizers, such as levosimendan, enhance cardiac contractility without actually increasing intracellular calcium levels. Levosimendan has been shown to improve cardiac output, increase lactate clearance, and reduce norepinephrine requirements in decompensated heart failure.[20] At least one meta-analysis has suggested it may reduce overall mortality in critically ill patients, although the data are mixed.[21] The SURVIVE trial compared levosimendan with dobutamine in acute decompensated heart failure, and found no difference in all-cause mortality at 6 months.[22]

Other Considerations

It should be noted that cardiogenic shock may develop iatrogenically, and up to three-quarters of all cases do not progress until after hospital presentation.[23] Drugs that may precipitate cardiogenic shock in the setting of acute MI include β-blockers, angiotensin-converting enzyme inhibitors, morphine, nitrates, and various classes of diuretics.[5] Although the use of many of these agents is considered standard of care, they should be used cautiously, and patients receiving these therapies should be monitored closely for hemodynamic deterioration. In particular, nitrates and diuretics should be avoided in patients with right ventricular dysfunction, because adequate preload is critical for preserving cardiac output.[9] Finally, it should be appreciated that endogenous catecholamine release itself is part of the "vicious cycle" of cardiogenic shock. When using inotropes to treat cardiogenic shock, practitioners are seeking a delicate balance between excessive myocardial oxygen demand and total cardiovascular collapse.

MECHANICAL SUPPORT

Efforts to augment a failing heart via mechanical intervention date back to the early 1960s, when Spyridon Moulopoulos and colleagues first pioneered the intra-aortic balloon pump (IABP). Since then, several improvements have been made on the original design, alongside the development of several novel treatment options (**Table 3**). Although not inserted by emergency physicians directly, these devices may be placed

Table 3		
Modes of mechanical support in cardiogenic shock (mechanism of action)			
Intra-aortic balloon pump placement (using counterpulsation principles)	Left-ventricular assistant devices (acting via centrifugal or axial flow augmentation)	Extracorporeal membrane oxygenation (continuously removing, oxygenating, and replacing blood volume)

in the emergency department while these critically ill patients await the intensive care unit, the catheterization laboratory, or the operating room. A basic understanding of their function is prudent.

Intra-aortic Balloon Pump

The IABP uses the principle of counterpulsation to augment systolic function and promote myocardial oxygen delivery. Specifically, the device is a polyethylene balloon that rapidly inflates during diastole and deflates during systole. First, the balloon inflates, enhancing blood flow through the coronary vessels via backpressure in the aorta. Next, the balloon rapidly deflates, effectively decreasing afterload on the heart by creating a vacuum and promoting forward blood. The cycle is repeated in sync with the native heartbeat in a 1:1 fashion, with increasing ratios used during weaning periods.

In principle, counterpulsation seems like a logical and effective way to manage cardiogenic shock. In practice, the data have not been entirely compelling. The SHOCK-II trial, among others, failed to demonstrate benefit when routinely used in the setting of cardiogenic shock and acute MI.[24] However, the BCIS-1 trial demonstrated a long-term mortality benefit in patients with severe cardiomyopathy undergoing PCI.[25] In certain patients, IABP may indeed be an effective therapy in cardiogenic shock, but the data do not clearly support its routine use.

Ventricular-Assist Device

Several different ventricular-assist devices (VADs) have been developed, but the most common type in current practice involves a continuous-flow pump that enhances output from the left ventricle (LVAD) (This is a jarring reality for novice practitioners who discover that these patients do not, in fact, have a pulse!). Less commonly, these devices can be used to augment the right ventricle, or even both ventricles. Implanted and percutaneous forms exist. The relatively small INTrEPID trial demonstrated significant morbidity and mortality benefits for patients ineligible for transplant who underwent LVAD placement versus medical therapy alone.[26]

The newest generation of VADs is percutaneous devices that use impeller-driven axial flow pumps, as opposed to the centrifugal flow seen in traditional implanted LVADs. Compared with IABP, these newer percutaneous models (such as the TandemHeart and Impella devices) have demonstrated improved hemodynamics, but no conclusive mortality benefit.[27]

Extracorporeal Membrane Oxygenation

Extracorporeal membrane oxygenation (ECMO) combines a centrifugal pump, a heat exchanger, and an oxygenator to provide cardiac and respiratory support. Venovenous and venoarterial forms exist; the former provides only pulmonary support, whereas the latter is true cardiopulmonary bypass. ECMO has been used in a variety of settings, including cardiogenic shock, acute respiratory distress syndrome, and the periarrest period.

There is evidence to suggest that ECMO may improve short- and long-term survival compared with conventional cardiopulmonary resuscitation in the setting of in-hospital cardiac arrest, particularly for patients with primary cardiac pathologies.[28,29] There is also a growing interest in initiating ECMO on emergency department arrival, with the hope that it can improve meaningful neurologic outcomes.[30] However, there are currently no randomized trials evaluating the use of ECMO in cardiogenic shock and acute MI, and its role remains unclear for patients not suffering from circulatory arrest.[31]

SUMMARY

Based on the evidence presented, the following treatment recommendations can be made:

1. Recognize that ACS most commonly precipitates cardiogenic shock; standard ACS therapies, such as aspirin and heparin administration, should not be overlooked.
2. Patients in cardiogenic shock should be promptly evaluated to determine if they are candidates for revascularization therapy, either via PCI or coronary artery bypass graft. The benefit of revascularization is time-dependent, and treatment within 12 hours of symptom onset may offer the greatest benefit.
3. Correction of hypovolemia with fluid resuscitation may be necessary, but care must be taken not to precipitate or worsen pulmonary edema.
4. Norepinephrine should be considered the treatment of choice in patients requiring pressors before adding dobutamine or milrinone as adjuncts. Pressors should be used judiciously, and infusion rates should be titrated as low as possible.
5. Patients who remain hemodynamically unstable despite pressors and fluid optimization may be candidates for mechanical augmentation, including IABP and LVAD placement.

REFERENCES

1. Rogers WJ, Frederick PD, Stoehr E, et al. Trends in presenting characteristics and hospital mortality among patients with ST elevation and non-ST elevation myocardial infarction in the national registry of myocardial infarction from 1990 to 2006. Am Heart J 2008;156(6):1026–34.
2. Harker M, Carville S, Henderson R, et al. Key recommendations and evidence from the NICE guideline for the acute management of ST-segment-elevation myocardial infarction. Heart 2014;100(7):536–43.
3. Jernberg T, Johanson P, Held C, et al. Association between adoption of evidence-based treatment and survival for patients with ST-elevation myocardial infarction. JAMA 2011;35(16):1677–84.
4. O'Flaherty M, Buchan I, Capewell S. Contributions of treatment and lifestyle to declining CVD mortality: why have CVD mortality rates declined so much since the 1960s? Heart 2013;99:159–62.
5. Reynolds HR, Hochman JS. Cardiogenic shock: current concepts and improving outcomes. Circulation 2008;117:686–97.
6. Pirrachio R, Parenica J, Rigon MR, et al. The effectiveness of inodilators in reducing short term mortality among patient with severe cardiogenic shock: a propensity-based analysis. PLoS One 2013;8(8):e71659.

7. Axler O. Low diastolic blood pressure as best predictor of mortality in cardiogenic shock. Crit Care Med 2013;41(11):2644–7.
8. Stout KK, Verrier ED. Acute valvular regurgitation. Circulation 2009;119(25):3232–41.
9. Ondrus T, Kanovsky J, Novotny T, et al. Right ventricular myocardial infarction: from pathophysiology to prognosis. Exp Clin Cardiol 2013;18(1):27–30.
10. Valente S, Lazzeri C, Vecchio S, et al. Predictors of in-hospital mortality after percutaneous coronary intervention for cardiogenic shock. Int J Cardiol 2007;114:176–82.
11. Mavrić Z, Zaputović L, Zagar D, et al. Usefulness of blood lactate as a predictor of shock development in acute myocardial infarction. Am J Cardiol 1991;67(7):565–8.
12. Sutton AG, Finn P, Hall JA, et al. Predictors of outcome after percutaneous treatment for cardiogenic shock. Heart 2005;91(3):339–44.
13. Carville S, Harker M, Henderson R, et al. Acute management of myocardial infarction with ST-segment elevation: summary of NICE guidance. BMJ 2013;347:f4006.
14. White HD, Assmann SF, Sanborn TA, et al. Comparison of percutaneous coronary intervention and coronary artery bypass grafting after acute myocardial infarction complicated by cardiogenic shock: results from the should we emergently revascularize occluded coronaries for cardiogenic shock (SHOCK) trial. Circulation 2005;112(13):1992–2001.
15. Gheorghiade M, Braunwald E. Reconsidering the role for digoxin in the management of acute heart failure syndromes. JAMA 2009;302(19):2146–7.
16. Gheorghiade M, Van veldhuisen DJ, Colucci WS. Contemporary use of digoxin in the management of cardiovascular disorders. Circulation 2006;113(21):2556–64.
17. Francis GS, Bartos JA, Adatya S. Inotropes. J Am Coll Cardiol 2014;63:2069–78.
18. De Backer D, Biston P, Devriendt J, et al. Comparison of dopamine and norepinephrine in the treatment of shock. N Engl J Med 2010;362:779–89.
19. Cuffe MS, Califf RM, Adams KF, et al. Short-term intravenous milrinone for acute exacerbation of chronic heart failure: a randomized controlled trial. JAMA 2002;287(12):1541–7.
20. Berry WT, Hewson RW, Langrish CJ, et al. Levosimendan: a retrospective single-center case series. J Crit Care 2013;28(6):1075–8.
21. Landoni G, Mizzi A, Biondi-zoccai G, et al. Levosimendan reduces mortality in critically ill patients. A meta-analysis of randomized controlled studies. Minerva Anestesiol 2010;76(4):276–86.
22. Mebazaa A, Nieminen MS, Packer M, et al. Levosimendan vs dobutamine for patients with acute decompensated heart failure: the SURVIVE randomized trial. JAMA 2007;297(17):1883–91.
23. Babaev A, Frederick PD, Pasta DJ, et al. Trends in management and outcomes of patients with acute myocardial infarction complicated by cardiogenic shock. JAMA 2005;294:448–54.
24. Thiele H, Zeymer U, Neumann FJ. Intraaortic balloon support for myocardial infarction with cardiogenic shock. N Engl J Med 2012;367(14):1287–96.
25. Perera D, Stables R, Clayton T, et al. Long-term mortality data from the balloon pump-assisted coronary intervention study (BCIS-1): a randomized, controlled trial of elective balloon counter pulsation during high-risk percutaneous coronary intervention. Circulation 2013;127(2):207–12.
26. Rogers JG, Butler J, Lansman SL, et al. Chronic mechanical circulatory support for inotrope-dependent heart failure patients who are not transplant candidates: results of the INTREPID trial. J Am Coll Cardiol 2007;50(8):741–7.

27. Cheng JM, den Uil CA, Hoeks SE, et al. Percutaneous left ventricular assist devices vs. intra-aortic balloon pump counterpulsation for treatment of cardiogenic shock: a meta-analysis of controlled trials. Eur Heart J 2009;30(17):2102–8.
28. Chen YS, Lin JW, Yu HY, et al. Cardiopulmonary resuscitation with assisted extracorporeal life-support versus conventional cardiopulmonary resuscitation in adults with in-hospital cardiac arrest: an observational study and propensity analysis. Lancet 2008;372(9638):554–61.
29. Shin TG, Choi JH, Jo IJ, et al. Extracorporeal cardiopulmonary resuscitation in patients with in-hospital cardiac arrest: a comparison with conventional cardiopulmonary resuscitation. Crit Care Med 2011;39(1):1–7.
30. Bellezzo JM, Shinar Z, Davis DP, et al. Emergency physician-initiated extracorporeal cardiopulmonary resuscitation. Resuscitation 2012;83(8):966–70.
31. Werdan K, Gielen S, Ebelt H, et al. Mechanical circulatory support in cardiogenic shock. Eur Heart J 2014;35(3):156–67.

Emergency Care of Patients with Pacemakers and Defibrillators

Michael G. Allison, MD[a,b], Haney A. Mallemat, MD[b],*

KEYWORDS

- Pacemaker • Implantable cardioverter-defibrillator • Electrical storm
- Cardiac arrest • Magnet

KEY POINTS

- The traditional categories of pacemaker malfunction (failure to pace, failure to capture, failure to sense) do not provide sufficient insight or description for the emergency care provider; in the emergency department, the focus needs to be on correcting hemodynamic instability.
- A magnet causes a pacemaker to go into an asynchronous mode and a defibrillator to stop delivering shocks without affecting the pacing function of the device.
- In patients with pacemakers and implantable cardioverter-defibrillators who present in cardiac arrest, defibrillation pads should be placed in an anterior-posterior configuration.
- Patients who present after the single discharge of a defibrillator can be sent home with close cardiology follow-up for device interrogation.
- Electrical storm is defined as more than 3 episodes of ventricular tachycardia in 24 hours. In refractory cases, β-blockers can be used to treat the malignant arrhythmia.

INTRODUCTION

Implantable cardiac devices are used to reduce morbidity and mortality among patients with, or at risk for, rhythm disturbances. Permanent pacemakers and implantable cardioverter-defibrillators (ICDs) can be lifesaving. The invasive nature of their insertion and the way they affect cardiac electrophysiology make troubleshooting problems

Funding sources: Nil.
Conflict of interest: Nil.
The article was copyedited by Linda J. Kesselring, MS, ELS, the technical editor/writer in the Department of Emergency Medicine at the University of Maryland School of Medicine.
[a] Division of Pulmonary and Critical Care Medicine, Department of Medicine, University of Maryland School of Medicine, 110 South Paca Street, 2nd Floor, Baltimore, MD 21201, USA;
[b] Department of Emergency Medicine, University of Maryland School of Medicine, 110 South Paca Street, 6th Floor, Baltimore, MD 21201, USA
* Corresponding author.
E-mail address: haney.mallemat@gmail.com

associated with these devices a necessary skill for emergency physicians. When problems with the devices arise, patients typically present to the emergency department (ED). Reports from the US Food and Drug Administration and device registries estimate 26.5 ICD malfunctions and 1.3 pacemaker malfunctions per 1000 person years (likely an underestimate of the true incidence of device malfunction).[1,2] All practicing emergency physicians should understand the possible problems associated with implantable cardiac devices and have a framework for addressing their malfunction.

PERMANENT PACEMAKERS

In 2009, more than 185,000 pacemakers were inserted in the United States.[3] Eighty-two percent of them were dual-chamber pacemakers, an increase of 20% compared with the previous 16 years. The North American Society of Pacing and Electrophysiology and the British Pacing and Electrophysiology Group settled on a common language to describe pacemaker terminology and settings (**Table 1**).[4] Pacemakers are fully described by a 5-position code. The first 3 positions define the function of the device and should be understood by every emergency physician. The first 3 positions of pacemaker code can be remembered by the mnemonic PaSeR. The first position (Pa) describes the pacing function of the device, the second position (Se) describes the sensing position of the device, and the third position (R) describes the pacemaker's response to sensing. Pacing and sensing can be set to one of 4 settings: ventricle (V), atrium (A), dual (D), or no pacing (O). Response to sensing can be set to one of 4 settings as well: inhibited (I), triggered (T), dual (D), or no response (O). The most common setting for dual-chamber devices is DDD. The pacemaker paces and senses the atria and the ventricle. If a native cardiac beat is sensed, the pacemaker is inhibited; if no native beat is sensed after a set interval, the pacemaker delivers a triggered beat.

INDICATIONS FOR PACEMAKER PLACEMENT

The indications for placement of permanent pacemakers are varied and complex. Professional societies have created guidelines to assist electrophysiologists in determining the need for these devices. Guidelines issued jointly by the American College of Cardiology Foundation (ACCF [formerly the ACC]), the American Heart Association (AHA), and the Heart Rhythm Society (HRS) were first published in 2008 and were updated in 2012.[5,6] The European Society of Cardiology (ESC) and the European Heart Rhythm Association (EHRA) have also published guidelines to assist clinicians.[7] Patients with persistent bradycardia, intermittent bradycardia, syncope with a bundle branch block, and reflex syncope with long sinus pauses can be considered for pacemakers in the right clinical context. The 2 sets of recommendations and levels of evidence for various cardiac rhythm disturbances are summarized in **Table 2**.

Table 1
Uniform pacemaker code

Position	I	II	III	IV	V
Function	Chamber Paced	Chamber Sensed	Response to Sensing	Programmability	Antitachycardia Function
Code	V	V	I	O: none	O: none
	A	A	T	P: simple programmable	P: pacing
	D	D	D	M: multiprogrammable	S: shock
	O	O	O	C: communicating	D: dual
				R: rate responsive	

Table 2
Indications for pacemaker placement

	ESC Guidelines	ACCF/AHA/HRS Guidelines
Persistent Blocks		
Sinus bradycardia, symptomatic	I B	I C
Sinus bradycardia, asymptomatic	III C	III C
AV block, second degree type II or third degree	I C	I C
AV block, second degree type I	IIa C, symptomatic III B, asymptomatic	I B, symptomatic III B, asymptomatic
Intermittent Blocks		
Sinus node disease (brady-tachy syndrome)	I B	I C
Paroxysmal AV block, second degree type II or third degree	I C	I C
Reflex asystolic syncope	IIa B	I C (if carotid sensitivity present)
Sinus arrest, pauses >6 s + syncope	IIa C	IIa C
Bundle Branch Blocks		
Alternating bundle branch block	I C	I C
Bundle branch block	I B, syncope and abnormal EPS IIb B, syncope and nondiagnostic EPS	No recommendation
Other Scenarios		
Situational syncope	No recommendation	III C
Unexplained syncope	III C	III C

Abbreviations: AV, atrioventricular; EPS, electrophysiology study.

PACEMAKER MALFUNCTION

Pacemaker failure can be divided into 3 categories: failure to pace, failure to capture, and failure to sense.[8–11] This traditional categorization has little value in the acute setting. The types of pacemaker malfunction overlap greatly (**Table 3**), and all of them are managed similarly in the emergency setting until the cause can be identified

Table 3
Traditional categories of pacemaker malfunction

Failure to Pace	Failure to Capture	Failure to Sense
Lead misplacement or fracture	Lead misplacement or fracture	Lead misplacement or fracture
Dead battery	Cardiac scarring	Cardiac scarring
Component Failure	Myocardial threshold changes	Low sensing threshold
Trauma	Improper programming	Dead battery
	Dying battery	Oversensing

by device interrogation and remedied by an electrophysiologist. Simply put, categorizing the type of pacemaker failure neither determines the work-up nor aids in the emergency treatment of device malfunction. The traditional categories are described, followed by a more useful framework for understanding pacemaker malfunction and how to treat it in the ED.

Failure to Pace

Failure to pace describes the condition in which the pacemaker does not trigger the myocardium to depolarize. The electrocardiogram (ECG) shows neither pacemaker spikes nor pacemaker-induced QRS complexes after an appropriate escape interval. The ECG therefore shows the native rhythm of the patient. If the patient has a pacemaker and the native rhythm is less than its set point, failure to pace should be suspected. Failure to pace can be caused by lead misplacement, fracture, or migration; a dead or dying battery; failure of the pulse generator or another component; or trauma.

Failure to Capture

Failure to capture describes the condition in which a pacemaker impulse is given but the impulse is unable to depolarize nonrefractory myocardial tissue. Pacemaker spikes are seen on the ECG, but there is no induced cardiac response to the pacemaker impulse. The causes of failure to capture include lead misplacement, fracture, or migration; cardiac scarring; delivery of energy below the depolarization threshold; or a dying battery. Electrolyte derangements and supratherapeutic drug levels can sometimes artificially increase the depolarization threshold, resulting in failure to capture.[12] Typically, the patient's native rhythm is seen on the ECG, with intermittent or continuous noncaptured pacemaker-generated spikes.

Failure to Sense: Oversensing and Undersensing

Failure to sense describes 2 conditions: oversensing and undersensing. Oversensing is a condition marked by improper interpretation of electrical activity, which is sometimes categorized as a failure to pace. The pacemaker misinterprets other signals as if they are QRS complexes, such as peaked T waves in hyperkalemia, or is affected by electromagnetic interference, which inhibits its response. Oversensing is typically a pacemaker inhibition problem. The pacemaker incorrectly interprets the native cardiac rate as faster than it actually is, which can result in unstable rhythms. The pacemaker does not depolarize the myocardium when it should be pacing.

Undersensing describes a condition in which the pacemaker is unable to correctly interpret the native cardiac activity. The pacemaker might not recognize a native P wave of atrial depolarization and therefore sends an impulse to the myocardium to stimulate ventricular contraction. Undersensing is typically an improper pacemaker triggering problem. Causes include lead misplacement, fracture, or migration; a low sensing threshold; cardiac fibrosis or scarring; electrolyte disturbances; and battery failure.

COMPONENTS OF THE PACEMAKER

The categorization of pacemaker failure presented earlier has some overlap in underlying causes and provides no substantial framework for management and treatment. The major components of a pacemaker and their contribution to pacemaker malfunction are discussed here. An understanding of how the individual parts of a pacemaker can result in failure leads to a rational approach to investigating pacemaker malfunction.

Pulse Generator

The pulse generator, which contains the battery, is implanted in the soft tissues or muscles of the anterior chest wall. Low battery or battery depletion remains one of the most common causes of pacemaker failure and can manifest clinically as failure to pace, failure to capture, or failure to sense.[2] Most pacemakers have a battery life of 5 to 10 years after implantation. The life of the pacemaker battery depends on how often the pacemaker is used to provide sensing and pacing functions and can be affected by certain programmable functions of the pacemaker, such as continuous ECG recording. Because battery life cannot be predicted more precisely, appropriate follow-up with a cardiologist or electrophysiologist is necessary to ensure timely replacement of a low battery. Pacemaker interrogation is the only accurate way to determine remaining battery life. The elective replacement indicator is the signal detected on interrogation that the battery is nearing the end of its life. When indicated, the battery should be replaced under sterile operative conditions by a cardiologist.

Other problems associated with the pulse generator include trauma and loose connections of the pacemaker leads. Blunt trauma to the chest can damage the pacemaker and cause it to fail.[13] Loose connections sometimes become apparent on chest radiography. These problems are picked up on routine interrogation of the pacemaker before an emergency situation arises. Improper connections require surgical correction.

Pacemaker Leads

Pacemaker leads connect the pulse generator to the myocardium. Typically, leads are placed in the right ventricle for single-chamber pacemakers; in the right atrium and right ventricle for dual-chamber pacemakers; and the right atrium, right ventricle, and coronary sinus for biventricular pacemakers. Fracture of the leads or breakdown in the insulated coating may lead to improper pacing or sensing functions of the pacemaker system. Trauma has been reported, although rarely, as a cause of lead failure.[14]

Detachment of the lead from the myocardium typically occurs soon after implantation. The clinical presentation might be failure to capture, failure to pace, or failure to sense. A late cause of lead detachment is twiddler's syndrome,[15,16] caused by manipulation and rotation of the pulse generator in the anterior chest wall by the patient. As the generator is rotated, the leads become detached from the myocardium. The syndrome can be diagnosed on routine chest radiography, and its management requires intervention by a cardiologist.

Pacemaker Lead/Myocardium Interface

The pacemaker leads interface with the heart at the myocardium. Alterations at this interface can result in failure to pace, capture, and sense. Changes to the myocardium may alter the threshold energy needed to depolarize the cardiac muscle. Within a few days after implantation, the leads induce a fibrous response in the surrounding myocardium. The classic electrolyte derangement that can increase the depolarization threshold is hyperkalemia.[12] Antiarrhythmic and other classes of drugs can cause changes in the myocardial depolarization threshold. Flecainide is the notorious cause, but even amiodarone can cause myocardial conduction changes.[17] The diagnosis is based on routine laboratory analysis and can be confirmed on device interrogation. Treatment involves changing the device threshold in patients with myocardial fibrosis at the lead implantation site or correcting the underlying cause in patients with electrolyte or toxic drug levels.

EMERGENCY DEPARTMENT APPROACH TO PACEMAKER MALFUNCTION
Investigation and Work-up

The history and physical examination should be directed toward determining whether the patient has any underlying problems or circumstances that could lead to pacemaker problems, such as acute coronary syndrome (ACS), trauma, medication changes, or recent device reprogramming. The physician should document the name of the device manufacturer and the date the device was implanted. Patients are given cards with this information to keep in their wallets, but these might not be available in the ED. If the patient is unaware of the manufacturer, an overpenetrated chest radiograph can be used to determine the device maker by identifying the company symbol (**Fig. 1**). The patient should be asked about the last time the pacemaker was checked; many patients with pacemakers have not seen a cardiologist for a long time and might not realize that their device's battery has run low.

The work-up of the patient with presumed pacemaker malfunction involves a few routine tests. All patients should have an ECG to determine whether an unstable bradycardia is present. Patients should have a chest radiograph to check for lead dislodgement, fracture, or pneumothorax. Patients should have electrolyte testing and serum measurements of any cardiotoxic drugs, especially those with a narrow therapeutic index. Depending on the patient's complaint and history of present illness, assessment of cardiac biomarkers can be considered but are not needed routinely in all cases.

Management

No matter the cause of pacemaker failure, ED management is dictated by the patient's symptoms and hemodynamic status. Transcutaneous pacing pads should be placed on the patient whenever malfunction is suspected. In the absence of hemodynamic compromise, early interrogation and admission to a monitored setting are appropriate. If a pacemaker-dependent patient is bradycardic with symptoms of hypoperfusion, standard advanced cardiac life support (ACLS) protocols should be followed. Transcutaneous pacing has a 77% success rate for electrical capture and 20.6% for

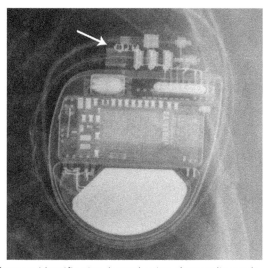

Fig. 1. ICD manufacturer identification (*arrow*) using chest radiograph.

mechanical capture.[18] In cases of failure of capture from transcutaneous pacing, emergent transvenous pacing might be necessary. In all cases, the patient's cardiologist or a hospital-based electrophysiologist should be involved early; local resources influence the consultation process. Admission to an intensive care unit or cardiac care unit for close monitoring might be warranted.

Emergency care providers should recognize that one cause of pacemaker failure can be remedied by placing a cardiac magnet over the pacemaker pocket. Oversensing by the pacemaker can lead to inappropriate inhibition of a pacing stimulus. If oversensing is thought to be causing an unstable rhythm, a magnet can be placed on top of the pacemaker device to change its settings. The magnet changes the pacemaker to a fixed, asynchronous pacing mode (typically VOO or DOO). This mode eliminates any sensing functionality of the pacemaker and allows pacing at a prefixed rate, which is typically set between 60 and 80 beats per minute.

Deciphering the true cause of device malfunction often requires device interrogation. A device representative or cardiologist experienced in interrogation usually does this testing, but a recent study showed that interrogation can also be performed in the ED by noncardiologists.[19] Interrogation yields information on battery life, sensing and pacing thresholds, integrity of the lead system, and recordings of cardiac rhythm. The results of interrogation might indicate the need for battery or lead replacement or threshold adjustment. A specialist needs to be involved in the care of many of these patients, but, with growing confidence among emergency care providers, interrogation will be conducted more often in the ED to identify the cause of pacemaker malfunction early in its presentation.

PACEMAKER-INDUCED DYSRHYTHMIAS AND SYNDROMES
Pacemaker-mediated Tachycardia

Pacemaker-mediated tachycardia (PMT) is a reentrant loop tachycardia that is unique to dual-chamber pacemakers that have atrial-sensing functionality. In patients with both atrial and ventricular leads, a premature ventricular contraction or paced ventricular depolarization is occasionally delivered to the atria in retrograde fashion, which stimulates atrial sensing, triggering another ventricular depolarization. An endless feedback loop of continuous ventricular discharges is created. The rate of this pacemaker-mediated dysrhythmia never exceeds the upper rate limit to which the pacemaker is set. With advances in pacemaker programming, PMT is encountered less frequently.[20]

Treatment of PMT involves interrupting the reentrant loop. One way of accomplishing this is by using a magnet to put the pacemaker in a temporary asynchronous pacing mode. This mode eliminates the sensing function of the atria and enables the pacemaker to pace at the predefined asynchronous rate. In the absence of a magnet, any medical therapy, such as adenosine, that increases the refractory period at the atrioventricular (AV) node can terminate the arrhythmia.[21] Similar success should be expected with calcium channel blockers and β-blockers.

Runaway Pacemaker

The runaway pacemaker is an often-discussed but infrequently encountered scenario of pulse generator failure. In this rare event, the central processing unit–based programming system of the pacemaker somehow becomes unpredictable and paces the patient at a rate considerably greater than any programming threshold. A runaway pacemaker is differentiated from PMT by virtue of the pacing rate being greater than the programmed upper limit. Reports of magnets being used to control the rate can be found in the literature, but usually the runaway pacemaker and its pulse generator cannot be reprogrammed to produce a stable output.[22,23] The option of last resort is to disconnect the pacemaker leads from the pulse generator, which involves cutting open the pocket to expose the components. In hemodynamically stable patients, this procedure can be accomplished by involving a surgeon or cardiology specialist, but in some cases it has been performed by emergency physicians.[24]

Pacemaker Syndrome

Patients with pacemakers can present with a myriad of complaints. Pacemaker syndrome is a term used to describe abnormal patient symptoms after all other causes of pacemaker malfunction have been ruled out. Furman[25] defined is as "the result of the hemodynamic and rhythmic deficiencies of incomplete restorations of the normal pattern of cardiac depolarization, the normal relationship of atrial and ventricular contraction at a physiological AV interval, or retrograde activation of the atrium and an inadequate response to physiologic need." Stated more simply, this syndrome arises as a consequence of AV dyssynchrony. Symptoms can run the spectrum from mild to severe and include shortness of breath, dizziness, fatigue, pulsations in the neck, anxiety, chest pain, palpitations, choking, and confusion.[26] Pacemaker syndrome tends to be a diagnosis of exclusion and has many symptoms that overlap with emergencies such as ACS. Careful evaluation of these patients and involvement of their cardiologists is key to management without overtesting.

ADVANCED CARDIAC LIFE SUPPORT

As pacemakers are implanted into an aging population with cardiac disease, emergency physicians will encounter those with unstable cardiac rhythms or in cardiac arrest more frequently. ACLS can be delivered according to the AHA guidelines, with a few extra considerations. Earlier pacemaker models had pulse generators that were reset when defibrillation was performed with the paddles or pads overlying the pacemaker pocket. It is now recommended that, whenever possible, an anterior-posterior configuration of defibrillation pads be used and that the pads never be placed over the cardiac device. The incidence of pulse generator reprogramming after defibrillation is lower with newer pacemakers, so device interrogation after defibrillation may not need to be routinely performed.[27]

IMPLANTABLE CARDIOVERTER-DEFIBRILLATORS

ICDs have decreased the mortality for patients with a history of, or risk factors for, cardiac arrhythmias and sudden cardiac death. These devices are inserted in a fashion similar to pacemakers, and most newly implanted ICDs have pacing functionality in addition to antitachycardia pacing and shock delivery. Patients often present to the ED after receiving one or more shocks. These defibrillations might be appropriate or inappropriate. This article discusses the general indications for placement of ICDs, the approach to patients with devices that have fired, how to manage patients in electrical storm, and how to approach ICD patients in cardiac arrest.

INDICATIONS FOR IMPLANTABLE CARDIOVERTER-DEFIBRILLATORS

ICDs are implanted for 2 reasons: the secondary prevention of sudden cardiac death in patients with unstable arrhythmias or the primary prevention of cardiac death in patients with risk factors for developing an unstable arrhythmia (eg, ischemic cardiomyopathy). The former group includes patients with congenital problems affecting the conduction of the heart, such as long-QT syndrome and Brugada syndrome; the latter group includes patients low systolic heart function from ischemic and nonischemic cardiomyopathy. Many trials have found that ICD implantation results in a survival benefit compared with antiarrhythmic medical therapy.[17] Indications for ICD placement are listed in **Table 4**. Current guidelines on ICD placement include a comprehensive list of indications, and levels of evidence are described in the 2008 ACC/AHA/HRS guidelines.[6]

APPROACH TO THE IMPLANTABLE CARDIOVERTER-DEFIBRILLATOR THAT HAS FIRED A SINGLE TIME

Some patients come to the ED after a single firing of their ICD, even though cardiologists advise them not to seek emergency care after receiving a single shock unless they have persistent or severe symptoms.[28] Patients who receive a single shock can be seen the next day by their cardiologist for urgent interrogation. However, when they come to the ED, they should have a medically appropriate work-up, including a focused history and physical. The practitioner should identify any symptoms that preceded the shock and any that lasted after the shock. Diagnostic testing should then be focused on the likely causes. An ECG, electrolyte studies, and a chest radiograph are appropriate tests to seek an underlying cause of the defibrillation. Interrogation should be arranged, through the patient's cardiologist, as an urgent outpatient appointment, or it can be performed in the ED if it can be arranged quickly.

APPROACH TO THE IMPLANTABLE CARDIOVERTER-DEFIBRILLATOR THAT HAS FIRED MULTIPLE TIMES

Patients presenting to the ED after multiple shocks should receive prompt evaluation and management of any ongoing tachydysrhythmia. Multiple ICD shocks can be

Table 4
Indications for ICD placement

Recommendation	ACCF/AHA/HRS Guidelines	Conditions That Must Be Met
Primary Prevention		
Coronary artery disease	I A	EF<35% and NYHA class II or III
Nonischemic cardiomyopathy	I B	EF<35% and NYHA class II or III
Nonischemic cardiomyopathy	IIb C	EF<35% and NYHA class I
Hypertrophic cardiomyopathy	IIa C	Requires 1 risk factor for SCD
Long-QT syndrome	IIb D	
Brugada syndrome	IIa C	—
Infiltrative diseases	IIa C	Sarcoidosis, giant cell myocarditis, Chagas disease
Secondary Prevention		
Coronary artery disease	I A	—
Nonischemic cardiomyopathy	I A	—
Hypertrophic cardiomyopathy	I B	—
Arrhythmogenic RV dysplasia	I A	—
Long-QT syndrome	IIa B	—
Syncope, inducible VF	I B	—

Abbreviations: NYHA, New York Heart Association; RV, right ventricle; SCD, sudden cardiac death; VF, ventricular fibrillation.

categorized as appropriate or inappropriate defibrillations. Early identification of the difference guides all subsequent management. All patients should have an ECG and a continuous rhythm strip that attempts to identify the cardiac dysrhythmia when the patient is symptomatic. Standard electrolyte and cardiac biomarker measurements should be obtained as well as a chest radiograph.

Inappropriate Shocks

Many ICD shocks are delivered for tachydysrhythmias that are not hemodynamically significant. An ICD determines whether to deliver a shock based on information about the heart rate and the duration of time spent at that rate. For this reason, many types of supraventricular tachycardia trigger inappropriate defibrillation. If a patient is diagnosed with supraventricular tachycardia, therapy should be initiated with medications that can treat it. If the defibrillations are persistent and distressing to the patient, a magnet can be placed over the ICD to temporarily disable tachyarrhythmia therapy. For all ICDs, when a magnet is applied, only the ability to defibrillate is disabled; the device maintains the ability to function as a pacemaker. Once the magnet is removed, the ICD, in most cases, resumes the ability to deliver therapy.[28] Because a cardiac magnet disables defibrillation functionality, and some defibrillators require reprogramming once the magnet is removed, all patients with a magnet in place should have external defibrillation pads placed on the chest and back.

Appropriate Shocks

Patients with ventricular dysrhythmias that result in multiple appropriate shocks should first be treated according to standard ACLS protocol. External defibrillation pads can be placed on the patient; the anterior-posterior configuration is preferred. Antiarrhythmic medications can be administered. A magnet should not be placed in this circumstance if the defibrillator is providing appropriate therapy to the patient. Patients with continued ventricular dysrhythmias are categorized as having electrical storm.

Electrical Storm

Electrical storm carries somewhat arbitrary diagnostic criteria. Patients receiving more than 3 distinct episodes of ventricular tachycardia or ventricular fibrillation in a 24-hour period are said to be in a state of electrical storm. Electrical storm has been reported in 10% to 40% of patients after receiving devices for secondary prevention of sudden cardiac death.[29] No reliable predictors of storm have been borne out in the literature.[30] It can be brought on by electrolyte abnormalities, heart failure, or noncompliance with medications; however, most cases occur without a precipitating event.[29,30] The pathophysiology is not well understood, but increased sympathetic outflow has been identified as both a contributor to onset and a possible target for medical therapy.

Treatment

Electrical storm is a highly morbid condition, with estimates of 1-year survival ranging from 5% to 35%.[31–33] Its treatment options are different from those recommended by ACLS guidelines. All patients should receive amiodarone as an initial antiarrhythmic. Some studies have found suboptimal outcomes with lidocaine and procainamide, but no head-to-head comparisons of the antiarrhythmics have been conducted.[34] In small studies, patients have done better with treatment designed to achieve sympathetic overstimulation. Stellate ganglion blockade by anesthesia and beta-blockade have been effective.[34] Intravenous metoprolol, propranolol, or esmolol can be used in addition to traditional antiarrhythmics. In many cases, specialized care by the elecrophysiologist with catheter-based ablation techniques may be needed.[35] Case reports have suggested that, when other measures fail, it may be reasonable to attempt general anesthesia.[28] Electrical storm is difficult to manage, and several different therapies might need to be initiated in close consultation with the electrophysiologist.

CHECKING CARDIAC BIOMARKERS AFTER DEFIBRILLATION

After defibrillation, evaluation of cardiac biomarkers can be difficult, especially when there is concern for possible ACS. Studies have shown that defibrillation can cause an increase in troponin levels.[36] There is some suggestion that troponins peak earlier in patients with ACS. An increased troponin level in the absence of ACS remains a predictor of morbidity for patients with ICDs. Cardiac biomarkers can be checked selectively in patients who present after a single defibrillation; only those with symptoms consistent with ACS preceding defibrillation should undergo such evaluation.

CARDIAC ARREST IN PATIENTS WITH IMPLANTABLE CARDIOVERTER-DEFIBRILLATORS

When a patient with an ICD presents in cardiac arrest, ACLS therapy should be instituted. Recommendations regarding pad placement, chest compressions, and use of magnets are discussed later.

Pad Placement

Defibrillation pads should be placed on the patient in the anterior-posterior orientation to avoid placing a pad directly over the ICD. External defibrillation should be used for any shockable rhythm, because patients with ICDs may have misplaced or malfunctioning leads.

Chest Compressions

Chest compressions should be provided with minimal interruptions. Rescuers can often feel cardiac defibrillation from ICDs when performing compressions.[37] There is no published evidence that rescuers have been harmed by performing defibrillation on patients with ICDs. Standard precautions should always be followed, and rescuers should wear gloves when providing chest compressions.

Use of Magnets

A magnet can be applied to the defibrillator to stop the ICD from delivering therapy. It is inadvisable to prevent the ICD from delivering appropriate shocks during cardiac arrest.

COMPLICATIONS ASSOCIATED WITH DEVICE INSERTION: PACEMAKERS AND IMPLANTABLE CARDIOVERTER-DEFIBRILLATORS
Pocket Hematoma

Bleeding is a common complication early after insertion of cardiac pacemakers and ICDs. The hematomas can be large enough to require surgical evacuation of the pocket. In a case series published in 1999, the rate of surgical evacuation of hematomas was 1% to 2% among patients who received implants.[38] Aspiration of bloody contents from the pocket is not recommended. This procedure is rarely effective and it runs the risk of damaging the pulse generator or the proximal portion of the pacemaker leads.

Pocket Infections

Infections of the ICD or pacemaker occur in up to 8% of patients. Infections that arise early after implantation typically stem from the surgical procedure and involve the pocket. Patients present with erythema, edema, fluctuance, and dehiscence of the surgical incision. The pocket might show erythema or fluctuance or be tender on examination. A formal diagnosis can be made through aspiration or culture of the device pocket; this is typically left to a physician experienced with the procedure to prevent damage to the components of the pacemaker or ICD system. The emergency physician can request laboratory studies (eg, complete blood count) and can obtain blood for culture, although these tests are typically low yield. Treatment with appropriate antibiotics should be initiated whenever infection is suspected. Because most infections are caused by *Staphylococcus aureus* and *Staphylococcus epidermidis*, empiric coverage with vancomycin or a similar antistaphylococcal with methicillin-resistant *S aureus* coverage should be initiated in the ED. Definitive care might require surgical removal by the physician who inserted the device.

Lead Infections

Infections that arise later after implantation tend to affect the pacemaker leads, leading to serious complications. Patients can present with bacteremia, lead vegetations, endocarditis, and septic pulmonary emboli. They are critically ill, with the signs and symptoms that define sepsis. Blood cultures and early antibiotics are the mainstay of therapy in the ED. Many of the causative bacteria are staphylococci, so grampositive coverage with vancomycin is recommended. Definite lead infection is an absolute indication for lead removal.

Pericardial Effusion

Perforation of the myocardium is a feared complication of lead implantation. Patients might present insidiously, typically in the early hours after device implantation, but perforation can also be a late complication.[39,40] As for other causes of pericardial effusion and tamponade, the clinical signs vary. Hypotension in a patient with a cardiac device should prompt the emergency physician to use ultrasonography to look for pericardial effusion. In a crashing patient with a pericardial effusion, emergency pericardiocentesis should be performed until the patient can be evaluated for pericardial window with myocardial repair.[41]

Pneumothorax

Placement of the pacemaker or ICD leads requires puncture of the subclavian vein and threading of the wires into the right atrium, right ventricle, or myocardium, depending on the type of device being inserted. The proximity of the subclavian vessels to the apical pleura of the lung makes pneumothorax a possible complication of device insertion. Pneumothorax occurs in about 1% of insertions. It can often be managed expectantly, but, if it is large enough, tube thoracostomy might be required. This complication usually occurs within the first 48 hours after insertion. It is rare in the ED and is most likely if a patient with a known pneumothorax had worsening dyspnea and lung collapse after expectant management and discharge.

Thrombosis/Superior Vena Cava Syndrome

Pacemaker and ICD lead systems enter the superior vena cava. Deep venous thrombosis (DVT) can develop soon after insertion or years after implantation. It is often reported that symptomatic venous thromboembolism occurs in 5% of patients, even though this number is taken from older literature. Changes have been made in the implantation technique and the types of leads that are implanted.[42] Patients can present with fever, upper extremity swelling, or facial swelling, depending on the location of the thrombus. When the face is involved, superior vena cava syndrome should be considered.[43] If thromboembolism occurs, pulmonary manifestations might predominate. Dyspnea, pleuritic chest pain, cough, and hemoptysis are classically described but not always present. DVT can be diagnosed with duplex ultrasonography or computed tomography venography if extensive disease is suspected. Treatment is early anticoagulation; further therapy is rarely required.[44] The lead is usually not removed, because removal risks a worsening of symptoms.

SUMMARY

Pacemakers and ICDs are inserted for a variety of cardiac conditions. Because these devices are becoming more common, it is imperative that emergency physicians understand how they work and under what conditions patients present for emergent evaluation. Basing treatment decisions on hemodynamic status associated with pacemaker malfunction ensures that patients receive timely and appropriate care. The approach to patients who come to the ED after receiving one or more shocks from their ICD varies depending on the presenting symptoms. Interventions for ICD patients in cardiac arrest can be performed with only modest modifications to ACLS protocols.

REFERENCES

1. Maisel WH, Moynahan M, Zuckerman BD, et al. Pacemaker and ICD generator malfunctions: analysis of food and drug administration annual reports. JAMA 2006;295:1901–6.
2. Maisel WH. Pacemaker and ICD generator reliability. JAMA 2006;295:1929–34.
3. Greenspon AJ, Patel JD, Lau E, et al. Trends in permanent pacemaker implantation in the United States from 1993 to 2009: increasing complexity of patients and procedures. J Am Coll Cardiol 2012;60:1540–5.
4. Bernstein AD, Daubert JC, Fletcher RD, et al. The revised NASPE/BPEG generic code for antibradycardia, adaptive-rate, and multisite pacing. North American Society of Pacing and Electrophysiology/British Pacing and Electrophysiology Group. Pacing Clin Electrophysiol 2002;25:260–4.
5. Epstein AE, DiMarco JP, Ellenbogen KA, et al. 2012 ACCF/AHA/HRS focused update incorporated into the ACCF/AHA/HRS 2008 guidelines for device-based therapy of cardiac rhythm abnormalities: a report of the American College of Cardiology Foundation/American Heart Association Task Force on Practice Guidelines and the Heart Rhythm Society. J Am Coll Cardiol 2013;61:e6–75.
6. Epstein AE, DiMarco JP, Ellenbogen KA, et al. ACC/AHA/HRS 2008 guidelines for device-based therapy of cardiac rhythm abnormalities: a report of the American College of Cardiology/American Heart Association Task Force on Practice Guidelines (writing committee to revise the ACC/AHA/NASPE 2002 guideline update for implantation of cardiac pacemakers and antiarrhythmia devices): developed in collaboration with the American Association for Thoracic Surgery and Society of Thoracic Surgeons. Circulation 2008;117:e50.
7. Brignole M, Auricchio A, Baron-Esquivias G, et al. 2013 ESC guidelines on cardiac pacing and cardiac resynchronization therapy: the Task Force on Cardiac Pacing and resynchronization Therapy of the European Society of Cardiology (ESC): developed in collaboration with the European Heart Rhythm Association (EHRA). Eur Heart J 2013;34:2281–329.

8. Cardall TY, Chan TC, Brady WJ, et al. Permanent cardiac pacemakers: issues relevant to the emergency physician, part I. J Emerg Med 1999;17:479–89.
9. Cardall TY, Brady WJ, Chan TC, et al. Permanent cardiac pacemakers: issues relevant to the emergency physician, part II. J Emerg Med 1999;17:697–709.
10. McMullan J, Valento M, Attari M, et al. Care of the pacemaker/implantable cardioverter defibrillator patient in the ED. Am J Emerg Med 2007;25:812–22.
11. Neuenschwander JF. Cardiac devices in emergency department heart failure patients. Heart Failure Clin 2009;5:63–73.
12. Schiraldi F, Guiotto G, Paladino F. Hyperkalemia induced failure of pacemaker capture and sensing. Resuscitation 2008;79:161–4.
13. Brown KR, Carter W Jr, Lombardi GE. Blunt trauma-induced pacemaker failure. Ann Emerg Med 1991;20:905–7.
14. Chen WL, Chen YJ, Tsao YT. Traumatic pacemaker lead fracture. J Trauma 2010;69:e34.
15. Bayliss CE, Beanlands DS, Baird RJ. The pacemaker-twiddler's syndrome: a new complication of implantable transvenous pacemakers. Can Med Assoc J 1968;99:371–3.
16. Nicholson WJ, Tuohy KA, Tilkemeier P. Twiddler's syndrome. N Engl J Med 2003;348:1726–7.
17. Van Herendael H, Pinter A, Ahmad K, et al. Role of anti-arrhythmic drugs in patients with implantable cardioverter defibrillators. Europace 2010;12:618–25.
18. Vukmir RB. Emergency cardiac pacing. Am J Emerg Med 1993;11:166–74.
19. Neuenschwander JF, Hiestand BC, Peacock WF. A pilot study of implantable cardiac device interrogation by emergency department personnel. Crit Pathw Cardiol 2014;13:6–8.
20. Oseran D, Ausubel K, Klementowicz PT, et al. Spontaneous endless loop tachycardia. Pacing Clin Electrophysiol 1986;9:379–86.
21. Conti JB, Curtis AB, Hill JA, et al. Termination of pacemaker-mediated tachycardia by adenosine. Clin Cardiol 1994;17:47–8.
22. Griffin J, Smithline H, Cook J. Runaway pacemaker: a case report and review. J Emerg Med 2000;19:177–81.
23. Makaryus AN, Patrick C, Maccaro P. A rare case of "runaway" pacemaker in a modern CPU-controlled pacemaker. Pacing Clin Electrophysiol 2005;28:993–6.
24. Campo A, Nowak R, Magilligan D, et al. Runaway pacemaker. Ann Emerg Med 1983;12(1):32–4.
25. Furman S. Pacemaker syndrome. Pacing Clin Electrophysiol 1994;17:1–5.
26. Ellenbogen KA, Gilligan DM, Wood MA, et al. The pacemaker syndrome - a matter of definition. Am J Cardiol 1997;79:1226–9.
27. Gammage MD. External cardioversion in patients with implanted cardiac devices: is there a problem? Eur Heart J 2007;28:1668–9.
28. Braunschweig F, Boriani G, Bauer A, et al. Management of patients receiving implantable cardiac defibrillator shocks: recommendations for acute and long-term patient management. Europace 2010;12:1673–90.
29. Hohnloser SH, Al-Khalidi HR, Pratt CM, et al. Electrical storm in patients with an implantable defibrillator: incidence, features, and preventive therapy: insights from a randomized trial. Eur Heart J 2006;27:3027–32.
30. Brigadeau F, Kouakam C, Klug D, et al. Clinical predictors and prognostic significance of electrical storm in patients with implantable cardioverter defibrillators. Eur Heart J 2006;27:700–7.

31. Sesselberg HW, Moss AJ, McNitt S, et al. Ventricular arrhythmia storms in posin-farction patients with implantable defibrillators for primary prevention indications: a MADIT-II substudy. Heart Rhythm 2007;4:1395–402.

32. Exner DV, Pinski SL, Wyse DG, et al. Electrical storm presages nonsudden death: the antiarrhythmics versus implantable defibrillators (AVID) trial. Circulation 2001; 103:2066–71.

33. Verma A, Kilicaslan F, Marrouche NF, et al. Prevalence, predictors, and mortality significance of the causative arrhythmia in patients with electrical storm. J Cardiovasc Electrophysiol 2004;15:1265–70.

34. Nademanee K, Taylor R, Bailey WE, et al. Treating electrical storm: sympathetic blockade versus advanced cardiac life support-guided therapy. Circulation 2000;102:742–7.

35. Carbucicchio C, Santamaria M, Trevisi N, et al. Catheter ablation for the treatment of electrical storm in patients with implantable cardioverter-defibrillators: short- and long-term outcomes in a prospective single-center study. Circulation 2008; 117:462–9.

36. Targett C. Towards evidence-based emergency medicine: best BETs from the Manchester Royal Infirmary. BET2: is there value in testing troponin levels after ICD discharge? Emerg Med J 2014;31:249–51.

37. Lechleuthner A. Electric shock to paramedic during cardiopulmonary resuscita-tion of patient with implanted cardiodefibrillator. Lancet 1995;345:253.

38. Kiviniemi M, Pirnes M, Eränen H, et al. Complications related to permanent pace-maker therapy. Pacing Clin Electrophysiol 1999;22:711–20.

39. O'Neill R, Silver M, Khorfan F. Pneumopericardium with cardiac tamponade as a complication of cardiac pacemaker insertion one year after procedure. J Emerg Med 2012;43:641–4.

40. Koyama S, Itatani K, Kyo S, et al. Subacute presentation of right ventricular perfo-ration after pacemaker implantation. Ann Thorac Cardiovasc Surg 2013;19:73–5.

41. Pavia S, Wilkoff B. The management of surgical complications of pacemaker and implantable cardioverter-defibrillators. Curr Opin Cardiol 2001;16:66–71.

42. Phibbs B, Marriott H. Complications of permanent transvenous pacing. N Engl J Med 1985;22:1428–32.

43. Mazzetti H, Daussaut A, Tentori C, et al. Superior vena cava occlusion and/or syn-drome related to pacemaker leads. Am Heart J 1993;125:831–7.

44. Barakat K, Robinson NM, Spurrell RA. Transvenous pacing lead-induced throm-bosis: a series of cases with a review of the literature. Cardiology 2000;93: 142–9.

Cardiac Arrest Resuscitation

Francis X. Guyette, MD, MPH[a], Joshua C. Reynolds, MD, MS[b],*,
Adam Frisch, MD, MS[c], Post Cardiac Arrest Service

KEYWORDS

- Cardiac arrest • Defibrillation • Chest compressions • Airway • Medications

KEY POINTS

- Pit crew–style cardiopulmonary resuscitation improves efficiency, communication, and is associated with improved outcomes.
- Large, randomized controlled trials are underway to address the optimal strategy for ALS resuscitation.
- No resuscitative medication has ever been shown to improve long-term survival or neurologic outcomes.
- The duration of the peri-shock pause is inversely associated with survival and neurologic outcomes.
- High-quality observational evidence suggests that routine prehospital advanced airway management is associated with worse outcomes; a well-conducted randomized trial is needed to address this question.
- Extracorporeal life support is an exciting new therapy that is gaining traction in the United States.

INTRODUCTION

Out-of-hospital cardiac arrest (OHCA) is a profound clinical and public health challenge, both in the United States and across the globe. The incidence of OHCA globally is highest in Australia (113 per year per 100,000 population), followed by North America (94 per year per 100,000 population), Europe (86 per year per 100,000 population), and Asia (55 per year per 100,000 population).[1] Cardiovascular disease is the most common cause of OHCA, and death caused by cardiovascular disease accounts

Disclosures: none.
[a] Department of Emergency Medicine, University of Pittsburgh, Suite 10028, Forbes Tower, Pittsburgh, PA 15260, USA; [b] Department of Emergency Medicine, Michigan State University College of Human Medicine, 15 Michigan Street Northeast, Suite 420, Grand Rapids, MI 49503, USA; [c] Department of Emergency Medicine, Albany Medical Center, 47 New Scotland Avenue, MC 139, Albany, NY 12208, USA
* Corresponding author.
E-mail address: reyno406@msu.edu

Emerg Med Clin N Am 33 (2015) 669–690
http://dx.doi.org/10.1016/j.emc.2015.04.010
0733-8627/15/$ – see front matter © 2015 Elsevier Inc. All rights reserved.

for one-third of annual deaths in the United States.[2] The incidence of OHCA from a presumed cardiac cause is highest in North America (55 per year per 100,000 population), followed by Australia (44 per year per 100,000 population), Europe (35 per year per 100,000 population), and Asia (32 per year per 100,000 population).[1] OHCA is more likely to be from a cardiac cause in patients older than 35 years and more likely to be from a noncardiac cause in patients younger than 35 years.[3] In fact, 83% of cardiac arrests occurring in patients younger than 19 years are noncardiac in origin.[4] Health care providers are notoriously inaccurate in predicting the cause of OHCA, often underestimating noncardiac causes.[5,6]

There is marked regional variation in outcomes from OHCA, as documented by a 10-site North American resuscitation research consortium with a total catchment population of 21.4 million.[7] The median survival to hospital discharge of emergency medical services (EMS)–treated patients with cardiac arrest was 8.4% (interquartile range: 5.4%–10.4%), with survival rates ranging from 3.0% to 16.3% across North America. Survival was markedly higher in patients with ventricular fibrillation (VF) as the initial rhythm. The median survival to hospital discharge in this subpopulation was 22.0% (interquartile range: 15.0%–24.4%), with survival rates ranging from 7.7% to 39.9% across the same geographic locales.

Resuscitation science has evolved greatly since the inception of cardiopulmonary resuscitation (CPR).[8] An internal body of experts, the International Liaison Committee on Resuscitation (ILCOR), updates the guidelines and recommendations for resuscitation by health care professionals every 5 years. ILCOR conducts hundreds of systematic reviews every 5 years to delineate the latest consensus on resuscitation science and provide treatment recommendations based on available evidence and expert opinion. ILCOR recommendations are then funneled through national or regional associations (eg, American Heart Association) and packaged as educational curricula (eg, Basic Life Support or Advanced Cardiac Life Support). The emergency provider must be aware of the source material for these curricula and understand the accumulated evidence behind the latest recommendations. In this section, the authors highlight the latest evidence and controversies surrounding key facets of cardiac arrest resuscitation.

GENERAL MANAGEMENT CONSIDERATIONS

Cardiac arrest is a dynamic disease. Few other clinical presentations strain the multitasking and leadership abilities of the emergency physician to the same degree. However, the astute clinician must realize that he or she is orchestrating only one portion of a larger series of events, each of which directly affects patient outcomes. Prehospital and/or emergency department resuscitation to achieve return of spontaneous circulation (ROSC) is only one small piece of the puzzle. Layperson recognition of cardiac arrest, activation of the EMS system, and provision of bystander CPR are equally important tasks. Likewise, the critical care, inpatient, and rehabilitation phases play crucial roles in attaining neurologically favorable survival. This larger view of cardiac arrest care is embodied in the success of bundled postresuscitation care packages that boost rates of neurologically favorable survival among patients attaining ROSC.[9]

Pit Crew Cardiopulmonary Resuscitation

Prompt and effective cardiac arrest management is often difficult in the hectic and potentially austere environments surrounding cardiac arrest. To orchestrate efficient and effective resuscitation, regimented training and good working relationships between providers are vitally important. One proposed way of managing the chaos of resuscitation is with pit crew CPR. This technique, similar to that used in auto racing, is centered on a core group of providers who each have preassigned roles in patient management. Each provider's role is determined by his or her physical location and proximity to the patient. For example, the provider at the head will always be in charge of the airway, and the provider near the patient's left shoulder will always be in charge of chest compressions. This concept is similar to that used by trauma resuscitation teams. Having these predetermined roles as part of a bundle of cardiac arrest management has been shown to improve outcomes in cardiac arrest care.[10]

CIRCULATORY SUPPORT
Mechanical Cardiopulmonary Resuscitation

Several devices currently exist that perform mechanical CPR. The most common devices use either a piston system or compression band system to decrease the volume of the thoracic cavity, pushing blood throughout the body. These devices are intended to deliver compressions comparable with manual CPR but in a mechanized fashion that is reliable and efficient. The devices are timed to either work in a 30:2 ratio or to deliver continuous compressions at rates suggested by the American Heart Association.

Several studies have been performed to evaluate these devices, but it should be noted that many of them are manufacturer sponsored. Studies evaluating CPR metrics, including end-tidal carbon dioxide measurements, cerebral blood flow, and coronary perfusion pressure, have shown better results with mechanical CPR devices when compared with manual CPR.[11–13] Despite this, randomized trials and a meta-analysis have found a slight trend toward higher rates of ROSC but have failed to show an outcome benefit between the two techniques.[14–17]

Application time of the mechanical device currently seems to be the biggest issue with its use.[18,19] For most devices, some amount of hands-off time is needed to apply the device; in the hands of an untrained rescuer, this could lead to significant time without compressions. All of the currently manufactured devices have some posterior component that necessitates halting compressions to allow for proper device placement.

Some device-related injuries have been reported, but these have not been associated with patient outcomes.[20] Not surprisingly, most injuries reported are similar to those seen with manual CPR: rib fractures, sternal fractures, liver lacerations, and pulmonary contusions. However, it should be noted that mechanical devices are typically applied after some duration of manual CPR. Therefore, it is difficult to attribute specific injuries to the mechanical device as opposed to the preceding manual compressions.

Mechanical devices seem to provide the most benefit in prolonged resuscitations when providers may tire,[21] in situations whereby manual CPR is dangerous or not feasible,[21] or as a bridge to percutaneous coronary intervention (PCI) or mechanical support.[22,23] Devices may also be helpful while transporting patients or in the prehospital setting where environmental conditions may make manual CPR techniques dangerous to patients and/or providers. Mechanical devices may also simplify the logistics of resuscitation, decrease the number of providers needed at the bedside, and allow providers to focus on other critical interventions. By removing one of the most physically demanding portions of cardiac arrest management, more time, energy, and focus may be allotted to other tasks and/or addressing the underlying cause for cardiac arrest.

Compression-Only Cardiopulmonary Resuscitation

Compression-only CPR refers to the use of only the chest compression portion of traditional CPR. CPR guidelines place a large emphasis on limiting interruptions in chest compressions. The American Heart Association now suggests the use of compression-only CPR for lay rescuers because it is technically simpler and better received by most laypersons.[24] Data for professional rescuers and hospital personnel are varied, and the current literature shows studies with mixed results on outcomes that may hinge on the cause of cardiac arrest. Some observational data suggest that patients who experience cardiac arrest from a noncardiac cause may do better with traditional CPR.[25–27] A recent meta-analysis of observational studies found no outcome difference between the two techniques.[28] Although there are inconsistent data on the need for rescue breaths during CPR, there is consensus on the need for prompt, effective chest compressions with limited interruptions.

Continuous Versus 30:2

The primary arguments for continuous chest compressions are similar to those for compression-only CPR. The term *continuous chest compressions* most often refers to the initial period of resuscitation, most notably during the first 4 to 6 minutes after loss of pulses. During this initial phase, myocardial and cerebral tissue may be most sensitive to decreased blood flow, and hypoperfusion during this sensitive window will lead to worse outcomes. It has been well demonstrated that any interruption in chest compressions, even those for ventilation, decreases coronary perfusion pressure and forward blood flow, which are vital to perfusing the heart and brain, respectively.[29] Not only do quality, uninterrupted compressions perfuse vital organs but they also improve the probability of successful defibrillation. The combination of uninterrupted compressions and a minimized preshock pause in compressions is associated with improved defibrillation success and neurologic outcomes in preclinical studies.[30] A multicenter randomized trial of continuous compressions and standard CPR is currently underway (ClinicalTrials.gov NCT01372748).

The other argument for the use of continuous compressions is that it prevents providers from performing advanced airway maneuvers or other interventions that, at worst, may be harmful to patients or may simply detract from the focus on quality, minimally interrupted compressions. Several studies have called into question the use of advanced airways in patients with prehospital cardiac arrest.[31] In large observational studies, the use of advanced airways is associated with worse outcomes.[32–34] Preclinical studies have found that even the 2 breaths given during a conventional 30:2 compression cycle cause increased intrathoracic pressures, decreased venous return to the chest, and decreased blood flow to the heart and brain.[35] Although there is still ongoing controversy over the best compression/breath ratio with a BLS/native airway, continuous compressions at a rate 100 or more per minute should be used after placement of an advanced airway.

DEFIBRILLATION
Energy Selection and Delivery Method

The original defibrillator was a simple pair of electrodes conducting a 110-V alternating current through the exposed heart. Modern external defibrillators are available in a variety of designs with proprietary waveforms (eg, biphasic truncated exponential, pulsed biphasic, rectilinear biphasic, damped sinusoid monophasic, and monophasic truncated exponential) specific to the manufacturer. Most defibrillators currently available on the market use biphasic waveforms, which are associated with lower energy requirements to terminate VF and improved first shock success.[36,37] A randomized clinical trial comparing monophasic and biphasic defibrillation did demonstrate improved first shock success and decreased time to ROSC with biphasic defibrillation but failed to find any difference in survival or neurologic outcomes.[38] Providers should be familiar with the defibrillator available to them and the manufacturer recommendations for its use. The recommended energy for biphasic defibrillation is manufacturer dependent, varying between 150 to 360 J.[39,40] Recently, concerns have arisen regarding the effectiveness of the recommended first shock energies, which have prompted some prehospital agencies to protocolize a highest-dose-first strategy. In some cases of refractory fibrillation, successful restoration of a perfusing rhythm has been achieved by double sequential defibrillation, which is the concurrent application of 2 defibrillators that are discharged nearly simultaneously. Double sequential defibrillation was originally described in the electrophysiology laboratory as a strategy for terminating persistent atrial fibrillation. Since then, it has been attempted with some success in out-of-hospital VF.[41,42]

Timing of Shock Delivery

Historically, early defibrillation has been a key link in the chain of survival and is important to minimize the elapsed interval until ROSC.[43] However, observational data suggests that defibrillation of a myocardium depleted of high energy phosphates resulted in higher incidence of post-defibrillation asystole.[44] This begged the following question: Should some period of chest compressions be performed before defibrillation to restore high-energy phosphates and prime the myocardium?[45,46] Three studies attempted to address this question and produced conflicting results: 2 failed to demonstrate any benefit of CPR before defibrillation, whereas a third showed improved survival in a subgroup of patients for whom EMS response exceeded 4 minutes.[47–49] In 2011, an international multicenter randomized controlled trial of nearly 10,000 patients failed to show a difference in survival with good neurologic outcomes between the two strategies.[50]

Preclinical data suggest that the VF waveform can be used to guide the optimal timing of defibrillation. Certain waveform characteristics (eg, amplitude, frequency, periodicity) are associated with coronary perfusion pressure and myocardial ATP concentration.[51–53] Several studies have suggested that defibrillation success can be predicted with quantitative analysis of the waveform. Clinically, some providers may be familiar with the practice of delaying shock delivery for fine VF to provide CPR, improve perfusion of the myocardium, and increase the coarseness of the waveform.[48,54,55] Real-time automated waveform analysis is not currently available, and no studies of provider interpretation have been conducted. Current recommendations are to perform 200 compressions of high-quality CPR before defibrillation. In addition, defibrillator placement and charging can be accomplished during uninterrupted compressions.

The Peri-Shock Pause

The peri-shock pause begins when compressions are stopped to allow for defibrillation and ends when compressions are resumed after defibrillation. Logistically, this period often includes rhythm assessment, charging the defibrillator, delivering the defibrillation, and waiting for instructions to resume chest compressions. The duration of the peri-shock pause is inversely associated with both ROSC and survival.[56] Reductions in the peri-shock pause, particularly the preshock component, (ie, rhythm analysis and defibrillator charging) increase survival.[57]

The pit crew–style CPR techniques endorsed by the American Heart Association directly address the peri-shock pause. Providers should communicate with each other, so that the defibrillator is simultaneously charging while a compression cycle is finishing. Additionally, use of a monitor defibrillator in the manual mode (as opposed to the automated external defibrillator [AED] mode) is associated with reduction in the preshock pause and improved rates of ROSC. The preshock pause should be minimized as much as possible.

The postshock pause primarily consists of rhythm and pulse checks after defibrillation. Myocardial stunning is very common in the period after ROSC.[58] Even if successfully defibrillated, patients may be initially hypotensive with weak/absent peripheral pulses. Furthermore, the interruption of compressions to perform pulse checks is associated with decreased survival.[59] Therefore, it is prudent to immediately follow a defibrillation attempt with an additional cycle (2 minutes) of chest compressions to minimize the postshock pause.[60] The pit crew techniques discussed earlier also inform this coordination of care between providers.

An alternative technique to eliminate the peri-shock pause altogether is hands-on defibrillation, which consists of continuous compressions throughout the defibrillation. A compelling study of patients undergoing elective cardioversion with a biphasic defibrillator demonstrated that rescuers, protected only by standard polyethylene gloves, could be in contact with the chest without exposure to dangerous levels of current.[61] Subsequent preclinical investigations have provided conflicting results about the amount of current the provider is exposed to,[62,63] and further study is necessary to determine the safety of this technique over the range of conditions encountered during resuscitation.

AIRWAY
Adjuncts

Oropharyngeal and nasopharyngeal airways are the two most commonly available airway adjuncts to health care providers. They have a long history of use, despite a lack of published data during human CPR. There are 2 case reports of inadvertent intracranial insertion of a nasopharyngeal airway in patients with basal skull fractures.[64,65]

Cricoid Pressure

Cricoid pressure was originally proposed to reduce gastric inflation during ventilation with a bag-valve mask. However, the original studies that demonstrated these findings used much higher tidal volumes than those currently recommended.[66,67] More recent data now show that cricoid pressure hampers the placement of both supraglottic and endotracheal airways. Cricoid pressure impairs both laryngeal mask airway placement and subsequent ventilation.[68–75] It also impairs tracheal intubation via multiple mechanisms: increased time to intubation, decreased success rate, and reduced laryngoscopic view.[68–83] Cricoid pressure should not be routinely performed during airway management in cardiac arrest.

Advanced Airways

Prehospital advanced airway management is a controversial topic beyond the scope of this article. However, there is no clear evidence for benefit[31]; the incidence of adverse events during intubation attempts become unacceptably high when providers do not receive active, continued training and skills maintenance.[84–89] The same can likely be said for all types of health care providers. Whether in the prehospital setting or in the emergency department, prolonged attempts at advanced airway management unnecessarily interrupt chest compressions, especially when there are acceptable alternatives.

There is mixed evidence to guide the optimal timing of advanced airway management during cardiac arrest resuscitation. Analysis of a large in-hospital cardiac arrest registry (25,000 patients) found that earlier airway management (less than 5 minutes) was associated with improved 24-hour survival.[90] In OHCA, intubations performed less than 12 minutes into the resuscitation were associated with improved survival, compared with intubations performed 13 or more minutes into the resuscitation.[91] However, a bundled care package of delayed intubation, passive oxygen delivery via a nonrebreather during CPR, and minimally interrupted chest compressions improved neurologically intact survival to hospital discharge in adult, witnessed, OHCA presenting with a shockable rhythm.[92]

Supraglottic airways represent an acceptable alternative to endotracheal intubation during cardiac arrest resuscitation. Ventilation through a variety of supraglottic devices results in similar arterial blood gas values, compared with traditional bag-valve-mask ventilation.[93,94] Additionally, ventilation through a laryngeal mask airway results in less regurgitation (3.5%) than ventilation with a bag-valve mask (12.4%).[95] Supraglottic airways perform as well as, or better than, endotracheal intubation in terms of insertion success, time to insertion, and ventilation parameters.[96–104] Supraglottic airways are also excellent rescue devices for difficult/failed intubations in cardiac arrest.[97,98,102,105–110] There are mixed data on the outcomes of patients in cardiac arrest that receive supraglottic airway devices. One retrospective study comparing endotracheal intubation with an esophageal-tracheal double lumen airway found no differences in ROSC or survival.[103] Another found that patients receiving a laryngeal mask airway had a higher rate of ROSC than a historical control group of patients that were endotracheally intubated.[105]

Confirmation of advanced airway placement is a crucial step in airway management. The best available standard is continuous waveform capnography, which has 100% sensitivity and 100% specificity in cardiac arrest.[111,112] If this is not available, then the combination of a colorimetric end-tidal carbon dioxide (CO_2) detector and clinical assessment is an acceptable alternative.

OXYGENATION

The current convention is to oxygenate with 100% fraction of inspired oxygen (Fio_2) during CPR. There are no studies of adult human cardiac arrest victims comparing 100% Fio_2 with titrated Fio_2 during CPR. Preclinical animal data suggest that 100% Fio_2 results in worse neurologic outcomes compared with 21% Fio_2.

Passive oxygenation during chest compressions is a proposed technique to minimize chest compression interruptions. It is predicated on cycles of successive chest wall compression and recoil that generate passive airflow while applying high-flow oxygen via a nonrebreather. If the tidal volumes generated are greater than the dead space, this moves oxygenated air into the lungs. If the tidal volumes generated are insufficient to overcome the dead space, the turbulent mixing of air may still result in molecular diffusion and subsequent gas exchange, similar to high-frequency oscillatory ventilation. In 2 human studies, passive oxygen delivery through a continuous positive airway pressure circuit at 15 L/min with ongoing chest compressions generated at least equal, if not improved, gas exchange and hemodynamics, compared with standard positive pressure oxygenation through an endotracheal tube; but there was no difference in clinical outcome.[113,114] However, a simplified cardiac arrest protocol consisting of passive oxygenation via a nonrebreather and continuous chest compressions resulted in improved neurologically intact survival to hospital discharge in adult, witnessed cardiac arrest with a shockable initial rhythm.[115–117]

VENTILATION

The sole human data on ventilation parameters during CPR are about respiratory rate. There are no data that address minute ventilation or peak inspiratory pressure. The ventilatory rate is frequently too high during cardiac arrest resuscitation, and the use of real-time CPR feedback devices results in delivered ventilation rates closer to those recommended in the guidelines.[48] Preclinical animal data suggest that hyperventilation is associated with diminished hemodynamics and survival,[35] but there is no human evidence that avoiding hyperventilation improves ROSC or survival.

End-tidal CO_2 monitoring represents one of the few modes of physiologic feedback available during resuscitation. Increases in end-tidal CO_2 typically herald ROSC.[118,119] Additionally, end-tidal CO_2 values greater than 10 mm Hg during CPR are associated with ROSC,[120] whereas values less than 10 mm Hg during CPR are associated with nonsurvival.[121–126] End-tidal CO_2 has not been evaluated specifically as a tool to guide resuscitation interventions in real time.

PHARMACOTHERAPY
Advanced Cardiac Life Support Drugs: General Principles

There is a shifting de-emphasis on pharmacologic intervention based on a growing body of literature that acknowledges short-term improvements in ROSC but has yet to demonstrate improved long-term or neurologically intact survival. This lack of treatment effect in clinical studies is in contrast to those benefits observed in preclinical animal trials.[127] Pharmacotherapy in cardiac arrest originated from a canine model of VF in the 1960s in which animals receiving epinephrine had improved survival. The use of epinephrine was primarily intended to improve systemic vascular resistance, leading to increased cardiac preload and, thus, augmenting the ability of CPR to produce coronary perfusion pressure[128] and end-organ perfusion. Human investigations have found the same improvements in ROSC or short-term survival, but no clinical trial of any resuscitation medication has ever found improvements in survival to hospital discharge or favorable neurologic outcome.

Epinephrine

Despite nearly 50 years of continuous clinical use, there is equipoise regarding epinephrine for cardiac arrest. A series of observational studies beginning in the 1990s demonstrated that administration of epinephrine was associated with lower survival and poor neurologic outcomes.[129–132] Speculations as to the cause of these unfavorable long-term effects center on compromised microvascular perfusion, beta-adrenergic–mediated toxicity, or the futility of transient survival in otherwise nonviable patients.[133] The first attempt to directly study the use of epinephrine was a 2009 randomized controlled trial of intravenous (IV) placement during resuscitation. This study randomized 916 patients to receive an IV or not. Those that received an IV had improved ROSC (40%) compared with those without an IV (25%); however, survival to discharge and 1-year survival did not differ between the groups.[134] Post hoc analysis of epinephrine administration yielded the same negative association between epinephrine and neurologic outcomes.[135] In 2011, a placebo controlled randomized trial of epinephrine administration was conducted but stopped before the enrollment goal. Of the 601 patients randomized, the epinephrine group had higher rates of ROSC and survival to hospital admission; but there was no difference in survival to hospital discharge or neurologic outcomes.[136] More recently, Hagihara and colleagues[137] conducted the largest observational study of epinephrine to date. A prospective propensity-matched population based study of more than 400,000 patients in Japan also found that prehospital epinephrine was associated with improved ROSC but decreased survival to hospital discharge and neurologic outcomes.

Critics of this work point out variability in the dosing of epinephrine, timing of administration, and postarrest care of resuscitated patients. The standard dose of epinephrine used in resuscitation (1 mg or 0.05–0.1 mg/kg) was originally derived from the study of 20- to 30-kg dogs. This dose is tremendously supraphysiologic and roughly 1000 times the maximum dose used as a vasopressor in the resuscitation of shock. Several studies in the 1990s explored even higher doses of epinephrine (3–5 mg).[138–141] Not surprisingly, most found no improvement in long-term survival. A lower epinephrine dose (<1 mg) may mitigate concerns regarding toxicity and microvascular compromise.[133] Two recent retrospective studies addressed the timing of epinephrine administration with a cohort of more than 3000 patients and stratified by receipt of epinephrine within the first 10 minutes of resuscitation. Those receiving epinephrine within the first 10 minutes had improved survival and neurologic outcomes compared with those after 10 minutes.[142] Similarly, Koscik and colleagues[143] found improved ROSC and survival if epinephrine was administered within 10 minutes after the onset of cardiac arrest. Although the original observational studies of epinephrine were conducted before the era of therapeutic hypothermia and protocolized postarrest care, follow-up studies have addressed these concerns with similar results.[135,136] A robust, well-designed, large, randomized, placebo-controlled trial of epinephrine in cardiac arrest is urgently warranted.

Vasopressin

Vasopressin, a potent vasoconstrictor, is associated with improved end-organ and cerebral blood flow in preclinical resuscitation studies and also lacks the beta toxicity associated with epinephrine. Despite this, vasopressin alone offers no survival advantage over epinephrine in head-to-head comparisons.[144–146] Furthermore, the combination of vasopressin and epinephrine offers no survival advantage over epinephrine alone.[147,148] In contrast, a recent trial of a cocktail of vasopressin, epinephrine, and methylprednisolone demonstrated improved survival and neurologic outcomes.[149,150] However, several confounders (protocolized postarrest care including stress-dose steroids) make it difficult to assess the treatment of vasopressin.

Atropine

At best, atropine offers no survival benefit[151–153]; at worst, it is associated with diminished survival.[154–156] (The authors humbly propose that death is an effective vagal nerve inhibitor and that atropine has no additional mechanistic advantage to offer during cardiac arrest resuscitation.)

Antiarrhythmics (Amiodarone or Lidocaine)

Current guidelines recommend the administration of an antiarrhythmic if VF or ventricular tachycardia (VT) persists after one defibrillation attempt and 2 minutes of CPR. Amiodarone is the preferred agent, but lidocaine may be given if amiodarone is unavailable. Two trials have demonstrated improved survival to hospital admission in patients receiving amiodarone versus lidocaine for refractory or recurrent VT/VT.[157,158] However, no study to date has demonstrated that either drug improves long-term survival or neurologic function. Furthermore, neither trial compared either agent with placebo. Subsequent work has also found no difference in long-term survival.[134,159] A 3-arm multicenter randomized trial of amiodarone, lidocaine, or placebo is currently underway (ClinicalTrials.gov NCT01401647).

DEVICES
Mechanical Chest Compression Devices

Mechanical chest compression devices are addressed earlier (see Circulatory support).

Active Chest Compression-Decompression

Active chest compression-decompression uses a handheld device with a suction cup to perform closed-chest cardiac massage. The operator applies a device to the mid-sternum to compress the chest and then uses the same device to actively decompress the chest after each compression. A recent Cochrane Review found no benefit from this technique.[160]

Impedance Threshold Device

The impedance threshold device was designed to decrease intrathoracic pressure, thereby improving venous return to the heart and subsequent cardiac output during CPR. It operates via a one-way valve that selectively impedes passive air entry during the decompression phase of CPR. Four randomized controlled trials have failed to show a benefit in survival to hospital discharge or neurologic outcomes.[161–164]

A UNIVERSAL TERMINATION OF RESUSCITATION RULE

In an attempt to establish universally applicable prehospital termination of resuscitation (TOR) rules, Morrison and colleagues[165] prospectively validated an established set of TOR rules for BLS providers in a cohort of 2145 patients with OHCA. These rules demonstrated 100% specificity for recommending transport of potential survivors and a positive predictive value of 100% for death. The predicted transport rate was 46%. This set of TOR rules recommended TOR when (1) there was no ROSC before transport, (2) no shock was given, and (3) the arrest was not witnessed by EMS personnel. A universal set of TOR rules could minimize practice variation among physicians providing online medical control. It could also improve resource utilization and EMS safety by reducing the number of patients transported to the hospital. However, reducing the number of patients transported may impede the development of new strategies and techniques for those patients currently deemed unable to resuscitate. Universal TOR rules also open the possibility for rare but occasional premature terminations of resuscitation (**Box 1**).

NOVEL FUTURE DIRECTIONS

A modern view of cardiac arrest resuscitation must look to novel resuscitation paradigms. Current examples include crowdsourcing first responders, mapping public AED locations with mobile media, and extracorporeal life support (ECLS).

Box 1
Validated universal set of prehospital TOR rules

Criteria for universal prehospital TOR rules

1. No ROSC before transport

2. No shock administered

3. Arrest not witnessed by EMS personnel

Dispatching Lay Rescuers Via Short Message Service (SMS) Mobile Phone Messages

Crowdsourcing is the process of outsourcing tasks to a distributed group of people. Scholten and colleagues[166] describe a prehospital dispatch system in the Netherlands that uses SMS alerts (ie, text messages) for crowdsourcing lay rescuers to suspected cardiac arrest victims while simultaneously dispatching traditional EMS providers. A total of 2168 lay rescuers enlisted and provided their home and work addresses. Based on these addresses, lay rescuers that lived or worked in a victim's vicinity were notified via SMS alert to proceed to the location of a suspected OHCA and begin CPR. Additional lay rescuers closer to a public AED were notified via SMS alert to obtain the AED and proceed to the patient's location. Over a 3-month period, this system was activated for 52 patients with suspected cardiac arrest. More than 3000 individual SMS alerts were sent to 2287 laypersons, and action was taken based on 579 alerts. Aid was provided for 47 patients. Laypersons started early CPR, performed early defibrillation, assisted EMS personnel, or took care of family members. Laypersons arrived before EMS personnel in 21 patients (45%), started CPR and/or performed defibrillation in 18 patients (38%), and assisted EMS personnel in 9 patients (19%).

Geographic Mapping of Automated External Defibrillators

The untrained public can effectively use AEDs. Of the 1 million AEDs sold in the United States over the past 20 years, the locations of many are unknown; there is no central registry of AED locations. AED registration is the responsibility of the device owner, and there are regional differences in the requirements for device registration. Bystanders may pass public AEDs during their daily activities but not remember where they are located when needed. Alternatively, bystanders may be completely unaware that an AED is nearby. Merchant and colleagues[167] describe an endeavor to create a central registry of public AEDs in Philadelphia, Pennsylvania. Through a public contest, participants took pictures of AEDs with mobile phones and submitted them to a central repository. A total of 1429 public AEDs were cataloged over 8 weeks by 313 teams and individuals. This central repository could be distributed in the form of a mobile phone application or other social media platform with a built-in mapping function.

Extracorporeal Life Support

ECLS, the incorporation of extracorporeal membranous oxygenation (ECMO) into cardiac arrest resuscitation, is a resource-intensive therapy that has been successfully deployed overseas to boost neurologically favorable survival in selected candidates with OHCA. One of the most sophisticated ECLS systems is in Japan.[168] Eligible patients have to satisfy the following criteria: aged 18 to 74 years, bystander-witnessed cardiac arrest, presumed cardiac cause, less than 15-minute estimated time interval from collapse until EMS arrival, shockable rhythm, and persistent cardiac arrest on arrival to the hospital. Eligible patients are percutaneously cannulated for ECMO in the emergency department with CPR in progress. Once ECMO is initiated, patients are rapidly cooled with the ECMO circuit while receiving urgent coronary angiography, if indicated, and intra-aortic balloon pumping. There is a clear, stepwise relationship between the outcome and quartiles of the collapse-to-ECMO and ECMO-to-34°C intervals. The optimal cutoff in the Japanese ECLS system is 55.5 minutes for the collapse-to-ECMO interval and 21.5 minutes for the ECMO-to-34°C interval. Survival with favorable neurologic outcome is 50% or greater when the ECMO-to-34°C interval is less than 21.5 minutes, regardless of the collapse-to-ECMO interval. A cumulative review of the Japanese ECLS literature through 2011 describes 1282 patients with OHCA between 1983 and 2008 who received ECLS.[169] Among the 516 patients with available outcome data, 27% survived to hospital discharge. Approximately half of the survivors had mild or no neurologic disability. In 2013, a propensity-adjusted analysis of ECLS in 162 patients with witnessed OHCA of cardiac cause found a 3-fold improvement in 3-month neurologically intact survival (29% vs 8%).[170] There is movement toward a randomized trial of ECLS compared with traditional resuscitation in Prague, Czech Republic.[171]

ECLS for OHCA has been slower to catch on the United States, although programs are commencing in select cities. Bellezzo and colleagues[172] described an emergency physician-led ECLS program in San Diego, California. Eligible patients had to satisfy the following criteria: any CPR initiated within 10 minutes of arrest, initial rhythm other than asystole, less than 10-minute approximate EMS transport time, less than 60 minutes total time in cardiac arrest, and lack of preexisting severe neurologic disease. The investigators use a tiered, 3-stage pathway for ECLS implementation, with the opportunity to exit the pathway at each stage. Over a 1-year period, 18 patients met the inclusion criteria, and ECLS was successfully initiated in 8 patients. Of these, 5 (63%) survived to hospital discharge with a good neurologic outcome.

In regional systems capable of this resource-intensive therapy, ECLS should be considered for select candidates with favorable prognostic characteristics that fail initial attempts at conventional resuscitation.[173]

REFERENCES

1. Sayre MR, Koster RW, Botha M, et al. Part 5: adult basic life support: 2010 international consensus on cardiopulmonary resuscitation and emergency cardiovascular care science with treatment recommendations. Circulation 2010; 122(16 Suppl 2):S298–324.
2. Writing Group Members, Roger VL, Go AS, et al. Heart disease and stroke statistics – 2012 update: a report from the American Heart Association. Circulation 2012;125:e2–220.
3. Herlitz J, Svensson L, Engdahl J, et al. Characteristics of cardiac arrest and resuscitation by age group: an analysis from the Swedish cardiac arrest registry. Am J Emerg Med 2007;25:1025–31.
4. Ong ME, Stiell I, Osmond MH, et al. Etiology of pediatric out-of-hospital cardiac arrest by coroner's diagnosis. Resuscitation 2006;68:335–42.
5. Kuisma M, Alaspaa A. Out-of-hospital cardiac arrests of non-cardiac origin: epidemiology and outcome. Eur Heart J 1997;18:1122–8, 52.
6. Kurkciyan I, Meron G, Behringer W, et al. Accuracy and impact of presumed cause in patients with cardiac arrest. Circulation 1998;98:766–71.
7. Nichol G, Thomas E, Callaway CW, et al. Regional variation in out-of-hospital cardiac arrest incidence and outcome. JAMA 2008;300(12):1423–31.
8. Reynolds JC, Bond MC, Shaikh S. Cardiopulmonary resuscitation update. Emerg Med Clin North Am 2012;30(1):35–49.
9. Sunde K, Pytte M, Jacobsen D, et al. Implementation of a standardised treatment protocol for post resuscitation care after out-of-hospital cardiac arrest. Resuscitation 2007;73(1):29–39.
10. Bobrow BJ, Vadeboncoeur TF, Stolz U, et al. The influence of scenario-based training and real-time audiovisual feedback on out-of-hospital cardiopulmonary resuscitation quality and survival from out-of-hospital cardiac arrest. Ann Emerg Med 2013;62:47–56.

11. McDonald JL. Systolic and mean arterial pressures during manual and mechanical CPR in humans. Ann Emerg Med 1982;11(6):292–5.
12. Ward KR, Menegazzi JJ, Zelenak RR, et al. Comparison of chest compressions between mechanical and manual CPR by monitoring end-tidal PCO2 during human cardiac arrest. Ann Emerg Med 1993;22(4):669–74.
13. Rubertsson S, Karlsten R. Increased cortical cerebral blood flow with LUCAS; a new device for mechanical chest compressions compared to standard external compressions during experimental cardiopulmonary resuscitation. Resuscitation 2005;65:357–63.
14. Rubertsson S, Lindgren E, Smekal D, et al. Mechanical chest compressions and simultaneous defibrillation vs conventional cardiopulmonary resuscitation in out-of-hospital cardiac arrest: the LINC randomized trial. JAMA 2014; 311(1):53–61.
15. Axelsson C, Nestin J, Svensson L, et al. Clinical consequences of the introduction of mechanical chest compression in the EMS system for treatment of out-of-hospital cardiac arrest—a pilot study. Resuscitation 2006;71(1):47–55.
16. Smekal D, Johansson J, Huzevka T, et al. A pilot study of mechanical chest compressions with the LUCAS device in cardiopulmonary resuscitation. Resuscitation 2011;82(6):702–6.
17. Westfall M, Krantz S, Mullin C, et al. Mechanical versus manual chest compressions in out-of-hospital cardiac arrest: a meta-analysis. Crit Care Med 2013; 41(7):1782–9.
18. Yost D, Phillips RH, Gonzales L, et al. Assessment of CPR interruptions from transthoracic impedance during use of the LUCAS mechanical chest compression system. Resuscitation 2012;83(8):961–5.
19. Ong ME, Annathurai A, Shahidah A, et al. Cardiopulmonary resuscitation interruptions with the use of a load-distributing band device during emergency department cardiac arrest. Ann Emerg Med 2010;56(3):233–41.
20. Krischer JP, Fine EG, Davis JH, et al. Complications of cardiac resuscitation. Chest 1987;92(2):287–91.
21. Bonnemeier H, Simonis G, Olivecrona G, et al. Continuous mechanical chest compression during in-hospital cardiopulmonary resuscitation of patients with pulseless electrical activity. Resuscitation 2011;82:155–9.
22. Fox J, Fiechter R, Gerstl P, et al. Mechanical versus manual chest compression CPR under ground ambulance transport conditions. Acute Card Care 2013; 15(1):1–6.
23. Grogaard HK, Wik L, Eriksen M, et al. Continuous chest compressions during cardiac arrest to facilitate restoration of coronary circulation with percutaneous coronary intervention. J Am Coll Cardiol 2007;50:1093–4.
24. Sayre MR, Berg RA, Cave DM, et al. Hands-only (compression only) cardiopulmonary resuscitation: a call to action for bystander response to adults who experience out-of-hospital sudden cardiac arrest: a science advisory for the public from the American Heart Association Emergency Cardiovascular Care Committee. Circulation 2008;117:2162–7.
25. Rea T, Fahrenbruch C, Culley L, et al. CPR with chest compression alone or with rescue breathing. N Engl J Med 2010;363:423–33.
26. Kitamura T, Iwami T, Kawamura T, et al. Bystander-initiated rescue breathing for out-of-hospital cardiac arrests of noncardiac origin. Circulation 2010;122:29309.
27. Japanese Circulation Society Resuscitation Science Study Group. Chest-compression-only bystander cardiopulmonary resuscitation in the 30:2 compression-to-ventilation ratio era. Circ J 2013;77:2742–50.

28. Yao L, Wang P, Zhou L, et al. Compression-only cardiopulmonary resuscitation vs standard cardiopulmonary resuscitation: an updated meta-analysis of observational studies. Am J Emerg Med 2014;32(6):517–23.

29. Mader TJ, Paquette AT, Salcido DD, et al. The effect of the preshock pause on coronary perfusion pressure decay and rescue shock outcome in porcine ventricular fibrillation. Prehosp Emerg Care 2009;13:487–94.

30. Kern KB, Ewy GA, Voorhees WD, et al. Myocardial perfusion pressure: a predictor of 24-hour survival during prolonged cardiac arrest in dogs. Resuscitation 1998;16:241–50.

31. Carlson JN, Reynolds JC. Does advanced airway management improve outcomes in adult out-of-hospital cardiac arrest? Ann Emerg Med 2014;64(2): 163–4.

32. McMullan J, Gerecht R, Bonomo J, et al, CARES Surveillance Group. Airway management and out-of-hospital cardiac arrest outcome in the CARES registry. Resuscitation 2014;85(5):617–22.

33. Hasegawa K, Hiraide A, Chang Y, et al. Association of prehospital advanced airway management with neurologic outcome and survival in patients with out-of-hospital cardiac arrest. JAMA 2013;309(3):257–66.

34. Shin SD, Ahn KO, Song KJ, et al. Out-of-hospital airway management and cardiac arrest outcomes: a propensity score matched analysis. Resuscitation 2012; 83(3):313–9.

35. Aufderheide TP, Sigurdsson G, Pirrallo RG, et al. Hyperventilation-induced hypotension during cardiopulmonary resuscitation. Circulation 2004;109: 1960–5.

36. Schneider T, Martens PR, Paschen H, et al. Multicenter, randomized, controlled trial of 150-J biphasic shocks compared with 200- to 360-J monophasic shocks in the resuscitation of out-of-hospital cardiac arrest victims. Optimized Response to Cardiac Arrest (ORCA) Investigators. Circulation 2000;102(15): 1780–7.

37. van Alem AP, Chapman FW, Lank P, et al. A prospective, randomised and blinded comparison of first shock success of monophasic and biphasic waveforms in out-of-hospital cardiac arrest. Resuscitation 2003;58(1):17–24.

38. Kudenchuk PJ, Cobb LA, Copass MK, et al. Transthoracic incremental monophasic versus biphasic defibrillation by emergency responders (TIMBER): a randomized comparison of monophasic with biphasic waveform ascending energy defibrillation for the resuscitation of out-of-hospital cardiac arrest due to ventricular fibrillation. Circulation 2006;114(19):2010–8.

39. Stiell IG, Walker RG, Nesbitt LP, et al. BIPHASIC trial: a randomized comparison of fixed lower versus escalating higher energy levels for defibrillation in out-of-hospital cardiac arrest. Circulation 2007;115(12):1511–7.

40. Walsh SJ, McClelland AJ, Owens CG, et al. Efficacy of distinct energy delivery protocols comparing two biphasic defibrillators for cardiac arrest. Am J Cardiol 2004;94(3):378–80.

41. Alaeddini J, Feng Z, Feghali G, et al. Repeated dual external direct cardioversions using two simultaneous 360-J shocks for refractory atrial fibrillation are safe and effective. Pacing Clin Electrophysiol 2005;28(1):3–7.

42. Leacock BW. Double simultaneous defibrillators for refractory ventricular fibrillation. J Emerg Med 2014;46(4):472–4.

43. European Resuscitation Council Guidelines 2000 for Automated External Defibrillation. A statement from the Monsieurs KG, Handley AJ, Bossaert LL; European Resuscitation Council. Resuscitation. Basic Life Support and Automated

External Defibrillation Working Group(1) and approved by the Executive Committee of the European Resuscitation Council 2001;48(3):207–9.

44. Weaver WD, Cobb LA, Dennis D, et al. Amplitude of ventricular fibrillation waveform and outcome after cardiac arrest. Ann Intern Med 1985;102(1):53–5.

45. Reynolds JC, Salcido DD, Menegazzi JJ. Conceptual models of coronary perfusion pressure and their relationship to defibrillation success in a porcine model of prolonged out-of-hospital cardiac arrest. Resuscitation 2012;83(7):900–6.

46. Reynolds JC, Salcido DD, Menegazzi JJ. Coronary perfusion pressure and return of spontaneous circulation after prolonged cardiac arrest. Prehosp Emerg Care 2010;14(1):78–84.

47. Cobb LA, Fahrenbruch CE, Walsh TR, et al. Influence of cardiopulmonary resuscitation prior to defibrillation in patients with out-of-hospital ventricular fibrillation. JAMA 1999;281(13):1182–8.

48. Wik L, Hansen TB, Fylling F, et al. Delaying defibrillation to give basic cardiopulmonary resuscitation to patients with out-of-hospital ventricular fibrillation: a randomized trial. JAMA 2003;289(11):1389–95.

49. Jacobs IG, Finn JC, Oxer HF, et al. CPR before defibrillation in out-of-hospital cardiac arrest: a randomized trial. Emerg Med Australas 2005;17(1):39–45 [Erratum in Emerg Med Australas 2009;21(5):430].

50. Stiell IG, Nichol G, Leroux BG, et al, Resuscitation Outcomes Consortium (ROC) Investigators. Early versus later rhythm analysis in patients with out-of-hospital cardiac arrest. N Engl J Med 2011;365(9):787–97.

51. Salcido DD, Menegazzi JJ, Suffoletto BP, et al. Association of intramyocardial high energy phosphate concentrations with quantitative measures of the ventricular fibrillation electrocardiogram waveform. Resuscitation 2009;80(8):946–50.

52. Reynolds JC, Salcido DD, Menegazzi JJ. Correlation between coronary perfusion pressure and quantitative ECG waveform measures during resuscitation of prolonged ventricular fibrillation. Resuscitation 2012;83(12):1497–502.

53. Callaway CW, Sherman LD, Mosesso VN Jr, et al. Scaling exponent predicts defibrillation success for out-of-hospital ventricular fibrillation cardiac arrest. Circulation 2001;103(12):1656–61.

54. Eftestøl T, Losert H, Kramer-Johansen J, et al. Independent evaluation of a defibrillation outcome predictor for out-of-hospital cardiac arrested patients. Resuscitation 2005;67(1):55–61.

55. Snyder DE, White RD, Jorgenson DB. Outcome prediction for guidance of initial resuscitation protocol: shock first or CPR first. Resuscitation 2007;72(1):45–51.

56. Cheskes S, Schmicker RH, Christenson J, et al, Resuscitation Outcomes Consortium (ROC) Investigators. Perishock pause: an independent prodictor of survival from out-of-hospital shockable cardiac arrest. Circulation 2011;124(1):58–66.

57. Cheskes S, Schmicker RH, Verbeek PR, et al, Resuscitation Outcomes Consortium (ROC) investigators. The impact of peri-shock pause on survival from out-of-hospital shockable cardiac arrest during the Resuscitation Outcomes Consortium PRIMED trial. Resuscitation 2014;85(3):336–42.

58. Zia A, Kern KB. Management of postcardiac arrest myocardial dysfunction. Curr Opin Crit Care 2011;17(3):241–6.

59. Eftestøl T, Sunde K, Steen PA. Effects of interrupting precordial compressions on the calculated probability of defibrillation success during out-of-hospital cardiac arrest. Circulation 2002;105(19):2270–3.

60. Rea TD, Helbock M, Perry S, et al. Increasing use of cardiopulmonary resuscitation during out-of-hospital ventricular fibrillation arrest: survival implications of guideline changes. Circulation 2006;114(25):2760–5.

61. Lloyd MS, Heeke B, Walter PF. Hands-on defibrillation: an analysis of electrical current flow through rescuers in direct contact with patients during biphasic external defibrillation. Circulation 2008;117(19):2510–4.

62. Neumann T, Gruenewald M, Lauenstein C, et al. Hands-on defibrillation has the potential to improve the quality of cardiopulmonary resuscitation and is safe for rescuers-a preclinical study. J Am Heart Assoc 2012;1(5):e001313.

63. Deakin CD, Lee-Shrewsbury V, Hogg K, et al. Do clinical examination gloves provide adequate electrical insulation for safe hands-on defibrillation? I: resistive properties of nitrile gloves. Resuscitation 2013;84(7):895–9.

64. Schade K, Borzotta A, Michaels A. Intracranial malposition of nasopharyngeal airway. J Trauma 2000;49:967–8.

65. Muzzi DA, Losasso TJ, Cucchiara RF. Complication from a nasopharyngeal airway in a patient with a basilar skull fracture. Anesthesiology 1991;74:366–8.

66. Petito SP, Russell WJ. The prevention of gastric inflation: a neglected benefit of cricoid pressure. Anaesth Intensive Care 1988;16:139–43.

67. Lawes EG, Campbell I, Mercer D. Inflation pressure, gastric insufflation and rapid sequence induction. Br J Anaesth 1987;59:315–8.

68. Asai T, Barclay K, Power I, et al. Cricoid pressure impedes placement of the laryngeal mask airway and subsequent tracheal intubation through the mask. Br J Anaesth 1994;72:47–51.

69. Asai T, Barclay K, Power I, et al. Cricoid pressure impedes placement of the laryngeal mask airway. Br J Anaesth 1995;74:521–5.

70. Ansermino JM, Blogg CE. Cricoid pressure may prevent insertion of the laryngeal mask airway. Br J Anaesth 1992;69:465–7.

71. Aoyama K, Takenaka I, Sata T, et al. Cricoid pressure impedes positioning and ventilation through the laryngeal mask airway. Can J Anaesth 1996;43:1035–40.

72. Brimacombe J, White A, Berry A. Effect of cricoid pressure on ease of insertion of the laryngeal mask airway. Br J Anaesth 1993;71:800–2.

73. Gabbott DA, Sasada MP. Laryngeal mask airway insertion using cricoid pressure and manual in-line neck stabilisation. Anaesthesia 1995;50:674–6.

74. Xue FS, Mao P, Li CW, et al. Influence of pressure on cricoid on insertion ProSeal laryngeal mask airway and ventilation function. Zhongguo Wei Zhong Bing Ji Jiu Yi Xue 2007;19:532–5 [in Chinese].

75. Li CW, Xue FS, Xu YC, et al. Cricoid pressure impedes insertion of, and ventilation through, the ProSeal laryngeal mask airway in anesthetized, paralyzed patients. Anesth Analg 2007;104:1195–8.

76. McNelis U, Syndercombe A, Harper I, et al. The effect of cricoid pressure on intubation facilitated by the gum elastic bougie. Anaesthesia 2007;62:456–9.

77. Harry RM, Nolan JP. The use of cricoid pressure with the intubating laryngeal mask. Anaesthesia 1999;54:656–9.

78. Noguchi T, Koga K, Shiga Y, et al. The gum elastic bougie eases tracheal intubation while applying cricoid pressure compared to a stylet. Can J Anaesth 2003;50:712–7.

79. Asai T, Murao K, Shingu K. Cricoid pressure applied after placement of laryngeal mask impedes subsequent fibreoptic tracheal intubation through mask. Br J Anaesth 2000;85:256–61.

80. Snider DD, Clarke D, Finucane BT. The "BURP" maneuver worsens the glottic view when applied in combination with cricoid pressure. Can J Anaesth 2005;52:100–4.

81. Smith CE, Boyer D. Cricoid pressure decreases ease of tracheal intubation using fibreoptic laryngoscopy (WuScope System). Can J Anaesth 2002;49: 614–9.
82. Heath ML, Allagain J. Intubation through the laryngeal mask: a technique for un-expected difficult intubation. Anaesthesia 1991;46:545–8.
83. Levitan RM, Kinkle WC, Levin WJ, et al. Laryngeal view during laryngos-copy: a randomized trial comparing cricoid pressure, backward-upward-rightward pressure, and bimanual laryngoscopy. Ann Emerg Med 2006;47: 548–55.
84. Bradley JS, Billows GL, Olinger ML, et al. Prehospital oral endotracheal intuba-tion by rural basic emergency medical technicians. Ann Emerg Med 1998;32: 26–32.
85. Sayre MR, Sakles JC, Mistler AF, et al. Field trial of endotracheal intubation by basic EMTs. Ann Emerg Med 1998;31:228–33.
86. Katz SH, Falk JL. Misplaced endotracheal tubes by paramedics in an urban emergency medical services system. Ann Emerg Med 2001;37:32–7.
87. Jones JH, Murphy MP, Dickson RL, et al. Emergency physician-verified out-of-hospital intubation: miss rates by paramedics. Acad Emerg Med 2004;11: 707–9.
88. Wirtz DD, Ortiz C, Newman DH, et al. Unrecognized misplacement of endotra-cheal tubes by ground prehospital providers. Prehosp Emerg Care 2007;11: 213–8.
89. Timmermann A, Russo SG, Eich C, et al. The out-of-hospital esophageal and en-dobronchial intubations performed by emergency physicians. Anesth Analg 2007;104:619–23.
90. Wong ML, Carey S, Mader TJ, et al. Time to invasive airway placement and resuscitation outcomes after inhospital cardiopulmonary arrest. Resuscitation 2010;81:182–6.
91. Shy BD, Rea TD, Becker LJ, et al. Time to intubation and survival in prehospital cardiac arrest. Prehosp Emerg Care 2004;8:394–9.
92. Bobrow BJ, Ewy GA, Clark L, et al. Passive oxygen insufflation is superior to bag-valve-mask ventilation for witnessed ventricular fibrillation out-of-hospital cardiac arrest. Ann Emerg Med 2009;54:656–62.e1.
93. Rumball CJ, MacDonald D. The PTL, combitube, laryngeal mask, and oral airway: a randomized prehospital comparative study of ventilatory device effec-tiveness and cost-effectiveness in 470 cases of cardiorespiratory arrest. Pre-hosp Emerg Care 1997;1:1–10.
94. SOS-KANTO Study Group. Comparison of arterial blood gases of laryngeal mask airway and bag-valve-mask ventilation in out-of- hospital cardiac arrests. Circ J 2009;73:490–6.
95. Stone BJ, Chantler PJ, Baskett PJ. The incidence of regurgitation during cardio-pulmonary resuscitation: a comparison between the bag valve mask and laryn-geal mask airway. Resuscitation 1998;38:3–6.
96. Frass M, Frenzer R, Rauscha F, et al. Ventilation with the esophageal tracheal combitube in cardiopulmonary resuscitation: promptness and effectiveness. Chest 1988;93:781–4.
97. Atherton GL, Johnson JC. Ability of paramedics to use the Combitube in preho-spital cardiac arrest. Ann Emerg Med 1993;22:1263–8.
98. Rabitsch W, Schellongowski P, Staudinger T, et al. Comparison of a conventional tracheal airway with the Combitube in an urban emergency medical services system run by physicians. Resuscitation 2003;57:27–32.

99. Rumball C, Macdonald D, Barber P, et al. Endotracheal intubation and esophageal tracheal Combitube insertion by regular ambulance attendants: a comparative trial. Prehosp Emerg Care 2004;8:15–22.

100. Samarkandi AH, Seraj MA, el Dawlatly A, et al. The role of laryngeal mask airway in cardiopulmonary resuscitation. Resuscitation 1994;28:103–6.

101. Staudinger T, Brugger S, Watschinger B, et al. Emergency intubation with the Combitube: comparison with the endotracheal airway. Ann Emerg Med 1993; 22:1573–5.

102. Staudinger T, Brugger S, Roggla M, et al. Comparison of the Combitube with the endotracheal tube in cardiopulmonary resuscitation in the prehospital phase. Wien Klin Wochenschr 1994;106:412–5 [in German].

103. Cady CE, Weaver MD, Pirrallo RG, et al. Effect of emergency medical technician-placed Combitubes on outcomes after out-of- hospital cardiopulmonary arrest. Prehosp Emerg Care 2009;13:495–9.

104. Verghese C, Prior-Willeard PF, Baskett PJ. Immediate management of the airway during cardiopulmonary resuscitation in a hospital without a resident anaesthesiologist. Eur J Emerg Med 1994;1:123–5.

105. Deakin CD, Peters R, Tomlinson P, et al. Securing the pre- hospital airway: a comparison of laryngeal mask insertion and endotracheal intubation by UK paramedics. Emerg Med J 2005;22:64–7.

106. Calkins TR, Miller K, Langdorf MI. Success and complication rates with prehospital placement of an esophageal-tracheal combitube as a rescue airway. Prehosp Disaster Med 2006;21:97–100.

107. Guyette FX, Wang H, Cole JS. King airway use by air medical providers. Prehosp Emerg Care 2007;11:473–6.

108. Tentillier E, Heydenreich C, Cros AM, et al. Use of the intubating laryngeal mask airway in emergency pre-hospital difficult intubation. Resuscitation 2008;77: 30–4.

109. Timmermann A, Russo SG, Rosenblatt WH, et al. Intubating laryngeal mask airway for difficult out-of-hospital airway management: a prospective evaluation. Br J Anaesth 2007;99:286–91.

110. Martin SE, Ochsner MG, Jarman RH, et al. Use of the laryngeal mask airway in air transport when intubation fails. J Trauma 1999;47:352–7.

111. Grmec S. Comparison of three different methods to confirm tracheal tube placement in emergency intubation. Intensive Care Med 2002;28:701–4, 131.

112. Silvestri S, Ralls GA, Krauss B, et al. The effectiveness of out-of-hospital use of continuous end-tidal carbon dioxide monitoring on the rate of unrecognized misplaced intubation within a regional emergency medical services system. Ann Emerg Med 2005;45:497–503.

113. Bertrand C, Hemery F, Carli P, et al. Constant flow insufflation of oxygen as the sole mode of ventilation during out-of- hospital cardiac arrest. Intensive Care Med 2006;32:843–51.

114. Saissy JM, Boussignac G, Cheptel E, et al. Efficacy of continuous insufflation of oxygen combined with active cardiac compression-decompression during out-of-hospital cardiorespiratory arrest. Anesthesiology 2000;92:1523–30.

115. Kellum MJ, Kennedy KW, Barney R, et al. Cardiocerebral resuscitation improves neurologically intact survival of patients with out-of-hospital cardiac arrest. Ann Emerg Med 2008;52:244–52.

116. Kellum MJ, Kennedy KW, Ewy GA. Cardiocerebral resuscitation improves survival of patients with out-of-hospital cardiac arrest. Am J Med 2006;119: 335–40.

117. Abella BS, Edelson DP, Kim S, et al. CPR quality improvement during in-hospital cardiac arrest using a real-time audiovisual feedback system. Resuscitation 2007;73:54–61.
118. Bhende MS, Thompson AE. Evaluation of an end-tidal CO2 detector during pediatric cardiopulmonary resuscitation. Pediatrics 1995;95:395–9.
119. Sehra R, Underwood K, Checchia P. End tidal CO2 is a quantitative measure of cardiac arrest. Pacing Clin Electrophysiol 2003;26(part 2):515–7.
120. Grmec S, Kupnik D. Does the Mainz Emergency Evaluation Scoring (MEES) in combination with capnometry (MEESc) help in the prognosis of outcome from cardiopulmonary resuscitation in a pre- hospital setting? Resuscitation 2003; 58:89–96.
121. Grmec S, Klemen P. Does the end-tidal carbon dioxide (ETCO2) concentration have prognostic value during out-of-hospital cardiac arrest? Eur J Emerg Med 2001;8:263–9.
122. Kolar M, Krizmaric M, Klemen P, et al. Partial pressure of end-tidal carbon dioxide successful predicts cardiopulmonary resuscitation in the field: a prospective observational study. Crit Care 2008;12:R115.
123. Levine RL, Wayne MA, Miller CC. End-tidal carbon dioxide and outcome of out-of-hospital cardiac arrest. N Engl J Med 1997;337:301–6.
124. Wayne MA, Levine RL, Miller CC. Use of end-tidal carbon dioxide to predict outcome in prehospital cardiac arrest. Ann Emerg Med 1995;25:762–7.
125. Ahrens T, Schallom L, Bettorf K, et al. End-tidal carbon dioxide measurements as a prognostic indicator of outcome in cardiac arrest. Am J Crit Care 2001; 10:391–8.
126. Sanders AB, Kern KB, Otto CW, et al. End-tidal carbon dioxide monitoring during cardiopulmonary resuscitation: a prognostic indicator for survival. JAMA 1989;262:1347–51.
127. Reynolds JC, Rittenberger JC, Menegazzi JJ. Drug administration in animal studies of cardiac arrest does not reflect human clinical experience. Resuscitation 2007;74(1):13–26.
128. Paradis NA, Martin GB, Rivers EP, et al. Coronary perfusion pressure and the return of spontaneous circulation in human cardiopulmonary resuscitation. JAMA 1990;263(8):1106–13.
129. Herlitz J, Ekström L, Wennerblom B, et al. Adrenaline in out-of-hospital ventricular fibrillation. Does it make any difference? Resuscitation 1995;29(3): 195–201.
130. Behringer W, Kittler H, Sterz F, et al. Cumulative epinephrine dose during cardiopulmonary resuscitation and neurologic outcome. Ann Intern Med 1998;129(6): 450–6.
131. Holmberg M, Holmberg S, Herlitz J. Low chance of survival among patients requiring adrenaline (epinephrine) or intubation after out-of-hospital cardiac arrest in Sweden. Resuscitation 2002;54(1):37–45.
132. Ong ME, Tan EH, Ng FS, et al, Cardiac Arrest and Resuscitation Epidemiology Study Group. Survival outcomes with the introduction of intravenous epinephrine in the management of out-of-hospital cardiac arrest. Ann Emerg Med 2007; 50(6):635–42.
133. Callaway CW. Epinephrine for cardiac arrest. Curr Opin Cardiol 2013;28(1): 36–42.
134. Olasveengen TM, Sunde K, Brunborg C, et al. Intravenous drug administration during out-of-hospital cardiac arrest: a randomized trial. JAMA 2009;302(20): 2222–9.

135. Olasveengen TM, Wik L, Sunde K, et al. Outcome when adrenaline (epinephrine) was actually given vs. not given - post hoc analysis of a randomized clinical trial. Resuscitation 2012;83(3):327–32.
136. Jacobs IG, Finn JC, Jelinek GA, et al. Effect of adrenaline on survival in out-of-hospital cardiac arrest: a randomised double-blind placebo-controlled trial. Resuscitation 2011;82(9):1138–43.
137. Hagihara A, Hasegawa M, Abe T, et al. Prehospital epinephrine use and survival among patients with out-of-hospital cardiac arrest. JAMA 2012;307(11):1161–8.
138. Brown CG, Martin DR, Pepe PE, et al. A comparison of standard-dose and high-dose epinephrine in cardiac arrest outside the hospital. The Multicenter High-Dose Epinephrine Study Group. N Engl J Med 1992;327(15):1051–5.
139. Gueugniaud PY, Mols P, Goldstein P, et al. A comparison of repeated high doses and repeated standard doses of epinephrine for cardiac arrest outside the hospital. European Epinephrine Study Group. N Engl J Med 1998;339(22):1595–601.
140. Callaham M, Madsen CD, Barton CW, et al. A randomized clinical trial of high-dose epinephrine and norepinephrine vs standard-dose epinephrine in prehospital cardiac arrest. JAMA 1992;268(19):2667–72.
141. Stiell IG, Hebert PC, Weitzman BN, et al. High-dose epinephrine in adult cardiac arrest. N Engl J Med 1992;327(15):1045–50.
142. Hayashi Y, Iwami T, Kitamura T, et al. Impact of early intravenous epinephrine administration on outcomes following out-of-hospital cardiac arrest. Circ J 2012;76(7):1639–45.
143. Koscik C, Pinawin A, McGovern H, et al. Rapid epinephrine administration improves early outcomes in out-of-hospital cardiac arrest. Resuscitation 2013;84(7):915–20.
144. Wenzel V, Krismer AC, Arntz HR, et al, European Resuscitation Council Vasopressor during Cardiopulmonary Resuscitation Study Group. A comparison of vasopressin and epinephrine for out-of-hospital cardiopulmonary resuscitation. N Engl J Med 2004;350(2):105–13.
145. Stiell IG, Hébert PC, Wells GA, et al. Vasopressin versus epinephrine for inhospital cardiac arrest: a randomised controlled trial. Lancet 2001;358(9276):105–9.
146. Aung K, Htay T. Vasopressin for cardiac arrest: a systematic review and meta-analysis. Arch Intern Med 2005;165(1):17–24.
147. Callaway CW, Hostler D, Doshi AA, et al. Usefulness of vasopressin administered with epinephrine during out-of-hospital cardiac arrest. Am J Cardiol 2006;98(10):1316–21.
148. Gueugniaud PY, David JS, Chanzy E, et al. Vasopressin and epinephrine vs. epinephrine alone in cardiopulmonary resuscitation. N Engl J Med 2008;359(1):21–30.
149. Mentzelopoulos SD, Zakynthinos SG, Tzoufi M, et al. Vasopressin, epinephrine, and corticosteroids for in-hospital cardiac arrest. Arch Intern Med 2009;169(1):15–24.
150. Mentzelopoulos SD, Malachias S, Chamos C, et al. Vasopressin, steroids, and epinephrine and neurologically favorable survival after in-hospital cardiac arrest: a randomized clinical trial. JAMA 2013;310(3):270–9.
151. Coon GA, Clinton JE, Ruiz E. Use of atropine for brady-asystolic prehospital cardiac arrest. Ann Emerg Med 1981;10:462–7.
152. Tortolani AJ, Risucci DA, Powell SR, et al. In-hospital cardiopulmonary resuscitation during asystole: therapeutic factors associated with 24-hour survival. Chest 1989;96:622–6.

153. Stiell IG, Wells GA, Hebert PC, et al. Association of drug therapy with survival in cardiac arrest: limited role of advanced cardiac life support drugs. Acad Emerg Med 1995;2:264–73.
154. Engdahl J, Bang A, Lindqvist J, et al. Can we define patients with no and those with some chance of survival when found in asystole out of hospital? Am J Cardiol 2000;86:610–4.
155. Engdahl J, Bang A, Lindqvist J, et al. Factors affecting short- and long-term prognosis among 1069 patients with out-of-hospital cardiac arrest and pulseless electrical activity. Resuscitation 2001;51:17–25.
156. van Walraven C, Stiell IG, Wells GA, et al. Do advanced cardiac life support drugs increase resuscitation rates from in-hospital cardiac arrest? The OTAC Study Group. Ann Emerg Med 1998;32(5):544–53.
157. Kudenchuk PJ, Cobb LA, Copass MK, et al. Amiodarone for resuscitation after out-of-hospital cardiac arrest due to ventricular fibrillation. N Engl J Med 1999; 341(12):871–8.
158. Dorian P, Cass D, Schwartz B, et al. Amiodarone as compared with lidocaine for shock-resistant ventricular fibrillation. N Engl J Med 2002;346(12):884–90 [Erratum in N Engl J Med 2002;347(12):955].
159. Glover BM, Brown SP, Morrison L, et al, Resuscitation Outcomes Consortium Investigators. Wide variability in drug use in out-of-hospital cardiac arrest: a report from the resuscitation outcomes consortium. Resuscitation 2012;83(11): 1324–30.
160. Reynolds JC. Does active chest compression-decompression cardiopulmonary resuscitation decrease mortality, neurologic impairment, or cardiopulmonary resuscitation-related complications after cardiac arrest? Ann Emerg Med 2014;64(2):190–1.
161. Plaisance P, Lurie KG, Vicaut E, et al. Evaluation of an impedance threshold device in patients receiving active compression-decompression cardiopulmonary resuscitation for out of hospital cardiac arrest. Resuscitation 2004;61: 265–71.
162. Plaisance P, Lurie KG, Payen D. Inspiratory impedance during active compression-decompression cardiopulmonary resuscitation: a randomized evaluation in patients in cardiac arrest. Circulation 2000;101:989–94.
163. Aufderheide TP, Pirrallo RG, Provo TA, et al. Clinical evaluation of an inspiratory impedance threshold device during standard cardiopulmonary resuscitation in patients with out-of-hospital cardiac arrest. Crit Care Med 2005;33:734–40.
164. Wolcke BB, Mauer DK, Schoefmann MF, et al. Comparison of standard cardiopulmonary resuscitation versus the combination of active compression-decompression cardiopulmonary resuscitation and an inspiratory impedance threshold device for out-of-hospital cardiac arrest. Circulation 2003;108: 2201–5.
165. Morrison LJ, Verbeek PR, Zhan C, et al. Validation of a universal prehospital termination of resuscitation clinical prediction rule for advanced and basic life support providers. Resuscitation 2009;80(3):324–8.
166. Scholten AC, van Manen JG, van der Worp WE, et al. Early cardiopulmonary resuscitation and use of automated external defibrillators by laypersons in out-of-hospital cardiac arrest using an SMS alert service. Resuscitation 2011; 82(10):1273–8.
167. Merchant RM, Asch DA, Hershey JC, et al. Abstract 57: a crowdsourcing, mobile media, challenge to locate automated external defibrillators. Circulation 2012;126:A57.

168. Nagao K, Kikushima K, Watanabe K, et al. Early induction of hypothermia during cardiac arrest improves neurological outcomes in patients with out-of-hospital cardiac arrest who undergo emergency cardiopulmonary bypass and percutaneous coronary intervention. Circ J 2010;74(1):77–85.

169. Morimura N, Sakamoto T, Nagao K, et al. Extracorporeal cardiopulmonary resuscitation for out-of-hospital cardiac arrest: a review of the Japanese literature. Resuscitation 2011;82(1):10–4.

170. Maekawa K, Tanno K, Hase M, et al. Extracorporeal cardiopulmonary resuscitation for patients with out-of-hospital cardiac arrest of cardiac origin: a propensity-matched study and predictor analysis. Crit Care Med 2013;41(5): 1186–96.

171. Belohlavek J, Kucera K, Jarkovsky J, et al. Hyperinvasive approach to out-of hospital cardiac arrest using mechanical chest compression device, prehospital intraarrest cooling, extracorporeal life support and early invasive assessment compared to standard of care. A randomized parallel groups comparative study proposal. "Prague OHCA study". J Transl Med 2012;10:163.

172. Bellezzo JM, Shinar Z, Davis DP, et al. Emergency physician-initiated extracorporeal cardiopulmonary resuscitation. Resuscitation 2012;83(8):966–70.

173. Reynolds JC, Frisch A, Rittenberger JC, et al. Duration of resuscitation efforts and functional outcome after out-of-hospital cardiac arrest: when should we change to novel therapies? Circulation 2013;128(23):2488–94.

APPENDIX

The Post Cardiac Arrest Service researchers are

Jon C. Rittenberger, MD, MS

Clifton W. Callaway, MD, PhD

Francis X. Guyette, MD, MPH

Ankur A. Doshi, MD

Cameron Dezfulian, MD

Joshua C. Reynolds, MD, MS

Adam Frisch, MD, MS

Postcardiac Arrest Management

Jon C. Rittenberger, MD, MS[a], Ankur A. Doshi, MD[a], Joshua C. Reynolds, MD, MS[b],*,
Post Cardiac Arrest Service

KEYWORDS

• Heart arrest • Resuscitation • Prognostication • Hypothermia • Critical care

KEY POINTS

- Following resuscitation from cardiac arrest, patients exhibit a sepsislike syndrome that affects multiple organ systems.
- Resuscitation and critical care interventions should be adapted to the unique neurologic injury patterns found in the postarrest population.
- Temperature management is a critical component of the critical care provided to this population.
- Neurologic recovery may require greater than 72 hours.

OVERVIEW AND GOALS OF CARE

Management of the postcardiac arrest patient is complex and addresses multiple key issues simultaneously: diagnosing and treating the cause, minimizing brain injury, managing cardiovascular dysfunction, and managing sequelae of global ischemia and reperfusion injury. During the initial minutes to hours after return of spontaneous circulation (ROSC), the most immediate threat to life is cardiovascular collapse. The astute practitioner will simultaneously address end-organ perfusion, oxygenation, ventilation, electrolyte abnormalities, and body temperature as well as concurrently search for the cause of cardiac arrest and initiate relevant treatments.[1]

DETERMINING THE CAUSE AND EXTENT OF INJURY AFTER CARDIAC ARREST
History and Physical Examination

Most patients are comatose after cardiac arrest resuscitation and are unable to provide a history of illness or medical conditions. Emergency Department (ED) providers

[a] Department of Emergency Medicine, University of Pittsburgh, Suite 10028, Forbes Tower, Pittsburgh, PA 15260, USA; [b] Department of Emergency Medicine, Michigan State University College of Human Medicine, 15 Michigan Street Northeast, Suite 420, Grand Rapids, MI 49503, USA
* Corresponding author.
E-mail address: reyno406@msu.edu

Emerg Med Clin N Am 33 (2015) 691–712
http://dx.doi.org/10.1016/j.emc.2015.04.011
0733-8627/15/$ – see front matter © 2015 Elsevier Inc. All rights reserved.

must turn to other sources of information, including family members, witnesses, Emergency Medical Services (EMS) personnel, and the medical record. In addition to routine medical history, medications, and drug allergies, there are several key pieces of information specific to the cardiac arrest and resuscitation to extract from these sources that are presented in **Box 1**.

Baseline Neurologic Examination

A baseline neurologic examination should be performed on all resuscitated patients. This examination helps to elucidate possible causes of cardiac arrest, estimate the patient's clinical course, and determine the target for temperature management. This examination should unequivocally be performed in the absence of confounding neuromuscular blockade and sedation. The baseline neurologic examination may be delayed if long-acting neuromuscular blockers or sedatives have already been administered. Sedation should be paused and train-of-4 testing should be considered to verify a valid neurologic examination. Optimizing hemodynamics and acid-base status is prudent before this examination.

Most postcardiac arrest patients are comatose and intubated. The Full Outline of Unresponsiveness (FOUR) score was developed by Wijdicks and colleagues[2] specifically to assess patients with impaired level of consciousness that may be intubated. It has been validated in both the ED[3] and the intensive care unit (ICU)[4] settings and has comparable interrater reliability to the Glasgow Coma Scale.[5] The FOUR score provides an excellent tool to quantify and systematically describe the level of consciousness and preserved brainstem reflexes in postcardiac arrest patients (**Table 1**).

Asymmetric or focal neurologic findings are unexpected in postcardiac arrest patients and suggest a focal intracranial lesion. At a minimum, ED providers should note the brainstem and motor components to the FOUR score, which include pupillary reactivity and symmetry, corneal reflexes, gag/cough reflex, flexor/extensor posturing, response to pain, and ability to follow commands. Providers should also pay particular attention to the motor component, because patients not following commands should be strongly considered for induced hypothermia.

Diagnostic Testing

The minimum initial diagnostic testing for the resuscitated cardiac arrest patient includes an electrocardiogram (EKG), laboratory tests, and imaging studies. The combination of results helps point toward the cause of cardiac arrest and assesses the degree of organ dysfunction and illness severity.

Electrocardiogram
Acute myocardial infarction, arrhythmia, and cardiomyopathy are common and correctable causes for cardiac arrest. A 12-lead EKG is mandatory to obtain after

---

Box 1
Salient pieces of information to obtain for the postcardiac arrest patient

Were there any prodromal symptoms (ie, chest pain, shortness of breath)?

Was the cardiac arrest witnessed?

Was bystander CPR provided?

What was the initial cardiac rhythm?

How long was CPR provided?

How many doses of advanced cardiovascular life support medications were administered?

Table 1
Full outline of unresponsiveness score

Action	Score
Eye response	
Opens eyes spontaneously, tracks, blinks to command	4
Opens eyes but does not track or blink to command	3
Eyes closed but open to loud voice	2
Eyes closed but open to painful stimulation	1
Eyes remain closed with painful stimulation	0
Motor response	
Obeys commands, makes sign (eg, "thumbs up")	4
Localizes painful stimulus	3
Flexes to painful stimulation	2
Extends to painful stimulation	1
No response to pain OR myoclonic status epilepticus	0
Brainstem reflexes	
Pupil and corneal reflexes present	4
One pupil wide and fixed	3
Pupil OR corneal reflexes absent	2
Pupil AND corneal reflexes absent	1
Absent pupil, corneal, and cough reflexes	0
Respiration	
Not intubated with regular breathing pattern	4
Not intubated with Cheyne-Stokes breathing pattern	3
Not intubated, irregular breathing pattern	2
Breathes more than the ventilator rate	1
Breathes at ventilator rate OR apnea	0

A numerical value is assigned for each component, and the results are added together for the total FOUR score.

ROSC. The EKG provides diagnostic clues to the cause of cardiac arrest and prompts urgent therapies. Providers should be vigilant for signs of ST-segment elevation myocardial infarction (STEMI) or other acute-appearing ischemic changes that require emergency reperfusion. However, the post-ROSC EKG has only limited predictive value in diagnosing acute coronary lesions among resuscitated patients. Zanuttini and colleagues[6] found an acceptable positive predictive value, but low negative predictive value, for ST-segment analysis to diagnose acute or presumed recent coronary lesions (85% and 67%, respectively). Metabolic derangements common in the post-arrest phase (electrolyte abnormalities and acidosis) can confound EKG interpretation. Furthermore, significant coronary artery disease is highly prevalent in out-of-hospital cardiac arrest patients, even in the absence of acute STEMI.[7–12] The incidence of coronary artery lesions is highest among patients with an initial shockable rhythm (ventricular fibrillation or pulseless ventricular tachycardia).[7,13] Emergent cardiac catheterization should be strongly considered in patients without STEMI, but who have a suggestive history (cardiac risk factors, and chest pain or shortness of breath that foreshadowed the cardiac arrest) or an initial shockable rhythm. Ongoing cardiogenic shock may be the sole manifestation of acute coronary syndrome in some patients. When available, bedside echocardiography to detect focal wall motion can help stratify patients at increased risk for acute coronary syndrome.

Providers should also evaluate the initial EKG for conduction abnormalities, electrical axis, and T-wave abnormalities. Predispositions toward primary arrhythmias should be considered, including Brugada syndrome, Wolff-Parkinson-White syndrome, and prolonged QTc syndrome. Other conduction abnormalities may suggest electrolyte derangements or accidental hypothermia. Signs of right heart strain suggest pulmonary embolism.

Laboratory testing

Laboratory tests help determine the cause of cardiac arrest and assess the extent of organ dysfunction following global ischemia/reperfusion. The most common abnormalities are electrolyte and acid-base disturbances; these require serial monitoring during on-going resuscitation of the postcardiac arrest patients.

Arterial blood gas (ABG) measurements should be obtained every 6 hours during induced hypothermia and rewarming to assess acid-base status and guide ventilator management. ABG measuring is critical if patients receive neuromuscular blockade to suppress shivering during temperature management because many patients demonstrate a metabolic acidosis, and attempted respiratory compensation is common. Serum electrolytes should also be obtained every 6 hours during induced hypothermia and rewarming. Rapid fluctuations in potassium occur from ischemia, acidosis, catecholamine administration, and core temperature changes. Induction of hypothermia results in a diuresis with concomitant potassium loss.[14] In the authors' experience, hyperkalemia during rewarming is rare when gradual rewarming is used in an adequately resuscitated patient with good urine output.

Baseline blood counts are useful to hematologic abnormalities. Profound anemia suggests blood loss as a factor contributing to cardiac arrest. Moderate leukocytosis ($10–20,10^3/\mu L$) is common after cardiac arrest and likely represents acute demargination and inflammatory response. Marked leukocytosis should be investigated for a cause other than cardiac arrest. Serum lactate should be measured every 6 hours until they normalize, because both initial lactate concentration and lactate clearance correlate with survival.[15,16] Higher lactate levels or levels that do not clear suggest on-going ischemia should prompt evaluation of the intra-abdominal and muscle compartments. Lactic acidosis is common after cardiac arrest, and lactate concentrations may increase to approximately 15 mmol/L. Specific toxicologic studies are indicated in patients with a history of drug ingestion, signs of a toxidrome, or clinical suspicion of poisoning.

Serum troponin levels should be measured every 8 to 12 hours to detect myocardial injury. If levels are elevated, testing should continue until there is a peak and decline. Mild increases in serum troponin (troponin I: 0–5 ng/mL) are common after cardiac arrest, cardiopulmonary resuscitation (CPR), and defibrillation; higher or rising levels suggest acute coronary syndrome or myocarditis.

Renal and hepatic injuries are common after cardiac arrest and reflect global ischemia/reperfusion. The presence of acute kidney injury will affect drug choices, drug dosing, and the use of intravenous contrast. Hepatic injury will also affect drug choices and drug dosing. Most renal and hepatic injuries improve with resuscitation and resolution of ischemia.[17]

Imaging

A baseline chest radiograph is required to confirm proper positioning of the endotracheal tube and central venous catheter. In addition, it provides a screening tool for pulmonary pathology. Pulmonary edema and aspiration are common findings after CPR and may be entirely unrelated to the cause of cardiac arrest. However, pneumothorax or mediastinal abnormalities require immediate attention and may prompt computed tomography (CT) imaging of the thorax.

Bedside emergency ultrasound provides an excellent screening tool for causes of cardiac arrest that represent an ongoing threat to life. These causes include pericardial tamponade, pneumothorax, massive pulmonary embolism, and intraperitoneal bleeding.[18–22] In addition, bedside ultrasound can provide estimates of ejection fraction[23] and volume status,[24] which provide useful information for titrating hemodynamic support.

Baseline unenhanced CT imaging of the brain is helpful in the postcardiac arrest patient. Intracranial hemorrhage should be excluded as a cause of cardiac arrest; one series noted a 4% incidence of intracranial hemorrhage that altered both prognosis and management, including the preclusion of anticoagulation.[25] In addition, unenhanced CT imaging detects early cerebral edema, which is helpful for neurologic prognostication and estimation of the patient's clinical course.[25–28]

In cases of suspected pulmonary embolism, CT angiography of the chest should be performed. CT angiography may be delayed in the setting of acute renal injury. Ancillary studies, such as echocardiography or ultrasonography of the lower extremities, may be performed while empiric anticoagulation is started. The high incidence of abnormalities on chest radiograph precludes the utility of V/Q scan in this population.[29] CT imaging of the abdomen and pelvis is indicated in the setting of traumatic mechanism, clinical findings of peritonitis, or markedly elevated lactate.

Postcardiac Arrest Illness Severity

The postcardiac arrest syndrome is a unique illness that combines global brain injury, myocardial dysfunction, and systemic global ischemia/reperfusion. Patients will exhibit a range of features of each of these components to varying degrees, depending on the extent of the anoxic insult. It is important to recognize the different phenotypes of postcardiac arrest patients, because clinical care should be tailored to the individual patient.

Several illness severity scores have been developed for the postcardiac arrest population.[30–35] The authors prefer the Pittsburgh Post-Cardiac Arrest Category (PCAC), because it uses bedside assessment and testing on hospital arrival rather than historical variables, thus providing early outcome prediction and facilitating risk-adjusted decision-making for hospital-based procedures and interventions. The PCAC is a validated, early postcardiac arrest illness severity score based on initial cardiopulmonary dysfunction (Sequential Organ Failure Assessment [SOFA] score: cardiovascular and respiratory components) and neurologic examination (FOUR score: motor and brainstem components).[00,00] It provides a 4-level stratification scheme that estimates in hospital mortality and discharge disposition. PCAC can be easily calculated during the initial patient assessment in the ED, provided there are no sedatives or neuromuscular blockers that will cloud the neurologic examination (**Fig. 1**, **Table 2**).

MANAGEMENT OF THE POSTARREST PATIENT

The initial management of the postarrest patient is multifaceted. Close attention must be paid to optimizing hemodynamic and ventilatory parameters while the search for underlying cause progresses. Following resuscitation from cardiac arrest, the most immediate life threat is hemodynamic collapse. Although optimizing hemodynamics is the first priority, the astute clinician will incorporate the unique needs of the brain-injured patient to their management strategy. Such an approach provides the optimal milieu for the brain to recover.

A

Category	FOUR Score Motor + Brainstem	SOFA Score Cardiovascular + Respiratory	Clinical Description
I	8	Any	Awake, follows commands
II	4-7	≤ 3	Moderate coma with preservation of some brainstem reflexes
III	4-7	≥ 4	Moderate coma with preservation of some brainstem reflexes and severe cardiopulmonary failure
IV	≤ 3	Any	Deep coma with loss of most or all brainstem reflexes

B

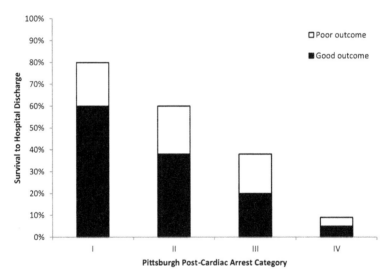

Fig. 1. Description (*A*) and prognostication (*B*) of the PCAC. Good outcome: discharge to home or acute rehabilitation facility. (*From* Reynolds JC, Rittenberger JC, Toma C, et al. Post Cardiac Arrest Service. Risk-adjusted outcome prediction with initial post-cardiac arrest illness severity: implications for cardiac arrest survivors being considered for early invasive strategy. Resuscitation. 2014;85(9):1232–9; with permission.)

Minimize Ongoing Brain Injury

Prevention of additional neuronal injury is critical. Following resucitation from cardiac arrest, the baroreceptor response in the brain is commonly impaired. Thus, many patients require a mean arterial pressure (MAP) of 80 mm Hg or more to maintain perfusion.[37] Lactic acidosis is common following cardiac arrest and a ventilatory compensation is frequently seen. However, the chemoreceptor response to $Paco_2$ remains intact; thus, hyperventilating may result in vasoconstriction and additional ischemia.[37] This response remains in effect for several hours following the initial resuscitation. Optimizing acid-base status and electrolyte abnormalities is the next focus

Table 2
Examination components needed to calculate the Pittsburgh Post Cardiac Arrest Category

FOUR Score	SOFA Score
Motor component	Cardiovascular component
4 points: Follows commands	4 points: Dop >15 OR Epi >0.1 OR Nor >0.1
3 points: Localizes to pain	3 points: Dop >5 OR Epi $\leq$0.1 OR Nor $\leq$0.1
2 points: Flexion response to pain	2 points: Dop $\leq$5 or Dob (any dose)
1 point: Extensor response to pain	1 point: MAP <70 mm Hg
0 point: No response to pain OR	
generalized myoclonic status	
Brainstem component	Respiratory component
4 points: Pupil AND corneal reflexes	4 points: Pao_2/Fio_2 <100 AND on ventilator
present	3 points: Pao_2/Fio_2 <200 AND on ventilator
3 points: Unilateral fixed/dilated pupil	2 points: Pao_2/Fio_2 <300
2 points: Pupil OR corneal reflexes absent	1 point: Pao_2/Fio_2 <400
1 point: Pupil AND corneal reflexes absent	
0 point: Pupil AND corneal AND cough	
reflexes absent	

Vasopressor doses are in μg/kg/min.
Abbreviations: Dob, dobutamine; Dop, dopamine; Epi, epinephrine; Nor, norepinephrine.

and frequently requires several hours to address. Managing temperature is also important and is discussed in detail later.

Neurologic Prognostication

During the first 24 hours following resuscitation, there are no clinical or imaging tests, used in isolation, that rule out the potential for neurologic recovery. Consequently, with the exception of those with active Do Not Resuscitate orders or an advanced directive, aggressive care should be considered for these patients. Many facilities have developed protocols delineating specific timelines for the consideration of withdrawal of life support because of poor neurologic prognosis. These protocols range from 3 to 7 days following resuscitation. A multimodal approach incorporating clinical examination, CT of the brain, electroencephalography, neurophysiology testing such as somatosensory-evoked potentials, and MRI should be incorporated to the prognostic workup in these patients.[25,38–43] Serum biomarkers, including neuronal specific enolase, S100b, and glial fibrillary acidic protein, have been evaluated; however, commonly agreed on cutoffs for determining a poor prognosis varies.[39,44,45] In addition, these tests are frequently a "send out" for most hospitals, limiting their utility as a marker to titrate care or guide prognostication. Thus, it is difficult to determine early on which patients will not recover.

Airway

Respiratory management of the postarrest patient should begin with an assessment of the patient's airway and ensuring maintenance of an adequate airway. An obstructed or inadequate airway can lead to recurrent cardiac arrest. Awake and alert patients may not require advanced airway intervention. Most of the survivors of cardiac arrest are neurologically injured, however, and will require the placement of an artificial airway. Often, during the initial resuscitation of the patient from cardiac arrest, an endotracheal tube is placed in the field. Endotracheal intubation can require a lengthy interruption in chest compressions,[46] and there is no good evidence to support routine prehospital advanced airway management in cardiac arrest.[47] In retrospective data sets, however, survival from cardiac arrest is associated with the fraction of time during which chest compressions are performed.[48,49] Therefore, some EMS services have begun favoring the use of rescue airways or other supraglottic airways that can be placed with chest compressions ongoing.[50–52] On arrival to the hospital, one of the first tasks for the emergency provider is an assessment of the adequacy of the airway. Because most comatose patients will require mechanical ventilation for at least 24 hours, and because a common complication of cardiac arrest is aspiration,[53,54] an existing rescue or supraglottic airway should be changed to an endotracheal tube as soon it can safely be done. Patients with aspiration may require frequent suctioning, and therefore, a large-caliber endotracheal tube may be useful.

Oxygenation

The next step in respiratory management of the postarrest patient involves ensuring adequate oxygenation to the brain and other vulnerable tissues. Early hypoxia is associated with poorer outcomes after cardiac arrest.[55] Early hyperoxia, in contrast, may or may not worsen neurologic outcomes.[56–58] Although this data are not robust, there is rarely a compelling reason to hyperoxygenate the postarrest patient. Providers should, therefore, use normoxia as the goal, while using adequate supplemental oxygen care to avoid arterial hypoxia. An initial ABG may be useful in defining the partial pressure of oxygen (Pa_{O_2}). If the peripheral pulse oximetry monitor correlates with the ABG, continuous monitoring of such can help the provider titrate supplemental oxygen appropriately.

Ventilation

Management of the partial pressure of carbon dioxide (Pa_{CO_2}) via assessment and support of ventilation is also important in the postarrest patient. Cerebrovascular autoregulation is related to the Pa_{CO_2}.[59] Hyperventilation, by decreased Pa_{CO_2}, causes cerebrovascular constriction, leading to a decrease in cerebral blood flow.[60,61] In addition, hyperventilation can increase intrathoracic pressure, leading to a decrease in cardiac preload and subsequent reduced cardiac output and coronary perfusion pressure.[62] Conversely, it is presently not known if hypercapnia from hypoventilation contributes to vasodilation, hyperemia, or cerebral edema. The authors recommend, therefore, adjusting mechanical ventilation settings to keep low intrathoracic pressures and the Pa_{CO_2} between 35 to 45 mm Hg.

Hemodynamic Considerations: End-Organ Perfusion

The postarrest patient will often require active maintenance of hemodynamic parameters to ensure adequate end-organ perfusion. After the ROSC from cardiac arrest, episodes of hypotension are common.[63] The shocklike state described in the postcardiac arrest syndrome is due to both a systemic ischemia/reperfusion response (analogous to sepsis) and myocardial dysfunction.[63] Even transient hypotension after cardiac arrest can cause secondary brain injury,[64] because cerebral autoregulation of perfusion is impaired.[65,66] MAP of less than 80 mm Hg is associated with a decline in brain perfusion. PET studies in postarrest patients have demonstrated that regional cerebral perfusion matches metabolic activity, however, when the MAP is adequate.[67,68] Therefore, the authors recommend frequent evaluation of the postarrest patients' MAP. At a minimum, noninvasive blood pressure checks should be done at least every 5 minutes until adequate perfusion is ensured, but ideally, arterial cannulation should be performed to monitor MAP continuously. The authors recommend maintenance of a MAP on the higher end of the normal range (80–100 mm Hg) during the postarrest period to prevent further central nervous system injury.[66]

Other parameters can be followed as surrogates of perfusion, such as adequate urine output (>0.5 mL/kg/h), central venous pressure (CVP) (8–12 mm Hg), and lactate clearance.

Because a significant component of hypotension in the postarrest patient is due to a sepsislike state, the authors recommend treatment of hypotension after cardiac arrest mirroring that of treatment of hypotension in sepsis. Volume replacement with isotonic crystalloids should be used until CVP reaches 8 to 12 mm Hg. Next, vasopressors can be titrated to reach the MAP goal of 80 to 100 mm Hg. As in sepsis, the authors recommend the use of norepinephrine (0.01–1 μg/kg/min) as first line over dopamine (5–20 μg/kg/min) because of the potential arrhythmogenic side effects of dopamine.[69]

Myocardial Dysfunction

Another common cause of hypotension in the postarrest patient is myocardial dysfunction. The postarrest myocardial dysfunction generally peaks at 8 to 24 hours after cardiac arrest[63] and is due to coronary reperfusion injury. This cellular damage leads to decreased cardiac stroke volume and decreased cardiac output.[70] Cardiac ionotropes (such as dobutamine [2–15 μg/kg/min] or milrinone [loading dose: 50 μg/kg over 10 minutes, then 0.375–0.75 μg/kg/min]) may be useful in the setting of isolated cardiogenic shock. However, because these agents can cause further hypotension from vasodilation, the authors recommend their use only when cardiogenic shock is confirmed (such as by global hypokinesis on echocardiogram or persistently low Svo_2 despite normalized MAP). In the authors' experience, patients requiring vasopressors or ionotropes after cardiac arrest often display labile hemodynamics during the first 24 hours with accompanying changes in dosing requirements. Therefore, they recommend invasive arterial blood pressure monitoring and admission to the ICU.

Patients after cardiac arrest may have arrhythmias. Some patients suffer their cardiac arrest from a primary arrhythmia. Despite this, there are no data to support the routine, prophylactic use of antiarrhythmic medications after cardiac arrest. A better strategy is for the treating team to identify and correct the cause of the arrhythmia.

Coronary Revascularization

Coronary angiography and percutaneous coronary intervention (PCI) when indicated are key components of systematic, multidisciplinary postcardiac arrest care, especially for patients with STEMI on EKG or clinical suspicion for coronary ischemia as the precipitating cause. In the absence of STEMI, patients with an initially shockable rhythm (ventricular fibrillation or ventricular tachycardia) carry a high incidence of coronary lesions as well.[9,13,71] Regardless of EKG findings, emergent left heart catheterization may be indicated for ongoing hemodynamic instability, cardiogenic shock, rising troponin levels, or focal wall-motion abnormalities on echocardiogram.

Adjusting for other factors, cardiac catheterization is associated with improved mortality and functional status at hospital discharge.[7–9] Given the high burden of coronary disease in this population and the benefits of timely reperfusion, catheterization should be performed in all patients without obvious noncardiac cause of arrest, with precise timing determined by EKG, trajectory of cardiac biomarkers, presence of shock, and competing needs of other procedures. Moreover, because neurologic stunning and coma may take days to resolve, life-saving cardiovascular procedures should not be delayed pending neurologic recovery. Early discussion with interventional cardiology is essential and should be initiated in the ED.

Interventional cardiologists may be reluctant to perform coronary interventions in patients whose prognosis is poor because of noncardiac complications. Specifically, patients resuscitated from cardiac arrest who are initially comatose are at risk of death from neurologic injury regardless of coronary intervention.[30,72] Unfortunately, most postprocedural mortality data in resuscitated cardiac arrest patients do not distinguish between different causes of in-hospital death. Performance reporting at PCI centers is tied to awards, reimbursement, recognition, public reporting of hospital performance, and physician decision-making.[73,74] Because appropriate, early catheterization has the unintended consequence of increasing total mortality at centers that perform high-volume, quality postarrest care, a recent American Heart Association advisory panel now recommends tracking cardiac arrest cases separately from other PCI cases. Alternatively, the PCAC can be used to risk-stratify patients and facilitate risk-adjusted outcome prediction for those patients being considered for early invasive strategy.[8]

Temperature Management

After the first 24 hours, withdrawal of life support due to neurologic injury is the most common cause of death in patients resuscitated from out-of-hospital cardiac arrest and contributes to mortality in the in-hospital cardiac arrest population as well.[30,72] During the first 48 hours following resuscitation, each degree in temperature more than 37°C has been associated with an increased risk of death. Timing of fever is important, as earlier fever has been associated with poor outcomes, whereas later onset of fever has not conferred the same detriment.[75] Lowering the body temperature between 32°C and 34°C for 12 to 24 hours has been associated with improved neurologic outcomes in 2 randomized controlled trials.[53,54] Multiple studies combining therapeutic hypothermia with a standardized postarrest care protocol have yielded similar results.[76–78] Recent data evaluating 33°C and 36°C have not demonstrated a difference in neurologic outcome.[42] When considered in total, these data demonstrate that active control of temperature is needed during the postarrest phase and fever must be avoided.

Indications and Contraindications

Patients who do not follow commands (ie, ability to squeeze fingers, move toes) following resuscitation from cardiac arrest should have their temperature managed. Exceptions include those with advanced directives refusing aggressive care. Although a window exists to induce hypothermia, early fever is associated with worse outcomes, adding urgency to management of this aspect of care.[75] Patients with active, noncompressible bleeding should not have induction of hypothermia. Coagulopathy secondary to hypothermia is more prevalent less than a temperature of 35°C. Thus, management at 36°C is reasonable in this cohort.[42] Importantly, hypothermia has been successfully used in pregnancy, during cardiac catheterization, following thrombolytic administration, and in hemodynamically unstable patients.[7,8,37,79–82] One retrospective review demonstrated lower doses of vasopressor agents in patients receiving therapeutic hypothermia.[82]

Timing, Goal, and Duration

Preclinical research demonstrates that a brief duration of cooling is effective if hypothermia is achieved before ROSC.[83] Induction of hypothermia after ROSC requires longer duration of therapy to derive benefit.[83–85] This window of opportunity extends for several hours after ROSC.[86]

Clinical trials of hypothermia arrived at goal temperature between 2 and 10 hours following resuscitation.[42,53,54] These studies demonstrated similar clinical outcomes, supporting the window of opportunity outlined. Recent studies have evaluated the role of early cooling on survival and good neurologic outcome. In a trial by Bernard and colleagues,[54] hypothermia was induced using ice packs while en route to the hospital, resulting in achievement of hypothermia a mean of 2 hours following ROSC.Three additional studies have evaluated induced hypothermia using cold saline in the prehospital arena. Each study demonstrated lower temperatures on arrival to the hospital, but generally remained above the goal temperature range of 32°C to 34°C.[87–89] One trial of intra-arrest cooling randomized 200 patients to intra-arrest cooling using a novel intranasal cooling device versus cooling at hospital. Interestingly, mean temperature at ROSC was not different between the intranasal cooling group and standard treatment group (35.5°C intervention vs 35.8°C control) groups. Clinical outcomes including survival and good neurologic outcome were similar between groups.[90]

The optimal temperature for management remains debatable. The HACA (Hypothermia After Cardiac Arrest Study Group) and Bernard trials used goal temperatures of 34°C and 32°C, resulting in rates of good neurologic outcome of 55% and 49%. Recent work by Nielsen and colleagues[42] (the Targeted Temperature Management [TTM] trial) randomized subjects to 33°C and 36°C, resulting in rates of good neurologic outcome of 46% and 48%, respectively. Each of these trials primarily recruited patients with witnessed arrests and a primary rhythm of ventricular fibrillation/ventricular tachycardia; this represents a minority of the out-of-hospital cardiac arrest cohort.[91] When considering nonshockable arrests, a systematic review of 2 randomized trials and 12 nonrandomized trials suggested a survival benefit for hypothermia (odds ratio [OR] of death 0.84, 95% confidence interval [CI] 0.78–0.92), but no difference in good neurologic outcome (OR of poor neurologic outcome 0.93, 95% CI 0.88–1.00).[92]

Hypothermia therapy durations of 12 and 24 hours have been studied. In the recent TTM trial, the intervention temperature was maintained until 28 hours following ROSC and fever avoidance until 72 hours after ROSC.[42] These data support active control of temperature after ROSC. At this time, temperatures should be controlled between 32°C and 34°C for 12 to 24 hours or 36°C for the first 24 hours after ROSC followed by slow (<0.5°C/h) rewarming. Tailoring temperature management (both temperature and duration) based on neurologic injury or other patient characteristics is a goal for the resuscitation community.

Methods for Induction/Maintenance

Monitoring core body temperature is required during the postarrest phase. The most accurate method is central venous temperature monitoring. However, esophageal, bladder, and rectal monitoring may also be used.[93] Esophageal monitoring is the most accurate method. Bladder temperature is limited by urine output. If urine output is less than 0.5 mL/kg/h, bladder temperature may be inaccurate. Rectal monitoring is less reliable because it may lag behind during acute temperature changes and can vary up to 1.5°C. Tympanic, oral, and axillary monitoring are inaccurate and should not be used.

Either surface or intravascular cooling may be used to induce and maintain temperature. Time to goal temperature, survival, and good neurologic outcome do not differ based on cooling method.[94] Most patients are mildly hypothermic after ROSC (35°C–35.5°C). Rapid intravenous infusion of 30 mL/kg cold (4°C) normal saline can drop core temperature by more than 2°C per hour.[95] However, pulmonary edema and diuretic use were higher in subjects receiving rapid infusion of normal saline for hypothermia induction.[89] Surface cooling methods result in a more gradual reduction in core temperature (0.5°C–1°C/h). In patients without heart failure, the authors commonly administer 1 to 2 L of cold saline during hypothermia induction. In addition, surface cooling using ice packs, cooling blankets, or cold water baths facilitates induction of hypothermia.

For the maintenance phase of hypothermia, either an intravascular or a surface thermostatic device can regulate temperature and provide real-time temperature adjustments to maintain goal temperature.[42,96]

Sedation and Shivering

Shivering is the body's natural response to cooling. It results in increased oxygen demand and will raise body temperature. Shivering is a common reason for failure to achieve goal temperature and may be subtle. Sedation is commonly used to prevent or suppress shivering; however, this does require titration of sedative medications to shivering rather than traditional sedation scales. High doses of medications or intermittent paralysis may be required. Many sedative medications can result in hypotension; thus, consideration of the patient's cardiovascular status will influence the sedative used. Boluses of medications may be used during induction, but continuous infusions are commonly needed to maintain shivering suppression.

In the hemodynamically stable patient, an infusion of propofol (up to 50 μg/kg/min) can be used to suppress shivering. Addition of fentanyl (0.1–0.5 μg/kg/h) may be used, either in bolus or in infusion form.[97] Dexmedetomidine has been used for shivering suppression, but is limited by its side effects of bradycardia and hypotension.

Continuous infusion of midazolam (2–10 mg/h) will suppress shivering with less cardiovascular effect, but may accumulate in adipose tissue.[98] Hypothermia decreases metabolism and excretion of midazolam in healthy individuals.[99] In addition, renal impairment is commonly encountered during the postarrest phase.[17] In combination, these may prolong the effect of midazolam and confound the neurologic examination.

Neuromuscular blockade will suppress shivering and is commonly used during hypothermia induction. Continuous infusion of paralytic agents may prevent recognition of seizures, which are common.[53,97,100] The authors recommend continuous electroencephalogram monitoring if continuous neuromuscular blockade is used.

Rewarming

Although induction can be done rapidly, rewarming should be done gradually. Rewarming should be done at no greater than 0.5°C per hour. The authors advocate a rate of 0.2°C to 0.25°C per hour. Rewarming at faster rates can result in hyperkalemia, cerebral edema, and seizures. Animal models demonstrated a reversal in protective effect from hypothermia in animals rapidly rewarmed.[101]

Both surface and intravascular devices have algorithms to facilitate rewarming at a set rate.[102,103] Shivering remains a concern and may be one cause of rapid rewarming. Thus, shivering suppression should be maintained during the rewarming process. Manual rewarming can be used when ice packs or a cooling blanket has been used. This method is more labor intensive and requires frequent temperature monitoring. Patients with ice packs can have packs added or removed based on the rate of rewarming. For those with a cooling blanket, one method is to increase the goal temperature by 0.5°C every 3 hours until the core temperature returns to normothermia. In patients who are difficult to rewarm, adjuncts include heating lamps, warming the ventilator air circuit, or applying a conductive heating device. Rather than using all methods simultaneously, the authors recommend the addition of one at a time to prevent rapid rewarming.

Side Effects

Hypothermia is a pleiotropic therapy and side effects may affect many organ systems. The most common cardiovascular side effect is bradycardia. Heart rates in the 30 to 40 range are common and do not require intervention if the blood pressure is acceptable. QT prolongation is also common because of slowing of cardiac conduction. Should ventricular tachycardia or ventricular fibrillation develop, defibrillation remains a first-line therapy. Preclinical models demonstrate a similar first shock success rate between 33°C and 37°C.[104]

Electrolyte shifts are common during hypothermia therapy. During hypothermia induction, glomerular blood flow increases, resulting in cold diuresis andpossibly in hypokalemia, hypovolemia, hypomagnesemia, and hypophosphatemia.[105,106] Patients treated at 33°C are more likely to experience hypokalemia.[42] Potassium also shifts into cells, resulting in hypokalemia. During rewarming, potassium will shift back out from cells, potentially resulting in hyperkalemia. This effect is uncommon in patients with normal renal function.

Hypothermia decreases leukocyte migration, increasing the risk of infection, and is most pronounced in patients treated with hypothermia for more than 24 hours. The rate of infection, including pneumonia, does not differ between patients treated at 33°C and 36°C.[42]

At temperatures less than 35°C, hypothermia slows the enzymes responsible for clotting and impairs platelet function.[107,108] Bleeding may occur in up to 20% of patients treated with hypothermia. This rate does not differ from patients not treated with hypothermia, and transfusions are rarely required.[29,42,53]

General Clinical Care

Standard ICU interventions also play a role in the management of the patient resuscitated from cardiac arrest. Elevation of the head of the bed to 30° can prevent aspiration and may decrease intracranial pressure. Providing H2 blocker or proton pump inhibition to prevent stress ulcers can also decrease the likelihood of gastrointestinal bleeding. During hypothermia, gastrointestinal motility is decreased. However, once rewarming is complete, enteral feeds may prevent bacterial translocation from the gut.[109] Standard therapies to prevent deep venous thrombosis are warranted. Similar to other critical illness states, tight glycemic management does not confer additional benefit in this population.[110] Finally, early physical and occupational therapy have been associated with improved outcomes in critical illness states and should be considered in this population.[111]

REGIONALIZATION OF CARE

Modern management of cardiac arrest and post-resuscitation care should occur at a regionalized cardiac arrest center. This model of care is not new for patients requiring time-sensitive interventions. Trauma, STEMI, and acute stroke all take advantage of established, regionalized systems of care that coordinate prehospital providers with receiving centers. Several case-control studies have highlighted the effectiveness of bundled post-resuscitation care, demonstrating improved outcomes compared with historical controls.[76–79,112–115] Typical hospital providers treat postcardiac arrest patients infrequently, given the low rates of resuscitation in individual communities. Regionalized cardiac arrest centers increase referral volumes, and thereby, provider experience.[116] There is a well-documented positive correlation between greater provider experience (or procedural volume) for complex diagnoses (or procedures) and better patient outcome.[117]

There is accumulating evidence for improved outcomes when cardiac arrest patients are treated at regionalized centers.[118] Wnent and colleagues[119] describe the influence of the prehospital emergency physician's choice of admitting hospital on patient outcome after cardiac arrest in an urban, German setting. A total of 434 patients were admitted to the hospital, 39% to PCI centers and 61% to hospitals without PCI capabilities. Adjusting for confounders, patients were more than 3 times as likely to survive with favorable neurologic outcome when transported to a PCI center. Cha and colleagues[120] describe more than 27,000 Korean patients transported to the hospital with CPR in progress. Even with longer transport intervals, patients transported to high-volume centers were more likely to survive to hospital discharge compared with low-volume centers. Regionalized centers can also offer organ donation and procurement services for patients that do not survive (**Box 2**).[121]

Box 2
Proposed clinical services for regionalized cardiac arrest centers

Neurologic services

   Induced hypothermia

   Continuous EEG monitoring

   Seizure management

   Neurology consultation

   Neurosurgical consultation

   Cerebral imaging (CT, MRI, perfusion studies)

   Neurophysiological testing (evoked potentials)

   Prognostication services

Critical care services

   Ventilator management

   Glucose control

   Goal-directed hemodynamic management

Cardiovascular services

   Cardiac catheterization/percutaneous coronary intervention

   Coronary artery bypass grafting

   Intra-aortic balloon pump

   Cardiovascular mechanical support devices

   Extracorporeal membranous oxygenation

   Transplant surgery consultation

   Electrophysiology consultation

   Implantable cardioverter defibrillator placement

Other services

   Physical medicine and rehabilitation consultation

   Physical and occupational therapy

   Social work

   Organ donation

   Outpatient physical and occupational therapy

   Outpatient neurologic rehabilitation

   Outpatient psychological services

One of the common barriers to implementation of regionalized cardiac arrest care is patient transport. Bypassing a local hospital to transport a cardiac arrest patient to a more distant resuscitation center is a controversial topic. However, 2 recent studies demonstrate that prehospital transport time does not independently impact patient outcome after cardiac arrest,[122,123] suggesting that a modest increase in transport interval from bypassing a local hospital en route to specialized care is feasible.

Interfacility transfer for post-resuscitation care is a related issue. Critically ill, recently resuscitated cardiac arrest patients are inherently at risk for deterioration en route. Hartke and colleagues[124] evaluated 248 resuscitated patients transported to tertiary care facilities. With a median transport time of 63 minutes (interquartile range: 51–81 minutes), they found that rearrest was uncommon (6%), and that critical events (hypotension or hypoxia) affected 23% of patients during transport. Most critical events occurred within the first hour of transport, and 27% occurred at the referring facility before departure. Patients on vasopressors were most likely to suffer critical events. The authors weighed the risk of transport against the overall survival rate of 53%, and the 29% survival rate of patients suffering a critical event. They proposed that resuscitated patients referred to a regional center from out-lying facilities derive benefit from transport to a cardiac arrest center, with an acceptable risk of decompensation en route.

SUMMARY

The management of the patient successfully resuscitated from cardiac arrest requires specific attention to neurologic injury. The clinical examination remains dynamic, and many patients will require more than 72 hours for an accurate neurologic prognosis to be determined.

REFERENCES

1. Reynolds JC, Lawner BJ. Management of the post-cardiac arrest syndrome. J Emerg Med 2012;42(4):440–9.
2. Wijdicks EF, Bamlet WR, Maramattom BV, et al. Validation of a new coma scale: the FOUR score. Ann Neurol 2005;58(4):585–93.
3. Stead LG, Wijdicks EF, Bhagra A, et al. Validation of a new coma scale, the FOUR score, in the emergency department. Neurocrit Care 2009;10(1):50–4.
4. Iyer VN, Mandrekar JN, Danielson RD, et al. Validity of the FOUR score coma scale in the medical intensive care unit. Mayo Clin Proc 2009;84(8):694–701.
5. Fischer M, Rüegg S, Czaplinski A, et al. Inter-rater reliability of the Full Outline of UnResponsiveness score and the Glasgow Coma Scale in critically ill patients: a prospective observational study. Crit Care 2010;14(2):R64.
6. Zanuttini D, Armellini I, Nucifora G, et al. Predictive value of electrocardiogram in diagnosing acute coronary artery lesions among patients with out-of-hospital-cardiac-arrest. Resuscitation 2013;84(9):1250–4.
7. Reynolds JC, Callaway CW, El Khoudary SR, et al. Coronary angiography predicts improved outcome following cardiac arrest: propensity-adjusted analysis. J Intensive Care Med 2009;24(3):179–86.
8. Reynolds JC, Rittenberger JC, Toma C, et al, the Post Cardiac Arrest Service. Risk-adjusted outcome prediction with initial post-cardiac arrest illness severity: implications for cardiac arrest survivors being considered for early invasive strategy. Resuscitation 2014;85:1232–9.
9. Dumas F, Cariou A, Manzo-Silberman S, et al. Immediate percutaneous coronary intervention is associated with better survival after out-of-hospital cardiac

arrest: insights from the PROCAT (Parisian Region Out of hospital Cardiac ArresT) registry. Circ Cardiovasc Interv 2010;3(3):200–7.

10. Hollenbeck RD, McPherson JA, Mooney MR, et al. Early cardiac catheterization is associated with improved survival in comatose survivors of cardiac arrest without STEMI. Resuscitation 2013;85:88–95.

11. Radsel P, Knafelj R, Kocjancic S, et al. Angiographic characteristics of coronary disease and postresuscitation electrocardiograms in patients with aborted cardiac arrest outside a hospital. Am J Cardiol 2011;108:634–8.

12. Gupta N, Kontos MC, Gupta A, et al. Clinical and angiographic characteristics of patients undergoing percutaneous coronary intervention following sudden cardiac arrest: insights from the NCDR [Abstract]. Circulation 2011;124:A10305.

13. Spaulding CM, Joly LM, Rosenberg A, et al. Immediate coronary angiography in survivors of out-of-hospital cardiac arrest. N Engl J Med 1997;336(23):1629–33.

14. Raper JD, Wang HE. Urine output changes during postcardiac arrest therapeutic hypothermia. Ther Hypothermia Temp Manag 2013;3(4):173–7.

15. Donnino MW, Miller J, Goyal N, et al. Effective lactate clearance is associated with improved outcome in post-cardiac arrest patients. Resuscitation 2007;75:229.

16. Donnino MW, Andersen LW, Giberson T, et al, for the National Post-Arrest Research Consortium. Initial lactate and lactate change in post-cardiac arrest: a multicenter validation study. Crit Care Med 2014;42:1804–11.

17. Yanta J, Guyette FX, Doshi AA, et al. Renal dysfunction is common following resuscitation from cardiac arrest. Resuscitation 2013;84(10):1371–4.

18. Moore CL, Copel JA. Point-of-care ultrasonography. N Engl J Med 2011;364:749.

19. Rose JS, Bair AE, Mandavia D, et al. The UHP ultrasound protocol: a novel ultrasound approach to the empiric evaluation of the undifferentiated hypotensive patient. Am J Emerg Med 2001;19:299.

20. Jones AE, Tayal VS, Sullivan DM, et al. Randomized, controlled trial of immediate versus delayed goal-directed ultrasound to identify the cause of nontraumatic hypotension in emergency department patients. Crit Care Med 2004;32:1703.

21. Scalea TM, Rodriguez A, Chiu WC, et al. Focused Assessment with Sonography for Trauma (FAST): results from an international consensus conference. J Trauma 1999;46:466.

22. Kirkpatrick AW, Sirois M, Laupland KB, et al. Hand-held thoracic sonography for detecting posttraumatic pneumothoraces: the Extended Focused Assessment with Sonography for Trauma (EFAST). J Trauma 2004;57:288.

23. McKaigney CJ, Krantz MJ, La Rocque CL, et al. E-point septal separation: a bedside tool for emergency physician assessment of left ventricular ejection fraction. Am J Emerg Med 2014;32(6):493–7.

24. Dipti A, Soucy Z, Surana A, et al. Role of inferior vena cava diameter in assessment of volume status: a meta-analysis. Am J Emerg Med 2012;30(8):1414–9.e1.

25. Metter RB, Rittenberger JC, Guyette FX, et al. Association between a quantitative CT scan measure of brain edema and outcome after cardiac arrest. Resuscitation 2011;82:1180.

26. Torbey MT, Selim M, Knorr J, et al. Quantitative analysis of the loss of distinction between gray and white matter in comatose patients after cardiac arrest. Stroke 2000;31(9):2163–7.

27. Yanagawa Y, Un-no Y, Sakamoto T, et al. Cerebral density on CT immediately after a successful resuscitation of cardiopulmonary arrest correlates with outcome. Resuscitation 2005;64(1):97–101.

28. Cristia C, Ho ML, Levy S, et al. The association between a quantitative computed tomography (CT) measurement of cerebral edema and outcomes in post-cardiac arrest - a validation study. Resuscitation 2014;85:1348–53.

29. Nielsen N, Hovdenes J, Nilsson F, et al. Outcome, timing and adverse events in therapeutic hypothermia after out-of-hospital cardiac arrest. Acta Anaesthesiol Scand 2009;53:926.

30. Rittenberger JC, Tisherman SA, Holm MB, et al. An early, novel illness severity score to predict outcome after cardiac arrest. Resuscitation 2011;82(11): 1399–404.

31. Gräsner JT, Meybohm P, Lefering R, et al, German Resuscitation Registry Study Group. ROSC after cardiac arrest–the RACA score to predict outcome after out-of-hospital cardiac arrest. Eur Heart J 2011;32(13):1649–56.

32. Ebell MH, Jang W, Shen Y, et al, Get With the Guidelines–Resuscitation Investigators. Development and validation of the Good Outcome Following Attempted Resuscitation (GO-FAR) score to predict neurologically intact survival after in-hospital cardiopulmonary resuscitation. JAMA Intern Med 2013;173(20):1872–8.

33. Adrie C, Cariou A, Mourvillier B, et al. Predicting survival with good neurological recovery at hospital admission after successful resuscitation of out-of-hospital cardiac arrest: the OHCA score. Eur Heart J 2006;27:2840–5.

34. Hunziker S, Bivens MJ, Cocchi MN, et al. International validation of the out-of-hospital cardiac arrest score in the United States. Crit Care Med 2011;39: 1670–4.

35. Ishikawa S, Niwano S, Imaki R, et al. Usefulness of a simple prognostication score in prediction of the prognoses of patients with out-of-hospital cardiac arrests. Int Heart J 2013;54(6):362–70.

36. Coppler PJ, Ahmed S, Sabedra A, et al. 534: validation of the Pittsburgh post-arrest illness severity score. Crit Care Med 2012;40:1–328.

37. Hovdenes J, Laake JH, Aaberge L, et al. Therapeutic hypothermia after out-of-hospital cardiac arrest: experiences with patients treated with percutaneous coronary intervention and cardiogenic shock. Acta Anaesthesiol Scand 2007; 51(2):137–42.

38. Wijdicks EF, Hijdra A, Young GB, et al, Quality Standards Subcommittee of the American Academy of Neurology. Practice parameter: prediction of outcome in comatose survivors after cardiopulmonary resuscitation (an evidence-based review): report of the Quality Standards Subcommittee of the American Academy of Neurology [review]. Neurology 2006;67(2):203–10.

39. Zandbergen EG, Koelman JH, de Haan RJ, et al, PROPAC-Study Group. SSEPs and prognosis in postanoxic coma: only short or also long latency responses? Neurology 2006;67(4):583–6.

40. Rittenberger JC, Sangl J, Wheeler M, et al. Association between clinical examination and outcome after cardiac arrest. Resuscitation 2010;81:1128–32.

41. Rossetti AO, Carrera E, Oddo M. Early EEG correlates of neuronal injury after brain anoxia. Neurology 2012;78(11):796–802.

42. Nielsen N, Wetterslev J, Cronberg T, et al, TTM Trial Investigators. Targeted temperature management at 33°C versus 36°C after cardiac arrest. N Engl J Med 2013;369(23):2197–206.

43. Young GB. Clinical practice. Neurologic prognosis after cardiac arrest. N Engl J Med 2009;361(6):605–11.

44. Calderon LM, Guyette FX, Doshi AA, et al, Post Cardiac Arrest Service. Combining NSE and S100B with clinical examination findings to predict survival after resuscitation from cardiac arrest. Resuscitation 2014;85:1025–9.

45. Zandbergen EG, Hijdra A, Koelman JH, et al, PROPAC Study Group. Prediction of poor outcome within the first 3 days of postanoxic coma. Neurology 2006; 66(1):62–8 [Erratum appears in Neurology 2006;66(7):1133].
46. Wang HE, Simeone SJ, Weaver MD, et al. Interruptions in cardiopulmonary resuscitation from paramedic endotracheal intubation. Ann Emerg Med 2009; 54(5):645–52.
47. Carlson JN, Reynolds JC. Does advanced airway management improve outcomes in adult out-of-hospital cardiac arrest? Ann Emerg Med 2013;64: 163–4.
48. Berg RA, Sanders AB, Kern KB, et al. Adverse hemodynamic effects of interrupting chest compressions for rescue breathing during cardiopulmonary resuscitation. Circulation 2001;104(20):2465–70.
49. Christenson J, Andrusiek D, Everson-Stewart S, et al, Resuscitation Outcomes Consortium Investigators. Chest compression fraction determines survival in patients with out-of-hospital ventricular fibrillation. Circulation 2009;120(13): 1241–7.
50. Bobrow BJ, Clark LL, Ewy GA, et al. Minimally interrupted cardiac resuscitation by emergency medical services for out-of-hospital cardiac arrest. JAMA 2008; 229(10):1158–65.
51. Kellum MJ, Kennedy KW, Barney R, et al. Cardiocerebral resuscitation improves neurologically intact survival of patients with out-of-hospital cardiac arrest. Ann Emerg Med 2008;52(3):244–52.
52. Gabrielli A, Layon AJ, Wenzel V, et al. Alternative ventilation strategies in cardiopulmonary resuscitation. Curr Opin Crit Care 2002;8(3):199–211.
53. HACA – Hypothermia after Cardiac Arrest Study Group. Mild therapeutic hypothermia to improve the neurologic outcome after cardiac arrest. N Engl J Med 2002;346(8):549–56.
54. Bernard SA, Gray TW, Buist MD, et al. Treatment of comatose survivors of out-of-hospital cardiac arrest with induced hypothermia. N Engl J Med 2002;346(8): 557–63.
55. Wright WL, Geocadin RG. Postresuscitative intensive care: neuroprotective strategies after cardiac arrest. Semin Neurol 2006;26(4):396–402.
56. Janz DR, Hollenbeck RD, Pollock JS, et al. Hyperoxia is associated with increased mortality in patients treated with mild therapeutic hypothermia after sudden cardiac arrest. Crit Care Med 2012;40(12):3135–9.
57. Kilgannon HN, Jones AE, Shapiro NL, et al. Association between arterial hyperoxia following resuscitation from cardiac arrest and in-hospital mortality. JAMA 2010;303(21):2165–71.
58. Bellomo R, Bailey M, Eastwood GM, et al. Arterial hyperoxia and in-hospital mortality after resuscitation from cardiac arrest. Crit Care 2011;15(2):R90–8.
59. Kågström E, Smith ML, Siesjö BK. Cerebral circulatory responses to hypercapnia and hypoxia in the recovery period following complete and incomplete cerebral ischemia in the rat. Acta Physiol Scand 1983;118(3):281–91.
60. Buunk G, van der Hoeven JG, Frölich M, et al. Cerebral vasoconstriction in comatose patients resuscitated from a cardiac arrest? Intensive Care Med 1996;22(11):1191–6.
61. Buunk G, van der Hoeven JG, Meinders AE. Cerebrovascular reactivity in comatose patients resuscitated from a cardiac arrest. Stroke 1997;28(8):1569–73.
62. Aufderheide TP, Lurie KG. Death by hyperventilation: a common and life-threatening problem during cardiopulmonary resuscitation. Crit Care Med 2004;32(9 Suppl):S345–51.

63. Neumar RW, Nolan JP, Adrie C, et al. Post-cardiac arrest syndrome. Circulation 2008;118(23):2452–83.
64. Mullner M, Sterz F, Binder M, et al. Arterial blood pressure after human cardiac arrest and neurologic recovery. Stroke 1996;27(1):59–62.
65. Nishizawa H, Kudoh I. Cerebral autoregulation is impaired in patients resuscitated after cardiac arrest. Acta Anaesthesiol Scand 1996;40(9):1149–53.
66. Sundgreen C, Larsen FS, Herzog TM, et al. Autoregulation of cerebral blood flow in patients resuscitated from cardiac arrest. Stroke 2001;32(1):128–32.
67. Rudolf J, Ghaemi M, Ghaemi M, et al. Cerebral glucose metabolism in acute and persistent vegetative state. J Neurosurg Anesthesiol 1999;11(1):17–24.
68. Schaafsma A, de Jong BM, Bams JL, et al. Cerebral perfusion and metabolism in resuscitated patients with severe post-hypoxic encephalopathy. J Neurol Sci 2003;210(1):2330.
69. Dellinger RP, Levy MM, Rhoades A, et al. Surviving Sepsis Campaign: international guidelines for management of severe sepsis and septic shock, 2012. Crit Care Med 2013;41(2):580–637.
70. Angelos MA, Menegazzi JJ, Callaway CW. Resuscitation from prolonged ventricular fibrillation bench-to-bedside. Acad Emerg Med 2001;8(9):909–24.
71. Bulut S, Aengevaeren WRM, Luijten HJE, et al. Successful out-of-hospital cardiopulmonary resuscitation: what is the optimal in-hospital treatment strategy? Resuscitation 2000;47(2):155–61.
72. Laver S, Farrow C, Turner D, et al. Mode of death after admission to an intensive care unit following cardiac arrest. Intensive Care Med 2004;30(11):2126–8.
73. Narins CR, Dozier AM, Ling FS, et al. The influence of public reporting of outcome data on medical decision making by physicians. Arch Intern Med 2005;165:83–7.
74. McMullan PW Jr, White CJ. Doing what's right for the resuscitated. Catheter Cardiovasc Interv 2010;76:161–3.
75. Gebhardt K, Guyette FX, Doshi AA, et al, Post Cardiac Arrest Service. Prevalence and effect of fever on outcome following resuscitation from cardiac arrest. Resuscitation 2013;84(8):1062–7.
76. Sunde K, Pytte M, Jacobsen D, et al. Implementation of a standardised treatment protocol for post resuscitation care after out-of-hospital cardiac arrest. Resuscitation 2007;73(1):29–39.
77. Rittenberger JC, Guyette FX, Tisherman SA, et al. Outcomes of a hospital-wide plan to improve care of comatose survivors of cardiac arrest. Resuscitation 2008;79:198–204.
78. Galeski DF, Band RA, Abella BS, et al. Early goal-directed hemodynamic optimization combined with therapeutic hypothermia in comatose survivors of out-of-hospital cardiac arrest. Resuscitation 2009;80:418–24.
79. Rittenberger JC, Kelly E, Jang D, et al. Successful outcome utilizing hypothermia after cardiac arrest in pregnancy: a case report. Crit Care Med 2008; 36(4):1354–6.
80. Chauhan A, Musunuru H, Donnino M, et al. The use of therapeutic hypothermia after cardiac arrest in a pregnant patient. Ann Emerg Med 2012;60(6):786–9.
81. Skulec R, Kovarnik T, Dostalova G, et al. Induction of mild hypothermia in cardiac arrest survivors presenting with cardiogenic shock syndrome. Acta Anaesthesiol Scand 2008;52(2):188–94.
82. Huynh N, Kloke J, Gu C, et al. The effect of hypothermia "dose" on vasopressor requirements and outcome aftercardiac arrest. Resuscitation 2013;84(2): 189–93.

83. Kuboyama K, Safar P, Radovsky A, et al. Delay in cooling negates the beneficial effect of mild resuscitative cerebral hypothermia after cardiac arrest in dogs: a prospective, randomized study. Crit Care Med 1993;21(9):1348–58.

84. Coimbra C, Wieloch T. Moderate hypothermia mitigates neuronal damage in the rat brain when initiated several hours following transient cerebral ischemia. Acta Neuropathol 1994;87(4):325–31.

85. Hicks SD, DeFranco DB, Callaway CW. Hypothermia during reperfusion after asphyxial cardiac arrest improves functional recovery and selectively alters stress-induced protein expression. J Cereb Blood Flow Metab 2000;20(3):520–30.

86. Che D, Li L, Kopil CM, et al. Impact of therapeutic hypothermia onset and duration on survival, neurologic function, and neurodegeneration after cardiac arrest. Crit Care Med 2011;39(6):1423–30.

87. Kim F, Olsufka M, Carlbom D, et al. Pilot study of rapid infusion of 2 L of 4 degrees C normal saline for induction of mildhypothermia in hospitalized, comatose survivors of out-of-hospital cardiac arrest. Circulation 2005;112(5):715–9.

88. Bernard SA, Smith K, Cameron P, et al, Rapid Infusion of Cold Hartmanns (RICH) Investigators. Induction of therapeutic hypothermia by paramedics after resuscitation from out-of-hospital ventricular fibrillation cardiac arrest: a randomized controlled trial. Circulation 2010;122(7):737–42.

89. Kim F, Nichol G, Maynard C, et al. Effect of prehospital induction of mild hypothermia on survival and neurological status among adults with cardiac arrest: a randomized clinical trial. JAMA 2014;311(1):45–52.

90. Castrén M, Nordberg P, Svensson L, et al. Intra-arrest transnasal evaporative cooling: a randomized, prehospital, multicenter study (PRINCE: Pre-ROSC IntraNasal Cooling Effectiveness). Circulation 2010;122(7):729–36.

91. Nichol G, Thomas E, Callaway CW, et al, Resuscitation Outcomes Consortium Investigators. Regional variation in out-of-hospital cardiac arrest incidence and outcome. JAMA 2008;300(12):1423–31.

92. Kim YM, Yim HW, Jeong SH, et al. Does therapeutic hypothermia benefit adult cardiac arrest patients presenting with non-shockable initial rhythms?: a systematic review and meta-analysis of randomized and non-randomized studies. Resuscitation 2012;83(2):188–96.

93. Robinson J, Charlton J, Seal R, et al. Oesophageal, rectal, axillary, tympanic and pulmonary artery temperatures during cardiac surgery. Can J Anaesth 1998;45:317.

94. Tømte Ø, Drægni T, Mangschau A, et al. A comparison of intravascular and surface cooling techniques in comatose cardiac arrest survivors. Crit Care Med 2011;39(3):443–9.

95. Kliegel A, Losert H, Sterz F, et al. Cold simple intravenous infusions preceding special endovascular cooling for faster induction of mild hypothermia after cardiac arrest–a feasibility study. Resuscitation 2005;64(3):347–51.

96. Merchant RM, Soar J, Skrifvars MB, et al. Therapeutic hypothermia utilization among physicians after resuscitation from cardiac arrest. Crit Care Med 2006;34(7):1935–40.

97. Rittenberger JC, Polderman KH, Smith WS, et al. Emergency neurological life support: resuscitation following cardiac arrest [review]. Neurocrit Care 2012;17(Suppl 1):S21–8.

98. Chamorro C, Borrallo JM, Romera MA, et al. Anesthesia and analgesia protocol during therapeutic hypothermia after cardiac arrest: a systematic review. Anesth Analg 2010;110:1328.

99. Hostler D, Zhou J, Tortorici MA, et al. Mild hypothermia alters midazolam pharmacokinetics in normal healthy volunteers. Drug Metab Dispos 2010;38:781.

100. Krumholz A, Stern BJ, Weiss HD. Outcome from coma after cardiopulmonary resuscitation: relation to seizures and myoclonus. Neurology 1988;38:401.

101. Suehiro E, Ueda Y, Wei EP, et al. Posttraumatic hypothermia followed by slow rewarming protects the cerebral microcirculation. J Neurotrauma 2003;20:381.

102. Heard KJ, Peberdy MA, Sayre MR, et al. A randomized controlled trial comparing the Arctic Sun to standard cooling for induction of hypothermia after cardiac arrest. Resuscitation 2010;81:9.

103. Pichon N, Amiel JB, François B, et al. Efficacy of and tolerance to mild induced hypothermia after out-of-hospital cardiac arrest using an endovascular cooling system. Crit Care 2007;11:R71.

104. Rhee BJ, Zhang Y, Boddicker KA, et al. Effect of hypothermia on transthoracic defibrillation in a swine model. Resuscitation 2005;65:79.

105. Polderman KH, Peerdeman SM, Girbes AR. Hypophosphatemia and hypomagnesemia induced by cooling in patients with severe head injury. J Neurosurg 2001;94:697.

106. Aibiki M, Kawaguchi S, Maekawa N. Reversible hypophosphatemia during moderate hypothermia therapy for brain-injured patients. Crit Care Med 2001;29:1726.

107. Michelson AD, MacGregor H, Barnard MR, et al. Reversible inhibition of human platelet activation by hypothermia in vivo and in vitro. Thromb Haemost 1994;71:633.

108. Reed RL 2nd, Bracey AW Jr, Hudson JD, et al. Hypothermia and blood coagulation: dissociation between enzyme activity and clotting factor levels. Circ Shock 1990;32:141.

109. Bjork RJ, Snyder BD, Campion BC, et al. Medical complications of cardiopulmonary arrest. Arch Intern Med 1982;142:500.

110. Oksanen T, Skrifvars MB, Varpula T, et al. Strict versus moderate glucose control after resuscitation from ventricular fibrillation. Intensive Care Med 2007;33:2093–100.

111. Schweickert WD, Pohlman MC, Pohlman AS, et al. Early physical and occupational therapy in mechanically ventilated, critically ill patients: a randomized controlled trial. Lancet 2009;373:1874–82.

112. Knafelj R, Radsel P, Ploj T, et al. Primary percutaneous coronary intervention and mild induced hypothermia in comatose survivors of ventricular fibrillation with ST-elevation acute myocardial infarction. Resuscitation 2007;74(2):227–34.

113. Wolfum S, Pierau C, Radke FW, et al. Mild therapeutic hypothermia in patients after out-of-hospital cardiac arrest due to ST-segment elevation myocardial infarction undergoing immediate percutaneous coronary intervention. Crit Care Med 2008;36(6):1780–6.

114. Oddo M, Schaller MD, Feihl F, et al. From evidence to clinical practice: effective implementation of therapeutic hypothermia to improve patient outcome after cardiac arrest. Crit Care Med 2006;34:1865–73.

115. Reynolds JC, Rittenberger JC, Callaway CW. Methylphenidate and amantadine to stimulate reawakening in comatose patients resuscitated from cardiac arrest. Resuscitation 2013;84(6):818–24.

116. Donnino MW, Rittenberger JC, Gaieski D, et al. The development and implementation of cardiac arrest centers. Resuscitation 2011;82(8):974–8.

117. Birkmeyer JD, Stukel TA, Siewers AE, et al. Surgeon volume and operative mortality in the United States. N Engl J Med 2003;349:2117–27.

118. Callaway CW, Schmicker RH, Brown SP, et al. Early coronary angiography and induced hypothermia are associated with survival and functional recovery after out-of-hospital cardiac arrest. Resuscitation 2014;85:657–63.

119. Wnent J, Seewald S, Heringlake M, et al. Choice of hospital after out-of-hospital cardiac arrest - a decision with far-reaching consequences: a study in a large German city. Crit Care 2012;16(5):R164.

120. Cha WC, Lee SC, Shin SD, et al. Regionalisation of out-of-hospital cardiac arrest care for patients without prehospital return of spontaneous circulation. Resuscitation 2012;83(11):1338–42.

121. Reynolds JC, Rittenberger JC, Callaway CW, Post Cardiac Arrest Service. Patterns of organ donation among resuscitated patients at a regional cardiac arrest center. Resuscitation 2014;85(2):248–52.

122. Spaite DW, Bobrow BJ, Vadeboncoeur TF, et al. The impact of prehospital transport interval on survival in out-of-hospital cardiac arrest: implications for regionalization of post-resuscitation care. Resuscitation 2008;79:61–6.

123. Spaite DW, Stiell IG, Bobrow BJ, et al. Effect of transport interval on out-of-hospital cardiac arrest survival in the OPALS study: implications for triaging patients to specialized cardiac arrest centers. Ann Emerg Med 2009;54:256–7.

124. Hartke A, Mumma BE, Rittenberger JC, et al. Incidence of re-arrest and critical events during prolonged transport of post-cardiac arrest patients. Resuscitation 2010;81(8):938–42.

APPENDIX

The Post Cardiac Arrest Service researchers are:

Jon C. Rittenberger, MD, MS

Clifton W. Callaway, MD, PhD

Francis X. Guyette, MD, MPH

Ankur A. Doshi, MD

Cameron Dezfulian, MD

Joshua C. Reynolds, MD, MS

Adam Frisch, MD, MS

Index

Note: Page numbers of article titles are in **boldface** type.

Emerg Med Clin N Am 33 (2015) 713–719
http://dx.doi.org/10.1016/S0733-8627(15)00050-4
0733-8627/15/$ – see front matter © 2015 Elsevier Inc. All rights reserved.

emed.theclinics.com